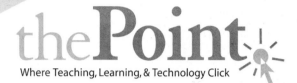
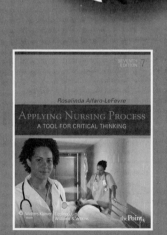

7th Edition

APPLYING NURSING PROCESS
A TOOL FOR CRITICAL THINKING

Rosalinda Alfaro-LeFevre, RN, MSN, ANEF
President
Teaching Smart/Learning Easy
Stuart, Florida
www.AlfaroTeachSmart.com

Wolters Kluwer | Lippincott Williams & Wilkins
Health
Philadelphia · Baltimore · New York · London
Buenos Aires · Hong Kong · Sydney · Tokyo

Acquisitions Editor: Jean Rodenberger
Senior Managing Editor: Helen Kogut
Director of Nursing Production: Helen Ewan
Senior Managing Editor / Production: Erika Kors
Production Manager: Debra Schiff
Art Director, Design: Joan Wendt
Art Director, Illustration: Brett McNaughton
Manufacturing Coordinator: Karin Duffield
Production Services / Compositor: Circle Graphics

7th Edition

9 8 7 6 5 4 3 2 1

Printed in the United States of America.

Library of Congress Cataloging-in-Publication Data

Alfaro-LeFevre, Rosalinda.
  Applying nursing process : a tool for critical thinking / Rosalinda Alfaro-LeFevre. — 7th ed.
      p. ; cm.
  Includes bibliographical references and index.
  ISBN 978-0-7817-7408-6
  1. Nursing—Handbooks, manuals, etc.   I. Title.
  [DNLM: 1. Nursing Process. WY 100 A385a 2010]
  RT51.A6255 2010
  610.73—dc22
                          2008047382

LWW.COM

About the Author

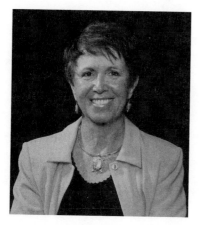

Known for making difficult content easy to understand, Rosalinda Alfaro-Lefevre, RN, MSN is an energetic presenter and an AJN Book of the Year and a Sigma Theta Tau Best Pick award recipient. She is a National League for Nursing Academy of Nursing Education Fellow. Rosalinda immigrated to the USA from Argentina via Canada at the age of 10, and is well known nationally and internationally. Her work is available in seven languages. She has more than 20 years' clinical experience (mostly in ICU, CCU, and ED) and has taught in associate degree and baccalaureate nursing programs. She currently is the president of Teaching Smart/Learning Easy in Stuart, Florida, a company dedicated to helping people to acquire the intellectual and interpersonal skills needed to deal with today's personal and workplace challenges. You can learn more about Rosalinda at www.AlfaroTeachSmart.com.

Rosalinda Alfaro-LeFevre, RN, MSN, ANEF
President
Teaching Smart/Learning Easy
Stuart, Florida
www.AlfaroTeachSmart.com

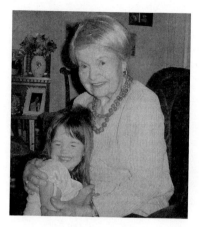

Doris Margaret Alfaro
(with great-granddaughter, Emma Riley)

June 14, 1920–December 13, 2005

My mother's first day of nursing school began during World War II with a 6-hour train ride from Blackpool to Derbyshire, England. Arriving at 4 pm, she was given a uniform and expected to be in charge of patients by 6 (she often said, "Can you imagine?"). Two years later, she met my father, Santiago, an Argentine who joined the British Army. Graduating in Chesterfield Royal Hospital's class of 1944, Mom spent most of her life at home raising six children—living in England, Argentina, Canada, and the United States. But, when the need arose, she put on a uniform and went back to doing something she loved to do: nursing.

Advisors and Reviewers

A Note of Thanks
Without the timely and insightful reviews and advice of the experts listed on these pages, this book would not have been possible. The author wishes to also acknowledge the translators of previous editions: Aiko Emoto and Kumiko Hongo (Japanese); Maria Teresa Luis (Spanish); and Maria Augusta Soares, Miriam de Abreu Almeida, and Valéria Giordani Araújo (Portuguese).

USA

Carolyn E. Adams, EdD, RN, NEA-BC
Professor and Director of the Graduate Program, Jefferson College of Health Sciences
Roanoke, Virginia.

Ledjie Ballard, CRNA, MSN
Independent Practitioner
Out Patient & Office Anesthesia
Affiliate Clinical Faculty
University of Washington
Seattle, Washington

Suzanne C. Beyea, RN, PhD, FAAN
Director of Nursing Research
Dartmouth-Hitchcock Medical Center
One Medical Center Drive
Lebanon, New Hampshire

Susan A. Boyer, MEd, RN
Director
Vermont Nurse Internship Project
Windsor, Vermont

Hilda Brito, RN, C, MSN
Director of Education
Kendall Regional Medical Center
Miami, Florida

Deanne A. Blach, MSN, RN
Nurse Educator
DB Productions
Green Forest, Arkansas

Susan Carper, RN, BS
Community Aging & Retirement Services
Port Richey, Florida

Bette Case, PhD, RN, BC
Chicago, Illinois

Darnell H. Cockram, EdD, RN
Educational Consultant
Martinsville, Virginia

Barbara J. Cohen, MsEd
Broomall, Pennsylvania

Bette Case Di Leonardi, PhD, RN, BC
Independent Consultant
Chicago, Illinois

Karen Elechko, RN, MSN
Golden Memory Clinic Coordinator
Veteran Affairs Medical Center Coatesville
Coatesville, Pennsylvania

Carol Ann Esche, DNP, RN, MA, CAN
Assistant Professor
University of Maryland School of Nursing
Baltimore, Maryland

Mark J. Fisher, MS, RN
Faculty Instructor
University of Oklahoma Health Sciences Center
College of Nursing
Oklahoma City, Oklahoma

Deborah L. Freyman, RN, MSN, MA
Nursing Faculty
National Park Community College
Hot Springs, Arkansas

Rebecca S. Frugé, RN, PhD
Director, Graduate Nursing Program
Universidad Metropolitana
San Juan, Puerto Rico

Pauline McKinney Green, PhD, RN
Associate Professor
Howard University
College of Nursing
Washington, DC

Cecelia G. Grindel, PhD, RN, CMSRN
Associate Director, Undergraduate Programs
Byrdine F. Lewis School of Nursing
Georgia State University
Atlanta, Georgia

Elizabeth E. Hand, MS, RN, CCRN
Acute Care Education Specialist
Hand-on Nursing, PLLC
Tulsa, Oklahoma

Ruth Hansten, PhD, FACHE, MBA, BSN
President
Hansten Healthcare
Port Ludlow, Washington

Dan Hankison
CONSULTING Dragons
Stuart, Florida

Cheryl Herndon, ARNP, CNM, MSN
Director Aesthetic Services
Women's Health Specialists,
Jensen Beach, Florida

Kim J. Herrington, RN, MSN
Associate Professor of Nursing
Louisiana State University at Alexandria
Alexandria, Louisiana

Robert Hess, RN, PhD, FAAN
Executive Vice President,
Continuing Education Programming
Nursing Spectrum CE
Gannett Healthcare Group
Falls Church, Virginia

Donna D. Ignatavicius, MS, RN, Cm
President, DI Associates, Inc.
Placitas, New Mexico

Frances J. Jessup, RN, BSN
Wound Care Specialist
Valdosta, Georgia

Sharon E. Johnson, MSN, RNC, CNA
Director, Home Health
Home Care Network
Jefferson Health System
Wayne, Pennsylvania

Suzanne Hall Johnson, MN, RN, CNS
Director
Hall Johnson Consulting
Lakewood, Colorado

Helen S. Joline, RN, BA
Duxbury, Massachusetts

Jackie H. Jones, EdD, RN, MSN
Assistant Professor, Department of Nursing
North Georgia College & State University
Dahlonega, Georgia

Elaine Bishop Kennedy, EdD, RN
Professor, Nursing
Wor-Wic Community College
Salisbury, Maryland

Nancy Konzelmann, MS, RN-BC, CPHQ
Nurse Education Specialist
St. Joseph's Healthcare System
Paterson, New Jersey

Corrine R. Kurzen, RN, MEd, MSN
Author and Consultant
Lafayette Hill, Pennsylvania

Heidi Pape Laird
Systems Designer
Partners HealthCare
Boston, Massachusetts

Sherry Lifsey, MSN, RN, BC
Manager, Clinical Education
Columbus Regional Medical Center
Columbus, Georgia

Marina Espiritu Lutz, MSN, RN
Faculty, Division of Nursing and Health Sciences
Neumann College
Aston, Pennsylvania

Angélica Y. Matos-Ríos, RN, DNS
Professor and Director
Graduate Dept. of Nursing
Medical Sciences Campus
University of Puerto Rico
San Juan, Puerto Rico

Patricia McCarthy, RN, MS
Associate Chief, Nursing Service for Education
VA Health Care System
Palo Alto, California

Marycarol McGovern, PhD, RN
Assistant Professor
College of Nursing
Villanova University
Villanova, Pennsylvania

Melani McGuire, RN, BSN
Staff Nurse, Emergency Dept.
Paoli Memorial Hospital
Paoli, Pennsylvania

Barbara N. McLaughlin, DNSc, RN, CNE
Associate Professor
Community College of Philadelphia
Philadelphia, Pennsylvania

Judith C. Miller, RN, MS
Nursing Tutorial & Consulting Services
Henniker, New Hampshire

Barbara A. Musinski, RN, C, BS
Independent Consultant
West Palm Beach, Florida

Jan Nash, RN, MS, PhD
Vice President, Patient Services
Paoli Memorial Hospital
Paoli, Pennsylvania

Charles L. Nola
Aerospace Engineer
Madison, Alabama

Nancy O'Donnell, RN, BSN, MSN
Interim Director, Nursing
J. Sargeant Reynolds Community College
Richmond, Virginia

Marilyn H. Oermann, PhD, RN, FAAN
Professor, College of Nursing
Wayne State University
Detroit, Michigan

Lourdes Maldonado Ojeda, EdD, RN
Dean, School of Health Sciences
Universidad Metropolitana
San Juan, Puerto Rico

Dawne DeVoe Olbrych, RN, MS
Instructor
Ellis Hospital School of Nursing
Schenectady, New York

Kathleen D. Pagana, PhD, RN
Professor Emeritus, Lycoming College
Pagana Seminars & Presentations
Williamsport, Pennsylvania

Terri Patterson, RN, MSN, CRRN, FIALCP
President
Nursing Consultation Services Ltd.
Plymouth Meeting, Pennsylvania

William F. Perry, MA, RN
Informatics Consultant
Creekspace Informatics
Beavercreek, Ohio

James Riley
JBR Advisors, LLC
Richmond, Virginia

Mathew Riley, BA
Therapeutic Staff Support
Chester County Regional Educational Services Inc
Downingtown, Pennsylvania

Michael Riley, LMSW, LPC, EMT-Paramedic
Safety Analyst
Praesidium Inc.
Arlington, Texas

Mary Anne Rizzolo, EdD, RN, FAAN
Senior Director of Professional Development
National League for Nursing
New York, New York

Tami J. Rogers, BSN, MSN, DVM
Professor or Nursing
Valencia Community College
Orlando, Florida

Karen Moore Schaefer, DNSc, RN
Director—Undergraduate Nursing
Temple University
Philadelphia, Pennsylvania

Rosalee J. Seymour, EdD, RN
Editor-in-Charge of Informatics Education OJNI
Associate Professor
Eastern Tennessee State University College of Nursing
Johnson City, Tennessee

Rose Sherman, Ed.D, RN, CNAA
Robert Wood Johnson Nurse Executive Fellow
Director, Nursing Leadership Institute
Christine E. Lynn College of Nursing
Florida Atlantic University
Boca Raton, Florida

Remedios A. Solarte, MSN, RN, NP
Nursing Faculty
Oakland Community College
Waterford, Michigan

Melva J. Solon, BSN, MSN, RN
Danville, Illinois

Maria Sophocles, MD
Princeton, New Jersey

Susanne Nancy Suchy, MSN, RN
Instructor, Nursing Department
Henry Ford Community College
Dearborn, Michigan

Carol Taylor, RN, PhD
Director, Center for Clinical Bioethics
Assistant Professor, Nursing
Georgetown University
Washington, DC

Brent W. Thompson, DNSc, RN
Associate Professor
Department of Nursing
West Chester University
West Chester, Pennsylvania

Joan Timalonis, RN, MSN
Assistant Professor of Nursing
Cedar Crest College
Allentown, Pennsylvania

Elizabeth M. Tsarnas, ARNP, BC
Clinical Director
Volunteers in Medicine Clinic
Stuart, Florida

Theresa M. Valiga, EdD, RN, FAAN
Director of the Institute for Educational Excellence
Duke University School of Nursing
Durham, North Carolina

Linda S. Weinberg, RN, MSN
Nursing Faculty
West Chester University
Community and Diabetes Educator
Chester County Hospital
West Chester, Pennsylvania

Gracie S. Wishnia, PhD, RN C (Gerontology)
Nursing Faculty
Spalding University School of Nursing
Louisville, Kentucky

Toni C. Wortham, RN, MSN
Professor, Nursing Department
Madisonville Community College
Madisonville, Kentucky

INTERNATIONAL

Miriam de Abreu Almeida, RN, PhD
Professor, School of Nursing
Federal University of Rio Grande do Sul
Porto Alegre, Brazil

Emilia Campos de Carvalho, RN, PhD
Professor, College of Nursing
University of São Paulo at Ribeirão Preto
Ribeirão Preto, Brazil

Dame June Clark, PhD, RN, FRCN
Professor Emeritus
School of Health Science
University of Wales Swansea
Wales, United Kingdom

Judy Boychuk Duchscher, RN, PhD
Executive Director, Nursing The Future
Faculty, Nursing Education
Saskatchewan Institute of Applied Science &
Technology (SIAST)
Saskatoon SK, Canada

Aiko Emoto
Professor Emeritus
Saniku Gakuin College
Chiba, Japan

Bernie Garrett, PhD, BA (Hons), RN
Assistant Professor
University of British Columbia
School of Nursing,
Vancouver, British Columbia, Canada

Maria Teresa Luis, RN
Professor of Medical-Surgical Nursing
University of Barcelona
Barcelona, Spain

Isabel Amélia Costa Mendes
Director
WHO Collaborating Center for Nursing Research
Development
Professor, College of Nursing
University of São Paulo at Ribeirão Preto
Ribeirão Preto, Brazil

Jeanne Michel, RN, MSN
Assistant Professor,
Department of Nursing
University of São Paulo
São Paulo, Brazil

Nico Oud, RN, MNSc, Dipl.N.Adm
Consultant and Trainer of Aggression Management
"CONNECTING"
Amsterdam, The Netherlands

Ann Paterson, RN, MA, MRCNA
Senior Lecture in Nursing & Midwifery
RMIT University
Bundoora West Campus
Melbourne, Australia

Joanne Profetto-McGrath, PhD, RN
Interim Dean and Associate Professor
Nursing Department
University of Alberta
Edmonton, Alberta, Canada

Yvonne Stillwell, RN, BA, PG Dip, MBS
Nurse Manager
Nursing Practice Development
MidCentral District Health Board
Palmerston North, New Zealand

Catherine Jean Thorpe, RN, RM, DipIC,
Health Nursing, BAdmin
Deputy Director, Nursing
Groote Schuur Hospital Observatory
Capetown, South Africa

Acknowledgments

I want to thank my husband, Jim, for his love, support, and sense of humor and fun; and the rest of my family for being behind me all the way.

I also want to thank the following people for their belief in me and their contribution to my personal and professional growth: Louise and Nat Rochester, Heidi Laird, Terri Patterson, Ledjie Ballard, Annette Sophocles, Maria Sophocles, Melani McGuire, Carol Taylor, Terry Valiga, Ruth Hansten, Barbara Cohen, Mary Anne Rizzolo, Lynda Carpenito-Moyet, Mary Jo Boyer, John Payne, Charlie and Nancy Lindsay, Becky Resh, Diane Verity, Nancy Flynn, Lorraine Locasale, Frank and Grace Nola, Chuck and Pat Morgan, the past and present nurses at Paoli Memorial, and the faculty of the Villanova College of Nursing.

My special thanks go to the Nursing Editorial division of Lippincott Williams & Wilkins, especially to Jean Rodenberger, Senior Acquisitions Editor; Helen Kogut, Senior Managing Editor; Brandi Spade, Editorial Assistant; and Debra Schiff, Senior Production Editor. I am in debt to Sheba Jalaluddin of O'Donnell & Associates who coached me through an ambitious schedule and stayed on task to make the project manageable. Finally, I want to thank the sales and marketing department whose efforts have helped make this book a bestseller.

Preface

Nursing Process: Out of the Box and Into the Information Age

Einstein once said, "The significant problems we face today can't be solved at the same level of thinking we were at when we created them." The necessary sweeping changes impacting on health care today require new thinking. For more than 20 years, this book—a past edition *Sigma Theta Tau Best Pick Award* winner—has been the one that students, teachers, and nurses turn to for help with learning how to use the nursing process in times of change. I'm happy to tell you that this edition gives you the new information and tools you need to be able to apply the nursing process to "think like a nurse" today.

As we move forward into the information age, where evidence-based practices are mandated, there are three main reasons that you need to have a strong foundation in the nursing process "in your head."

1. **American Nurses Association (ANA) practice standards stress** that the nursing process underpins virtually all care models, forms the foundation for decision-making, and serves as a critical thinking model to promote a competent level of nursing care.[1] While there are other useful tools for critical thinking, learning nursing process principles *first* helps you to comply with nursing standards and builds the foundation you need to learn other models.
2. **The National Council Licensure Examinations (NCLEX)** and most other advanced credentialing exams are based on the nursing process—without knowing basic rules and principles, you won't be able to think your way through these tests.
3. **As electronic charting and decision support systems that "do a lot of the thinking for you" become the norm,** you still need highly developed thinking skills—based on the nursing process—to be able to make decisions at the bedside and to be able to "think *with* the computer." Computers are important tools that can improve your ability to think critically. But they can't think *for* you. You've got to do a lot of independent thinking to ensure that the data you enter into the computer is factual and complete. You've got to discriminate about what information applies to each particular situation and therefore needs to be entered into the computer. Also, keep in mind that computers assume that the data you enter is *correct,* making YOU "the first in line to make or break" the accuracy of all subsequent information displayed by the computer. If you use computers and standard plans without learning principles of critical thinking and nursing process, it's like using a calculator without understanding what it means to add, subtract, multiply, or divide. You're like a "calculator cripple." Only in this case, you're "a care cripple," giving task-oriented rather than thought-oriented care. Without understanding the reasoning behind the process, you're unable to individualize approaches safely and effectively. You put patients at risk, and you put yourself in legal jeopardy. There's also another question: What will you do when the computer goes down (as it surely will)?

Who Should Read This Book?

If you need to do any of the following, this book is for you.

1. If you need an update on how to use the nursing process as a tool for critical thinking, within the context of current ANA Standards;
2. If you want to work in Magnet status hospitals—hospitals recognized by the American Nurses Credentialing Center (ANCC) to attract and retain quality employees—you must be thoroughly familiar with each phase of the nursing process;[2]
3. If you're an instructor and want everyone to be "on the same page," with clarity about the relationship between nursing process and critical thinking;
4. If you're a student and want to:
   - Be more confident and competent in new clinical situations.
   - Demonstrate critical thinking to your instructor.
   - Know how to think your way through NCLEX.

What's New?

You get new information on:

❑ Nurses' increased responsibilities related to medical diagnoses, nursing diagnoses, error prevention, early warning systems, and activating the chain of command
❑ Characteristics of the nursing process that promote critical thinking (what you have to *do* to use the nursing process as a tool for critical thinking)
❑ How to prioritize your thinking and do quick priority assessments (QPA) to identify and prevent major patient problems *early*
❑ How developing a culture of safety and Institute of Medicine (IOM) competencies impact on your ability to be a safe and effective nurse
❑ Evidenced-based Critical Thinking Indicators—behaviors that promote critical thinking—are spelled out for each phase of the nursing process.
❑ Nurses' roles in coordinating and delegating care
❑ The importance of using active—rather than passive—communication, using "Read Back" and "Repeat Back" rules
❑ How to use structured tools such as the SBAR approach to improve hand-off communication
❑ What to expect on NCLEX in context of each step of the nursing process.
❑ How the shift in thinking from "diagnose and treat" to "predict, prevent, manage, and promote" requires nurses to be proactive, focusing on identifying risk factors, screening for common health problems, and predicting potential complications, as well as treating actual problems
❑ How to use mapping and diagramming to determine relationships and better understand problems
❑ How to use the 4-Circle CT Model (pages 35–36) to improve your ability to think critically

❏ The need to develop healthy workplace and learning environments, including getting agreement on a code of conduct and commitments to patients, organizations, and one another
❏ Numerous new rules, tools, and strategies are highlighted throughout
❏ The need to promote collaborative practice, empowered partnerships, shared decision-making, and nursing wellness
❏ In-depth information on documentation and the use of computers, decision support systems, and informatics to facilitate care management and research
❏ The impact of real and simulated experiences on your ability to develop critical thinking skills
❏ The importance of "thinking ahead, thinking in action, and thinking back (reflecting on thinking)"

New Teaching and Learning Tools

❏ To help you develop study sheets, presentations, and course syllabi you can download teaching/learning materials in Word format from thePoint at http://www.thePoint.lww.com. These materials give you all major chapter headings, learning outcomes, and direct links that you can click on to take you to all URLs listed in this book.
❏ You can download additional handouts and tools to reinforce content from www.AlfaroTeachSmart.com. These tools are free for personal use.
❏ New maps and the use of brain-based learning principles (strategies that help you get your brain "plugged in" to learning mode) make it easier than ever to learn.

What's the Same?

To ensure a sound approach that's based on current standards, each chapter has been evaluated against requirements addressed in *Nursing Scope and Standards of Performance and Standards of Clinical Practice.*[3]

You also get:

❏ Lots of examples to make content relevant and easy to understand—the goal continues to be to give you a concise, engaging, user-friendly book.
❏ A "big-picture" summary of how to use the nursing process as a tool for critical thinking (inside front cover)
❏ A list of common complications associated with medical diagnoses, treatments, or diagnostic modalities (inside back cover and facing page)
❏ A *Nursing Diagnoses Quick Reference Section* that gives easy access to information on frequently seen diagnoses accepted for clinical testing by NANDA International.

❏ Practical information on the use and misuse of standard nursing languages such as North American Nursing Diagnosis Association (NANDA) International, Nursing Intervention Classification (NIC), and Nursing Outcome Classification (NOC)

❏ **More on:**
  • Nurses' roles in homes, communities, and multidisciplinary practice
  • Ethical, legal, cultural, and spiritual implications
  • The impact of cost-containment and insurance requirements
  • How nurses' roles as diagnosticians and case managers continue to evolve
  • How to use critical pathways and standard plans to promote critical thinking
  • The importance of acquiring communication, interpersonal, and technical skills to promote critical thinking

How to Use This Book

Great pains have been taken to make this a user-friendly book that helps you to move around the text as you please. The following elements promote critical thinking, enhance motivation to learn, and are integrated throughout:

1. Learning outcomes written at the cognitive level of analysis precede each chapter.
2. Advance organizers and "What's in this chapter?" precede content.
3. Relevant terms are defined in the glossary, and more difficult terms are clarified in the text by definition, discussion, and use within context.
4. Illustrations are placed throughout to establish relationships and clarify text.
5. Analogies, examples, and case studies are used to clarify information and demonstrate relevance of content.
6. Rationales are highlighted in illustrations and integrated as needed in other parts of the text.
7. Questioning at the analysis level is used:
   • During content presentation to stimulate curiosity and give clues to what's important
   • After the content (in Critical Thinking Exercises) to reinforce key points and provide the opportunity to test and refine knowledge
8. Content is presented in such a way that those who need structure have it, without restricting those who require more creative freedom.
9. "Try This on Your Own" sessions are offered to allow for practice without concern about being evaluated by others.
10. Summaries are given at the end of each chapter.

Other content and features retained from the previous edition include:

❏ **Think About It** boxes ("food for thought" to stimulate thinking and reinforce content)

❏ *Voices* boxes (quotes from nurses that are inspirational or exemplary of best practices)

❏ **HMO (Help Me Out)®** cartoons highlight content in a humorous way. HMO® is based on real experiences. If you have an experience you think would make a good cartoon, please contact me at www.AlfaroTeachSmart.com.

❑ **Critical Thinking Exercises** are highlighted throughout. You can find example responses in the back of the book beginning on page 241.

❑ **Try This On Your Own** exercises encourage you to learn more deeply through application and meaningful learning. These exercises don't have example responses in the back of the book because they're very individualized and would be too lengthy to cover.

A Word About "Patient/Client," "He/She," and Stakeholder

Whenever possible, I use a fictitious name or "someone," "person," "consumer," or "individual" instead of "client" or "patient" to help us keep in mind that each client or patient is an individual who has unique needs, values, perceptions, and motivations. "He" and "she" are used interchangeably to avoid the awkwardness of using "he/she" over and over. The term *stakeholder* is used when describing *all* the people who are impacted by how care is given and what outcomes are achieved (eg, patients, families, care providers, and insurance companies).

Comments and Suggestions Welcomed

I welcome and appreciate suggestions for improvement—often the most significant changes are made based on student and faculty suggestions.

Rosalinda Alfaro-LeFevre, RN, MSN
www.AlfaroTeachSmart.com

References

1. American Nurses Association. (2004). *Nursing scope and standards of performance and standards of clinical practice.* Washington, DC: American Nurses Publishing.
2. American Nurses Credentialing Center. (2005). *ANCC Magnet Program–Recognizing excellence in nursing services.* Silver Spring, MD: Author.
3. American Nurses Association. *Op. cit.*

Contents

3

Diagnosis

4

Planning

5

Implementation

6

Evaluation

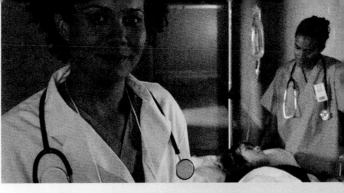

chapter 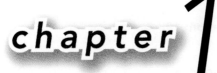1

Nursing Process Overview

what's in this chapter?

In this chapter, you get an overview of the nursing process and find out the answers to questions like, What do we have to know? What do we have to do first? and Why do we have to do it? You learn that there are five main reasons for studying the nursing process: (1) It's the first tool you need to learn to begin to "think like a nurse"; (2) American Nurses Association (ANA) Standards mandate its use; (3) It underpins virtually all care models and provides a tool for critical thinking and decision-making; (4) It forms the foundation for advanced certification and NCLEX exams; and (5) Understanding nursing process *principles* is the key to practicing safely in today's computer-driven world. To help you apply what you learn from this chapter when you go to the clinical setting, you're exposed to key factors in today's health care that impact on your role as a nurse—including new information on national safety goals, your responsibilities related to activating the chain of command, and competencies that you must develop to be a safe and effective nurse. Stressing the importance of having good communication skills and knowing how to form partnerships with patients, families, and colleagues, this chapter helps you understand how to apply ethical principles to give outcome-focused, patient-centered care. Finally, you gain an understanding of *critical thinking indicators* (behaviors that promote critical thinking) and consider the importance of: (1) developing critical thinking characteristics; (2) gaining theoretical and experiential knowledge; (3) acquiring interpersonal and technical skills; and (4) being willing and able to care.

critical thinking exercises

expected learning outcomes

After studying this chapter, you should be able to:

- Explain the relationships among the 5 nursing process steps (*Assessment, Diagnosis, Planning, Implementation,* and *Evaluation*).
- Give at least four benefits of using the nursing process.
- Address how standards, policies, laws, and ethics codes affect how you apply the nursing process as a tool for critical thinking.
- Explain why you need to understand nursing process *principles* to be able to safely use standard and electronic plans.
- Discuss the relationship between the nursing process and the care approaches of other disciplines (eg, medicine and physical therapy).
- Begin to develop the communications skills (speaking, listening, and writing) you need to communicate effectively with patients, families, and other staff (eg, peers, supervisors, educators, and doctors).
- Address how national safety goals and Institute of Medicine (IOM) competencies impact on your ability to be a safe and effective nurse.
- Discuss your responsibilities related to medical diagnoses, nursing diagnoses, and activating the chain of command.
- Explain the meaning of *"Assess, Re-assess, Revise, and Record"* and *"Think Ahead, Think-in-Action, and Think Back."*
- Discuss how real and simulated experiences impact on your ability to develop critical thinking skills.
- Describe what's required to develop healthy workplaces and learning environments in context of a culture of safety.

(continued on next page)

What Is the Nursing Process and Why Learn About It?
What Is It?
Why Learn About It?

Steps of the Nursing Process

Relationships Among the Steps of the Nursing Process
Assessment and Diagnosis
Diagnosis and Planning
Planning and Implementation
Implementation and Evaluation
Evaluation and the Other Nursing Process Steps

What Are the Benefits of Using the Nursing Process?

Nursing Process in Context of Today's Clinical Setting

Patient Safety Is Top Priority

Ethics: Advocating for Patients' Rights
Seven Ethical Principles
Following ANA Ethics Code

Including Patient Partners While Following HIPAA Rules

What's the Difference Between Nursing Process and Critical Thinking?
How to Become a Critical Thinker
Using the Four-Circle CT Model

Willingness and Ability to Care
Willingness to Care
Being Able to Care

After studying this chapter, you should be able to:

- Explain how to apply the seven ethical principles in this chapter to advocating for patients' rights.
- Address how to include patient partners in care, while staying within Health Insurance Portability and Accountability Act (HIPAA) guidelines.
- Determine at least five Critical Thinking Indicators (CTIs) you want to develop or improve.
- Use the 4-Circle CT Model on page 36 to identify skills you need to develop.
- Start to develop the interpersonal skills needed for critical thinking.
- Explain what it takes to be willing and able to demonstrate caring behaviors.
- Begin to use the nursing process as a tool for critical thinking in clinical, classroom, and testing situations.

What Is the Nursing Process and Why Learn About It?

Let's start to examine the nursing process: What is it and why do you need to learn about it?

What Is It?

The nursing process consists of five interrelated steps—***Assessment, Diagnosis, Planning, Implementation,*** and ***Evaluation.**** The steps are cyclical, rather than linear, as you'll see in this chapter.

Applying principles from each of the five steps helps you:

1. Organize and prioritize your patient care
2. Keep the focus on what's important—the patient's health status and quality of life
3. Form thinking habits that help you gain the confidence and skills you need to think critically in clinical, theoretical, and testing situations.

Nursing Process Characteristics That Promote Critical Thinking

Let's look at how using the nursing process promotes critical thinking. Think about the following characteristics:

Purposeful, Organized, and Systematic. Each step is designed to achieve a specific purpose. For example, *Assessment* aims to *gather* the facts you need to determine health status. *Diagnosis* aims to *analyze* those facts to identify the problems and risks involved. The steps guide you to think in a systematic, organized way, helping you to avoid missing anything important.

Humanistic. Based on the belief that we must consider patients' unique interests, values, needs, and culture, the nursing process guides you to focus holistically on the body, mind, and spirit. It pushes you to consider health problems *in context of how they impact on sense of well-being and ability to be independent.* For example, suppose "Bob" has severe arthritis. You work to understand how it impacts on his ability to work, to do desired activities, to sleep, and to function in his role as father of three young children.

Step-By-Step, Cyclic, and Dynamic. While there are specific steps, the nursing process is actually a cycle. You begin by assessing the patient, and when you do the fifth step, *Evaluation,* you come back to *Assessment* to determine patient responses to care. When you're a novice or in unfamiliar situations, you need to work in a strict step-by-step way to be sure that you don't miss anything important. For example, you *assess* carefully and completely before you *diagnose.* When you are in familiar situations—and after the *steps* become like second nature—you use the nursing process in dynamic ways. For example, experienced ICU nurses can take one look at their patients and know that something's wrong. Their eyes flash to the monitor—checking

Purposeful, Organized, and Systematic.

Humanistic.

Step-By-Step, Cyclic, and Dynamic.

---

*ANA Standards address six standards, considering *Outcome Identification* separately after *Diagnosis,* and before *Planning.* The NCLEX exam uses five steps, as we do in this book. We examine *Outcome Identification* as a key part of Step 4, *Planning.*

heart rate and rhythm. They may jump to the *Intervention* phase, raising or lowering the head of the bed depending on instincts, before completing *Diagnosis*. At same time, they talk with the patient and grab a blood pressure cuff to continue *Assessment.*

Outcome-Focused and Cost-Effective. Applying nursing process principles helps you figure out how to achieve the best results (outcomes) in the most efficient and cost-effective way.

Proactive. The nursing process stresses the need to not only treat *problems,* but also prevent them by managing risk factors and encouraging healthy behaviors, such as walking and deep breathing.

Evidence-Based. It mandates that judgments, decisions, and actions be based on the best evidence. Strict documentation requirements ensure that we have the data we need to manage care and to help researchers study care practices and improve them.

Intuitive and Logical. Principles of nursing process push you to acknowledge patterns and intuitive hunches, then to look for evidence that supports your intuition.

Reflective, Creative, and Improvement-Oriented. It stresses the need for ongoing evaluation, requiring us to continually reflect on both patient responses (outcomes) and our practice (how we give care), so that we can make corrections early. It requires us to work to continually improve nursing care, encouraging us to think creatively about how to get better results in easier, more efficient, less costly ways.

Outcome-Focused and Cost-Effective.

Proactive.

Evidence-Based.

Intuitive and Logical.

Reflective, Creative, and Improvement-Oriented.

> **NOTE: There are many helpful web links throughout this book.** To get worksheets and direct links to the online references and resources in this book, go to http://thePoint. lww.com/Alfaro7e. **Also realize that this book is written using brain-based learning principles.** Brain-based learning centers on using strategies that help your brain get "plugged in to learning mode."[1,2,3] Think about this: (1) You learn best when you're engaged by a conversational style and get lots of examples, strategies, and exercises to help you connect with how content applies to the "real world"; and (2) Humor reduces your stress and helps you learn.

Why Learn About It?

The nursing process is the first tool you need to learn to "think like a nurse." It gives you an organized, systematic way of thinking about nursing care. It also gives a standard frame of reference that promotes effective communication among nurses. American Nurses Association (ANA) practice standards—which nurses are accountable for maintaining—state that the nursing process underpins virtually all care models, providing a model for critical thinking and forming the foundation for decision-making.[4] The nursing process provides the basis for NCLEX* and other certification tests you need to pass to get your nursing license and advanced certification. To receive Magnet status—to be recognized by the American Nurses Credentialing Center (ANCC) as a health organization that attracts and retains quality employees—the health organi-

---

*National Council Licensure Examination (see www.ncsbn.org/nclex.htm)

zation's nurses must be very familiar with each phase of the nursing process. Most importantly, remember the following rule:

> **R U L E**
>
> **To use standard and electronic plans safely, learn the *principles* behind the nursing process.** If you don't understand the purpose of each step, the relationship among the steps, and how each step is accomplished, it would be like using a calculator without ever having learned what it means to add, subtract, multiply, or divide. To be an independent thinker who's able to give safe, effective care and improve current practices, understand the *reasoning* behind the nursing process.

Ultimate Goals of Nursing

An important starting point for using the nursing process is having a good understanding of the ultimate goals of nursing. At the big picture level, we aim to:

❏ Prevent illness and promote, maintain, or restore health (in terminal illness, the goal is a peaceful death)
❏ Maximize sense of well-being, independence, and ability to function in desired roles (as defined by the patient)
❏ Provide cost-effective, efficient care that pays attention to individual biological, social, spiritual, and cultural needs
❏ Continually work to improve patient outcomes, care practices, and consumer satisfaction

> **R U L E**
>
> **Communication skills (knowing how to listen, speak, and chart effectively) is the foundation of all the steps of the nursing process.** Your ability to communicate well with patients, families, peers, and other professionals makes the difference between competent, efficient care and care that's sloppy, unprofessional, and prone to errors.

Steps of the Nursing Process

Here's a brief description of what you do during each step of the nursing process:

1. **Assessment.** Collect and record all the information you need to:
   • Predict, detect, prevent, and manage actual and potential health problems
   • Promote optimum health, independence, and well-being
   • Clarify expected outcomes (results)
2. **Diagnosis.** Analyze the data you gathered, draw conclusions, and determine whether there are:
   • Risks for safety or infection transmission (deal with these immediately)
   • Signs or symptoms that need evaluation by a more qualified professional (report these immediately)
   • Actual and potential health problems requiring nursing or medical management
   • Risk factors requiring nursing or medical management
   • Issues that aren't quite clear, but require further investigation

- Learning needs that must be addressed
- Patient resources, strengths, and use of healthy behaviors
- Health states that are satisfactory but could be improved

> **R U L E**
>
> **Unless you're an Advanced Practice Nurse (APN)*, state laws prohibit you from making medical diagnoses independently.** You are, however, **accountable** for giving high priority to assessing for—and reporting—signs and symptoms that may indicate the need for attention from a professional more qualified than you are.[5] For example, if your patient has signs and symptoms of a myocardial infarction (eg, chest pain and shortness of breath), you're accountable for: (1) suspecting that this could be the problem; (2) recognizing that it is a high priority; (3) doing what you can to address the problem (eg, raise the head of the bed); and (4) reporting it immediately. **This is called "Activating the Chain of Command" (follow policies and procedures for getting help; be persistent—stay with the problems until your patient gets the qualified help they need).**

---

3. **Planning.** Clarify expected outcomes (expected results), set priorities, and determine interventions (nursing actions). The interventions are designed to:
   - Detect, prevent, and manage health problems and risk factors
   - Promote optimum function, independence, and sense of well-being
   - Achieve the expected outcomes safely and efficiently
4. **Implementation.** Put the plan into action:
   - Assess the patient to determine current status—decide whether the patient is ready and the interventions are still appropriate.
   - Perform the interventions (nursing actions)
   - Reassess the patient to determine end results (outcomes)
   - Make immediate changes as needed
   - Chart nursing actions and patient responses

> **R U L E**
>
> **Remember "Assess, Re-assess, Revise, Record."** *Assess* patients before you perform nursing actions. *Re-assess* them to determine their responses immediately *after* you perform nursing actions. *Revise* your approach as indicated. *Record* patient responses and any changes you made in the plan.

---

5. **Evaluation.** Do a comprehensive assessment of the patient to decide whether expected outcomes have been met or whether new problems have emerged.
   - Decide whether to modify or terminate the plan.
   - Plan for ongoing continuous assessment and improvement

Table 1.1 compares the Nursing Process and the Problem-Solving Method** Notice how the problem-solving method begins when you encounter a problem. The proactive

---

*For more information, see Appendix A (Advanced Practice Nurses' Roles).

**Throughout this book, *medical problem* refers to diseases or trauma diagnosed by primary care providers: physicians, physician's assistants, or advanced practice nurses.

table 1.1 Nursing Process Versus Problem-Solving Method

Nursing Process	Problem-Solving Method
Assessment: Continuously collecting data about health status to monitor for evidence of health problems and risk factors that may contribute to health problems (eg, smoking).	**Encountering a problem:** Collecting data about the problem.
Diagnosis: Analyzing data to clearly identify actual and potential health problems, risk factors, and strengths.	**Analyzing data** to determine exactly what the problem is.
Planning: Determining desired outcomes (benefits expected to be seen in the patient after care is done) and identifying interventions to achieve the outcomes.	**Making a plan** of action.
Implementation: Putting the plan into action and observing initial responses.	**Putting the plan into action.**
Evaluation: Determining how well the outcomes have been met and deciding whether changes need to be made. Looking for ways to make things better.	**Evaluating the results.**

nursing process stresses the need for continuous assessment for risk factors (even when no problems exist).

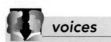 **voices**

Why We Have Two Hands
"God gave us two hands: One to help others and the other to help ourselves."
—*Eileen Lupton, RN, BSN*

Relationships Among the Steps of the Nursing Process

The steps of the nursing process are fluid and overlapping, as described in the following section.

Assessment and Diagnosis

The following diagram shows *Assessment* and *Diagnosis* as overlapping steps.

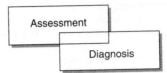

Assessment and Diagnosis are closely related and overlap for two reasons:

1. Accurate diagnosis depends on accurate and complete assessment.
2. As you gather information during *Assessment,* you start to analyze and interpret what it means before you have a complete "diagnostic picture." For example: You are interviewing Mrs. King as part of a preadmission assessment for surgery. You notice a rash on her arms and legs and make a tentative diagnosis (Mrs. King may have some sort of skin or allergy problem) as you focus your assessment to get more information.

Diagnosis and Planning

The following diagram shows *Diagnosis* and *Planning* overlapping.

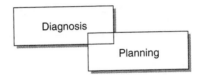

Diagnosis and Planning are related for several reasons:

1. Accurate planning requires accurate diagnosis. If you miss problems or misunderstand them, you waste time developing a plan to solve the wrong problems. The real problems may go undetected and become worse due to neglect or incorrect treatment.
2. To achieve the overall desired outcome of care—that is, that the person is able to be as independent as possible—you must develop specific outcomes for each problem or diagnosis that must be managed to stay on track for expected discharge. For example, if *constipation* is a major problem, one outcome might be the person has a soft bowel movement at least every other day.
3. The interventions you identify during *Planning* must be designed to prevent, resolve, or manage the problems identified during *Diagnosis.* For example, for *constipation,* you plan interventions to promote bowel regularity (eg, teaching the need for adequate hydration, dietary roughage, and so forth).
4. There are times when you have to act quickly, implementing a plan of action, before you identify all the problems. For example, if you encounter life-threatening problems, take immediate action. After the situation is under control, complete the *Diagnosis* phase by analyzing all of the data in depth.

5. It's important to incorporate the resources and strengths you identify during *Diagnosis* into the plan. For example, if you learn that someone is unable to plan meals but has relatives who are willing to help, use the relatives as a resource (eg, teaching relatives how to include high-roughage foods in the diet).

Planning and Implementation

The following diagram shows *Planning* and *Implementation* overlapping.

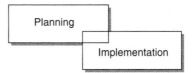

Planning and **Implementation** are related and overlap for two main reasons:

1. The plan guides interventions performed during *Implementation.*
2. As you implement the plan, you often need to fine-tune it to get the results you need. Sometimes, you even have to go back and check whether your assessment and diagnosis information is correct.

Implementation and Evaluation

The following diagram shows *Implementation* and *Evaluation* overlapping.

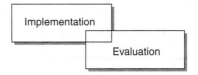

Implementation and **Evaluation** overlap for an obvious reason: **Evaluation** is an important *part* of **Implementation**. As you implement the plan, you evaluate your patients' responses carefully, and make changes early as needed.

Evaluation and the Other Nursing Process Steps

The following diagram shows that the nursing process is a *cycle* that begins with Assessment, goes *on through the other steps to Evaluation,* then back to *Assessment* (you assess the patient to determine current status and evaluate outcome achievement). The shading of the *Planning* and *Evaluation* boxes indicates the important relationship between *Evaluation* and *Planning:* Assuming that your diagnoses are accurate and your outcomes are appropriate, the ultimate question to be answered during *Evaluation* is, "Have we achieved the outcomes determined during *Planning?*"

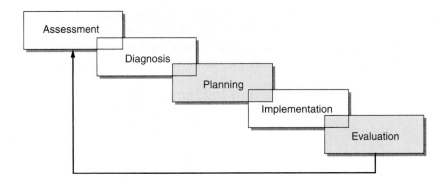

Comprehensive evaluation involves examining what happened in all of the other steps, as shown in the following diagram.

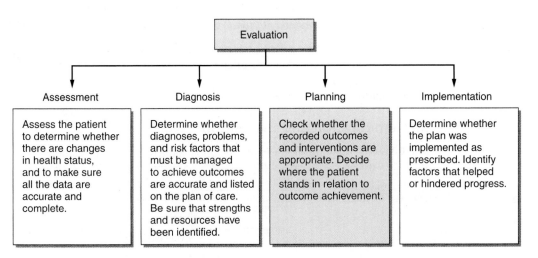

Assessment	Diagnosis	Planning	Implementation
Assess the patient to determine whether there are changes in health status, and to make sure all the data are accurate and complete.	Determine whether diagnoses, problems, and risk factors that must be managed to achieve outcomes are accurate and listed on the plan of care. Be sure that strengths and resources have been identified.	Check whether the recorded outcomes and interventions are appropriate. Decide where the patient stands in relation to outcome achievement.	Determine whether the plan was implemented as prescribed. Identify factors that helped or hindered progress.

RULE

In the clinical setting, remember the importance of thinking ahead, thinking in action, and thinking back (reflecting).[6,7] **Think ahead** (be proactive—anticipate what might happen and how you can be prepared). **Think in action** (pay attention to what's going on in your head as you "think on your feet," gathering and putting information together). **Think back** (reflect on your thinking to decide what you can learn from what happened, what influenced your thinking, and what you can do better next time—this usually requires dialogue with others or journaling to make your thoughts explicit).

To increase your understanding of the nursing process, review the following case scenario.

CASE SCENARIO

Applying the Steps of the Nursing Process to Caring for an Elderly Man at Home

Assessment. Mr. Martin is 80 years old and lives alone. He wants to be independent and keeps a clean home. However, today he has a cold, is weak, and states that he is feeling very tired. Other than that, his health is unchanged.

Diagnosis. You analyze the above data and realize that Mr. Martin's fatigue puts him at risk for falls. You recognize that his desire for independence is a strength, but you also know that it might be a weakness because he may not ask for help. You tell him that you'd like him to have some extra help while he's ill because you're concerned that his weakness puts him at risk for falls.

Planning. Together with Mr. Martin, you agree on the following outcome: Mr. Martin will be free of injury with reduced risk factors for falls. You then develop a plan to prevent falls (eg, you arrange furniture so things are out of the way or easy to grasp for balance, you stress the importance of adequate nutrition and hydration with a cold, and you ask who might be able to come and help for a few days). You plan to monitor his blood pressure, because you know that low blood pressure is a risk factor for falls.

Implementation. You monitor him closely, checking vital signs, monitoring food and fluid intake, and finding out if he has help each day. Knowing of his desire for independence, you stress the importance of accepting help from others. You encourage him to keep up his strength by avoiding being in bed all day.

Evaluation. You assess Mr. Martin to determine whether he is free from injury and whether the risk factors for falls are still present. If he has regained his strength, encourage him to continue his usual independent lifestyle. If not, reassess his health status and decide whether to make changes in the plan.

What Are the Benefits of Using the Nursing Process?

The nursing process complements what other health care professionals do by focusing on both the medical problems* and on the *impact* of medical problems and treatment plans on patients' lives (human responses). For example, if someone has a broken leg, the physician focuses on treating the broken bones, and the physical therapist focuses on promoting muscle strength and balance. You, as the nurse, follow the medical treatment plan, but focus on the *whole person*—for example, how to manage pain holistically, whether there's a risk for injury or problem with skin integrity, and what inconveniences the patient has.

---

*Throughout this book, the term *medical problem* refers to diseases or trauma diagnosed by primary care providers such as physicians or advanced practice nurses (see Appendix A, page 247). The term *medical order* refers to interventions (treatments) prescribed by primary care providers to treat medical problems.

This holistic focus helps to ensure that interventions are tailored to the *individual,* not just the disease. Can you think what it would be like if you were hospitalized with a head laceration, a fractured arm, and a bruised kidney and everyone focused only on your medical problems? Can you imagine lying there with daily visits from a surgeon to check your head, an orthopedist to look at your arm, a urologist to check your kidney, and no one there to be concerned with how *you* are doing—to ask about you (what things would help you be more independent and comfortable)?

Consider the following example of the difference between how a physician and a nurse might analyze the same patient's data.

E x a m p l e

Physician's data (disease focus): "Mrs. Garcia has pain and swelling in all joints. Diagnostic studies indicate that she has rheumatoid arthritis. We will start her on a course of anti-inflammatory drugs to treat the rheumatoid arthritis." (Focus is on treating the arthritis.)

Nurse's data (holistic focus, considering both problems and their effect on the person's ability to function independently): "Mrs. Garcia has pain and swelling in all joints, making it difficult for her to feed and dress herself. She has voiced that it's difficult to feel worthwhile when she can't even feed herself. She states that she is depressed because she misses seeing her two small grandchildren. We need to develop a plan to help her with her pain, to assist her with feeding and dressing, to work through feelings of low self-esteem, and for special visitations with the grandchildren." (Focus is on Mrs. Garcia.)

Box 1.1 summarizes the benefits of using the nursing process.

---

box 1.1 Benefits of Using the Nursing Process

❏ Speeds up diagnosis and treatment of actual and potential health problems, reducing the incidence of (and length of) hospital stays.
❏ Requires nurses to identify patient-centered outcomes (the benefits expected to be seen in the patient after care is done).
❏ Creates a plan that's cost-effective.
❏ Has precise documentation requirements designed to:
  • Improve communication and prevent errors, omissions, and unnecessary repetitions.
  • Leave a "paper trail" that later can be followed for evaluating patient care and for the purpose of doing studies to advance nursing and improve the quality and efficiency of health care.
❏ Prevents clinicians from losing sight of the importance of the human factor. Promotes independence and quality of life.
❏ Promotes flexibility and independent thinking.
❏ Tailors interventions for the individual (not just the disease).
❏ Helps:
  • Patients and significant others realize their input is important and strong points are assets.
  • Nurses have the satisfaction of getting results.

table 1.2 Comparison of Nursing Process and Medical Process

Nursing Process	Medical Process
Broad, holistic approach that assesses body, mind, and spirit and aims to maximize people's ability to do activities that are important to them.	Comparatively narrow approach that focuses on anatomy, physiology, and pathophysiology.
Mainly considers how peoples' lives are *affected by* problems with organ and system function (human responses).	Mainly considers problems with organ and system function.
Focuses on maximizing function and independence.	Focuses on treating diseases and trauma.
Manages medical problems under physician's orders or protocols. Prevents medical problems through proactive nursing care.	Manages medical problems independently.

Table 1.2 compares the nursing process and the medical process.

Nursing Process in Context of Today's Clinical Setting

To help you know what to expect when you apply the nursing process "at the bedside," this section summarizes key issues and trends that affect patient care today. For example, in the past, we were very involved with developing plans "from scratch." Today, in many cases we *adapt* standard plans already developed for specific conditions. To reflect these changes, throughout this book, we'll approach using the nursing process from two perspectives:

1. How to create a comprehensive plan of care from beginning to finish using the five steps of *Assessment, Diagnosis, Planning, Implementation, and Evaluation.* Studying each of the steps in depth will help you gain insights needed to be able to move on to using the nursing process in dynamic ways.
2. How to adapt existing plans to make them appropriate for each unique individual.

Read on to get a sense of other major things you need know.

Institute of Medicine (IOM) Outlines Core Competencies.* The IOM—an organization that provides unbiased, evidence-based information to policy-makers,

---

*For more information on the IOM, go to http://www.iom.edu.

professionals, leaders, and the general public—identifies five core competencies that healthcare professionals *must* develop (see following box). You can expect that you will need to focus on developing these competencies to pass NCLEX and work safely in clinical settings.

(IOM) Core Competencies

To function safely and effectively, learn to:

1. **Provide patient-centered care.** Identify, respect, and care about patients' unique values, preferences, and needs; communicate clearly; teach patients; make shared decisions; and promote wellness by preventing disease and promoting healthy lifestyles.
2. **Work in interdisciplinary teams.** Collaborate, communicate, and integrate care in teams to ensure that care is continuous and reliable.
3. **Employ evidence-based practice (EBP).** Apply research and determine *the best evidence* that supports your approaches. EBP means more than simply "applying research." It means integrating the *best research,* with *expert opinions* and *patient values* to achieve the best outcomes (this is addressed in detail in later chapters). The IOM also stresses that you must be able to participate in learning and research activities as much as feasible and determine *the best evidence* that supports your approaches. EBP means more than simply "applying research." It means integrating the *best research,* with *expert opinions* and *patient values* to achieve the best outcomes.
4. **Apply quality improvement.** Identify errors and hazards; understand and implement basic safety design principles, such as standardization and simplification; design and test interventions to change processes and systems of care to improve care, and continually measure care quality in terms of structure, process, and outcomes (discussed on page 211).
5. **Use informatics (use computers to manage information).** Know how to use computers to manage information, support decision-making, and reduce the incidence and effects of errors. See Box 1.2 for detailed list of required skills.

Importance of Developing Healthy Work and Learning Environments Stressed. Leaders recognize the importance of providing a climate that's respectful, healing, humane, and safe (For links for healthy workplace, violence and injury, prevention, and other topics go to www.cdc.gov/).

Stakeholders Included in Decisions. We know the importance of including key stakeholders—those who are most affected by the plan of care, for example, patients, families, care-givers, and third-party payers—early in the planning process.

Maintaining Privacy Is Law. Patient privacy is guarded by the Health Insurance Portability and Accountability Act (HIPAA) of 1996. (For frequently asked HIPAA questions and links to other helpful web pages, go to http://www.hhs.gov/news/facts/privacy.html.)

box 1.2 Diverse Skills Required to be a Nurse Today*

You must be able to

❏ **Be flexible and adapt** to different settings and circumstances, identifying new knowledge, skills, and perspectives needed to practice proficiently.

❏ **Solve problems, think critically and creatively,** and respond to clinical complexity.

❏ **Make independent and shared decisions,** considering costs and involving clients and their families as partners.

❏ **Meet deadlines,** demonstrating responsibility, self-esteem, self-confidence, self-management, sociability, and integrity.

❏ **Collaborate** with professionals, peers, patients, families, and other health care workers by cultivating communication, interpersonal, and group-thinking skills.

❏ **Think holistically,** looking after the entire patient, considering both disease process and the impact of the disease and associated problems on individual lifestyles.

❏ **Promote wellness** through education, health screening, reduction of risk factors, and control of symptoms and causative factors.

❏ **Make ethical decisions** based on ethical principles.

❏ **Teach and learn efficiently** by taking advantage of individual learning style preferences.

❏ **Assess and respond to the diverse needs** and values of various cultural and ethnic groups, as well as to reach out to diverse personalities through personality sensitivity.

❏ **Advocate for clients and families,** with the ability to present a case and listen to needs of others and a commitment to promote access to health care for all people, regardless of ability to pay.

❏ **Lead, supervise, and listen to and grasp** the needs of followers.

❏ **Manage information,** and organize and maintain files using computers to assist in interpretation and processing of information.

❏ **Use technology:** select equipment and tools, maintain and troubleshoot equipment, apply technology to tasks, and evaluate the appropriateness of complex and costly equipment.

❏ **Use resources: allocate time, money, materials, space, and human resources** in the development of programs and delivery of care.

❏ **Assess social and organizational systems;** monitor and correct performance; design or improve systems.

❏ **Determine the role of community services** in health care delivery, providing support as needed.

❏ **Provide customer service** with a clear understanding of what's important to consumers.

*This is a compilation of skills addressed in the following publications: U.S. Department of Labor. (1992). Washington, DC: Author; *Learning a Living: A blueprint for high performance, a SCANS report for America 2000; A Vision for Nursing.* [2000]. Retrieved September 1, 2000, from *http://nln.org/info-vision.htm*

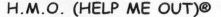

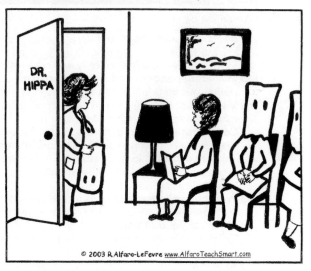

"Take this bag and put it over your head....
It's our way of ensuring privacy."

Partnerships Nurtured. To ensure common goals, professional, teacher–learner, and nurse–patient relationships are more equal. Patients are encouraged to speak up and take an active role in all nursing care (See Box 1.3).

Patients' Rights and Cultural and Spiritual Needs Addressed. Standards require that patients have the right to have their cultural, communication, and spiritual needs addressed. Statements of patients' rights (see page 20) must be given to clients; nurses must assess cultural influences such as beliefs, values, and spiritual orientation. You can download a detailed brochure on Patients' Rights in English and Spanish from http://www.jointcommission.org/PatientSafety/SpeakUp/.

Diverse Responsibilities. Nurses at all levels in hospitals, homes, skilled nursing facilities, nursing homes, and communities are more accountable for diagnosis, prevention, and management of various health problems. Other responsibilities include primary health care, patient education, health promotion, rehabilitation, self-care, and alternative methods of healing. In many cases, nurses are responsible for overseeing care given by unlicensed workers.

Nursing Roles in Collaborative Practice Expand. Nurses increasingly diagnose and manage problems that once were in the medical domain, depending on competency (knowledge, skills, and credentials) and authority (what's allowed based on laws and facility policies). For example, in critical care units, nurses diagnose and treat hypertension, congestive heart failure, and numerous other problems using well-defined clinical protocols. There's an increased demand for advanced practice nurses (APNs), who are prepared at the master's or doctorate level and who have

box 1.3 Improve Safety: Urge Your Patients To Speak Up®

Encourage your patients to be active, involved, and informed participants on the health care team. Tell them that the following simple steps are based on research which shows that patients who take part in making decisions about their health care are more likely to have better outcomes.

Speak up if you have questions or concerns, and if you don't understand, ask again. It's your body and you have a right to know.

Pay attention to the care you are receiving. Make sure you're getting the right treatments and medications by the right health care professionals. Don't assume anything.

Educate yourself about your diagnosis, the medical tests you are undergoing, and your treatment plan.

Ask a trusted family member or friend to be your advocate.

Know your medications and why you take them. Medication errors are the most common health care errors.

Use a hospital, clinic, surgery center, or other type of health care organization that has undergone a rigorous on-site evaluation against established state-of-the-art quality and safety standards, such as that provided by the Joint Commission.

Participate in all decisions about your treatment. You're the center of the health care team.

Summarized from http://www.jointcommission.org/PatientSafety/SpeakUp

specialized skills to function in clinical, educational, research, and management roles (see Appendix A, page 247).

Monitoring Role Stressed. The importance of having skilled nurses present to monitor signs and symptoms to detect, prevent, and treat potential complications early is stressed. Patients express that caring means being skilled and vigilant, and closely monitoring their status.

Nurses Must Prove Value. Regulatory requirements stress that nurses must prove their value to both consumers and their employers, showing how they impact on patient outcomes (eg, how they promote health and independence, how they reduce health care costs). As health care facilities cut costs by hiring unlicensed workers, nurses are challenged to develop new frameworks for evaluating and showing their impact on patient care and consumer satisfaction (Box 1.5, page 21).

Nurses' Roles as Advocates, Leaders, and Managers Are Key. Nurses play a central role in efficient management of scarce resources (staff, supplies, and equipment). Leadership, critical thinking, delegation, supervision, and organizational and communication skills are required for both new and seasoned nurses.

Shared Governance and Collaborative Decision-Making. We know that shared governance (the inclusion of nurses in making decisions about rules, procedures, and other aspects of care) gets the best results. (See the Forum for Shared Governance at http://sharedgovernance.org/.)

New Illnesses and Treatments Emerge. International travel is common, increasing concerns about the spread of diseases. Experts throughout the world respond quickly to emerging illnesses to prevent world-wide spread of disease.

box 1.4 Patients' Rights*

PATIENTS RIGHTS*

Dear Consumer:

State law requires that your health care provider or facility recognize your rights while receiving medical care and that you respect their right to expect certain behavior on the part of patients. You may request a copy of the full text of this law from your health care provider or facility.

YOU HAVE THE RIGHT TO:

❏ Be treated with courtesy and respect with appreciation of dignity and protection of your need for privacy.
❏ Prompt and reasonable response to questions and requests.
❏ Be informed of:

> who is providing medical services and who is responsible for your care.
> what patient support services are available, including whether an interpreter is available if you have communication problems.
> your diagnosis, planned course of treatment, alternatives, risks, and prognosis.
> whether treatment is for purposes of experimental research (and to give or refuse your consent to participate in such research).

❏ Refuse treatment, except as otherwise provided by law.
❏ Have impartial access to medical treatment or accommodations, regardless of race, national origin, religion, physical handicap, or source of payment.
❏ Be given treatment for any emergency condition that will deteriorate from failure to receive treatment.
❏ Express any grievances about any violation of your rights as stated by state law, through the grievance procedure of your health care provider or facility and appropriate state licensing agency.

❏ File complaints against a health care professional, hospital, or ambulatory surgical center with the Agency for Health Care Administration. (Appropriate information for how to reach each state's agency must be listed here.)
❏ Receive (upon request):

> full information and necessary counseling on the availability of financial recourses for your care.
> a reasonable estimate of charges for medical care before treatment.
> information about whether your health care provider or facility accepts the Medicare assignment rate before treatment.

❏ Be given a copy of a reasonably clear and understandable, itemized bill, and upon request, to have charges explained.

YOU HAVE THE RESPONSIBILITY TO:

❏ Provide your health care provider, to the best of your knowledge, accurate and complete information about your complaints, past illnesses, hospitalizations, medications, and other matters relating to your health.
❏ Follow the treatment plan recommended by your provider.
❏ Report unexpected changes in your condition to the health care provider.
❏ Keep appointments. And, if you're unable to do so for any reason, notify your provider or facility.
❏ Assure that the financial obligations of your health care are fulfilled as soon as possible.
❏ Comply with health care provider and facility rules and regulations affecting patient conduct.

---

* This is an example form and summary of rights. Rights may vary from state to state. Forms may vary from facility to facility.

---

box 1.5 Promoting Consumer Satisfaction

To promote consumer satisfaction, consider the following:

❏ **Symptom Severity:** Whether symptoms improve or worsen in frequency, duration, and intensity.

❏ **Level of Functioning:** Ability to perform activities of daily living (impact on physical, psychosocial, and cognitive function).

❏ **Therapeutic Alliance:** Degree of positive relationship between consumer and nurse.

❏ **Use of Services:** Quantity and appropriateness of nursing services used.

❏ **Client Satisfaction:** Consumer's satisfaction with various aspects and outcomes of the nurse–client experience.

❏ **Risk Reduction:** Type and quality of positive behaviors adopted by consumers and caregivers to reduce risk of illness, injury, and disease complication or progression.

❏ **Protective Factors:** Type and consistency of changes in the patient's or caregiver's environment that prevent deterioration in health.

Concern for prevention of new and resistant bacteria grows. For example, incidences of MRSA (methicillin-resistant *Staphylococcus aureus*) infections increase. Hand sanitizing in all settings is required. Experts voice concern about the overuse of antibiotics.

Bioterrorism and Other Terrorist Attacks Require Being Alert and Prepared. Health care professionals must have plans in place for detecting and responding to bioterrorism, radiation terrorism, and other terrorist attacks early.

Shortage of Nurses and Educators Threatens Patient Care. More demands with fewer nurses threaten patient care. Some state laws require more staff for certain types of patients.[8] Nursing and other key players in health care begin to actively recruit people into the profession and find ways to make nurses' jobs better. Nurse educators are especially in demand, as older educators retire with few young educators to replace them.

Preceptors and Mentors Are Valuable Teachers. We recognize the importance of having novices work closely with preceptors and mentors. Preceptors and mentors are experienced nurses with exemplary skills who take the role of teaching and nurturing novices in the clinical setting.

Increasingly Diverse U.S. Population, Nurses, and Students. Many patients, nurses, and students who learned English as a Second Language (ESL) struggle to understand American ways of interacting and learning. Schools and hospitals respond by developing help programs and bringing together those who use ESL and those who use English as a First Language (EFL) to facilitate learning.[9]

Lifelong Learning Required. Speed of change requires commitment to lifelong learning and professional development. Nurses must be knowledgeable workers who are able to make complicated clinical judgments. Independent learning, often through the use of computers and the Internet, is the norm.

Health Care Driven by Consumer and Community Needs. Services must be driven by consumer needs and customer satisfaction. Insurance companies and consumers want to know that they get the best value for their dollar.

Healthy People 2010. National health promotion and disease prevention initiatives bring together national, state, and local government agencies; nonprofit, voluntary, and professional organizations; businesses; communities; and individuals to take major steps to improve the nation's health (Box 1.6).

Evidence-Based Care and Best Practices Stressed. Now that we have more research data and know the importance of expert opinion, we continually work to develop the best ways (best practices) to manage specific conditions from outcome and cost perspectives. Today's consumer wants to know the answer to, "What evidence do you have that this is the best approach for me?" Box 1.7 addresses the Agency for Healthcare Research and Quality (AHRQ), which leads the nation in evidence-based care practices.

Case Management, Disease Management, and Telehealth Care Expand. With more people at home and in remote areas with chronic illnesses and complicated treatment regimens, nurses and physicians manage care from a distance, through the use of telephones, television monitors, and other communications technologies. More nurses are involved in disease management and case management (care delivery models that aim to keep costs down by helping people with chronic illnesses improve their health status through close monitoring, early intervention, and use of resources).

---

box 1.6 Healthy People 2010*

What is It? *Healthy People 2010* is a set of national health objectives designed to identify the most significant preventable threats to health and to establish national goals to reduce these threats by 2010. It challenges us all (individuals and professionals—national, state, and local government agencies—nonprofit, voluntary, and professional organizations—businesses and communities) to collaborate to take specific steps to ensure that good health and long life are enjoyed by people of all ages, regardless of culture or socioeconomic status.

How Will We Measure Progress? The Leading Health Indicators (LHIs), listed below, will be used to measure the health of the nation over the next 10 years. The LHIs—which are areas that we will monitor to show progress—were selected on the basis of their ability to motivate action; the availability of data to measure progress; and their importance as public health issues.

Leading Health Indicators

Physical Activity	Mental Health
Overweight and Obesity	Injury and Violence
Tobacco Use	Environmental Quality
Substance Abuse	Immunization
Responsible Sexual Behavior	Access to Health Care

*Data from: U.S. Dept. of Health and Human Services. *Healthy People 2010.* Retrieved from http://www.healthypeople.gov

---

box 1.7 What Is the Agency for Healthcare Research and Quality (AHRQ)?*

The AHRQ is the nation's lead Federal agency for research on health care quality, costs, outcomes, and patient safety. It is the health services research arm of the U.S. Department of Health and Human Services (DHHS) and complements the biomedical research mission of its sister agency, the National Institutes of Health.

The AHRQ is a science partner working with the public and with private sectors to build the knowledge base for what works—and does not work—in health and health care and to translate this knowledge into everyday practice and policymaking.
On the AHRQ home page (http://www.ahrq.gov/), **you can find:**

1. **Links to the homes of the following research centers:**
   ❑ Quality improvement and patient safety
   ❑ Outcomes and effectiveness of care
   ❑ Clinical practice and technology assessment
   ❑ Health care organization and delivery systems
   ❑ Primary care (including preventive services)
   ❑ Health care costs and sources of payment
2. **Links to programs and information on the impact of AHRQ research on the following topics:**
   ❑ Children With Chronic Illness and Disabilities
   ❑ Chronic Disease in Adults
   ❑ Disparities in Health Care
   ❑ Health Care for Women
   ❑ HIV Disease
   ❑ Improving Health Care for Americans with Disabilities
   ❑ Long-Term Care
   ❑ Men's Health Care
   ❑ Mental Health
   ❑ Patient Safety
   ❑ Pharmaceutical Research Highlights
   ❑ Prevention Research Highlights
   ❑ Rural Health Care
3. **Links to Patient Safety Indicators**

---

*Data from: Agency for Healthcare Research and Quality. Retrieved from http://www.ahrq.gov/

Refinement of Critical Paths and Protocols. Critical paths (also known as critical pathways, clinical pathways, and care maps), which are standard multidisciplinary plans used to predict and determine care for specific problems, are refined and improved (see example on pages 173–176). As we continue to track treatment and outcome data, we have more evidence-based protocols. For example, if you have pneumonia, you'll be likely to receive a specific antibiotic proven to be effective from human and cost perspectives.

More Elderly and Chronically Ill. People live longer with diseases and disabilities. Nurses must focus on promoting health in spite of existing health problems; for example, how to help people with lung disease maximize exercise tolerance. They also must be equipped to deal with patients with multiple health problems; for example, a patient who has diabetes, hypertension, chronic lung disease, and arthritis.

H.M.O. (HELP ME OUT) ®

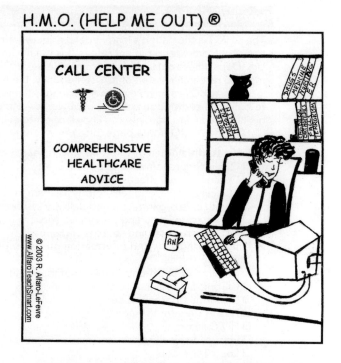

"Take two aspirin, drink lots of fluids, apply heat, get
lots of rest, and bury a potato in the back yard."

Computers and Technology Change Health Care Delivery. New technology facilitates diagnosis, decision-making, and research. Although these technologies create constant learning challenges, the ultimate improvements save time and improve care quality. More documentation is done directly through computers, often at patients' bedsides. Wireless handheld computers enable doctors and nurses to be close at hand, even when far away. Personal digital assistants (PDAs) and other electronic organizers help students and nurses access information and manage time. Electronic medical records (EMR) and On-Line Patient Records (OLPR) allow for patient care and health management across long distances.

Efforts to Standardize Language Continue. To improve communication and prevent errors, facilities must keep "do not use lists," so that staff doesn't use confusing abbreviations and terms. To create a standard language for computers to use, several organizations work to standardize terms. (This subject is discussed in detail in Chapter 3, pages 99–102).

New Ethical Concerns. Advances in infertility treatment and disease management challenge traditional values regarding conception, birth, death, and dying. Society is very concerned with the ethics of palliative care (care that alleviates pain and suffering and promotes a sense of physical and spiritual well-being, but doesn't cure). Nurses must know how to apply principles of ethics to help patients and families make informed decisions.

Wellness Centers, Holistic and Alternative Therapies. There's a greater focus on promoting health and triggering the body's natural healing powers through holistic and alternative therapies (eg, diet, exercise, acupuncture, massage, and other ways to manage stress, such as meditation and aromatherapy).

Nurse Wellness Stressed. Many workplaces recognize the need to help nurses stay healthy, giving nurses stress-reduction classes and free (or reduced-cost) wellness center memberships. A healthy nurse is central to safe, efficient nursing care. Concerns about long shifts, patient overloads, and stressful work environments get more attention. New approaches, regulations, and laws continue to address problems like poor nurse–patient ratios, and mandatory overtime.

Educated Consumers. Nurses help consumers at both ends of the "knowledge spectrum," from those who are illiterate to those who surf the Internet, becoming experts on the latest information about their problems. Many consumers today are well-informed— often knowing more about their problems than many of those who look after them.

Patient Safety Is Top Priority

Following a report by the Institute of Medicine (IOM), *To Err Is Human,*[10] which states that as many as 98,000 deaths per year in the United States may be due to medical errors, preventing errors and keeping patients safe has become top priority. The IOM stresses that to reduce errors, we need to change "cultures of blame" to "cultures of safety." In a culture of blame, those who make mistakes are personally blamed and punitive actions are taken against them. In a culture of safety, the emphasis is on identifying *all the contributing factors.* We examine errors carefully to determine the root (main) causes. For example, the root cause of medication errors may not be knowledge errors, but system failures, such as look-alike drugs being stored side by side. Other examples of system problems that contribute to mistakes include lack of IV pumps to prevent rapid infusion, nurses who are overworked or placed in positions that require knowledge and skills beyond their capabilities, and inconvenient hand sanitation stations. In a culture of safety, when errors happen, a root-cause analysis is done to study both the individual's role *and* the system's role in the mistake. Only then can we identify comprehensive strategies and procedures to prevent future errors.

> **R U L E**
>
> **Keep patients safe—move from a "culture of blame"** (where workers hide mistakes due to fear of punitive actions) **to a "culture of safety"** (where high priority is given to reporting mistakes, identifying systems that are error-prone, and working together to develop systems that keep patients safe).

The following shows key national organizations aiming to prevent errors and promote a culture of safety.

Key Organizations Focusing on Error Prevention

- Institute of Medicine (IOM): http://www.iom.edu
- The Joint Commission: www.jointcommission.org/ (Here, you find current national safety goals for ambulatory care, assisted living, behavioral health care, hospital care, disease-specific care, home care, long-term care, office-based surgery, and more.)
- Leapfrog Group: http://www.leapfroggroup.org
- National Center for Patient Safety: http://www.patientsafety.gov/
- National Patient Safety Foundation: http://www.npsf.org/
- Quality Interagency Coordination Task Force (QuIC): http://www.quic.gov/

Examples of National Safety Goals

1. Eliminate wrong-site, wrong-patient, and wrong-procedure surgery.
2. Reduce infections through improved hand washing, use of user-friendly protective barriers, and universal precautions.
3. Improve the:
   - accuracy of patient identification.
   - effectiveness of communication among caregivers.
   - safety of using high-alert medications and IV pumps.
   - effectiveness of clinical alarm systems.

(See above Web sites for up-to-date goals.)

Ethics: Advocating for Patients' Rights

To advocate for your patients and give ethical care, you need to have a good understanding of the following principles.

Seven Ethical Principles

Autonomy.

Autonomy. People have the right to make decisions based on:

❏ their own values and beliefs
❏ adequate information given free from coercion
❏ sound reasoning that considers all the alternatives

Beneficence.
Justice.
Fidelity.
Veracity.
Accountability.
Confidentiality.

Beneficence. Aim to do good and avoid harm.
Justice. Treat people fairly; aim for equality.
Fidelity. Keep promises and don't make promises you can't keep.
Veracity. Tell the truth. Be honest with patients, families, and peers.
Accountability. Take responsibility for the consequences of your actions.
Confidentiality. Keep information private (this is also law).

Following ANA Ethics Code

Think about your responsibilities in relation to the following key points, summarized from the ANA's *Code of Ethics for Nurses*[11]:

Choosing to be a nurse means making the commitment to:

❑ **Practice with compassion and respect for each person's dignity, worth, and unique individuality.** This applies to patients, families, and co-workers, regardless of the nature of their health problems, socioeconomic status, or culture. Understand that human beings have the right to self-determination—to make their own decisions based on adequate information and guided by their own values and beliefs.

❑ **Keep your primary commitment to consumers (patient, family, group, or community).** It's your responsibility to promote, advocate, and protect the health, safety, privacy, and rights of consumers. Recognize conflict of interests (when your own values and beliefs are at odds with those of patients' or other care givers). Advocate in patients' best interest.

❑ **Maintain a professional relationship.** Although giving care is personal, often requiring a friendly attitude, maintain professional boundaries. You're the professional and patients aren't your friends.

❑ **Ensure safe, effective, efficient, ethical care by collaborating with others.** Get second opinions. Delegate tasks as needed. Involve patients and key care givers to make decisions and establish shared goals. Recognize when you have an ethical dilemma that requires input from qualified ethicists. Get informed consent from patients involved in research studies.

❑ **Respect your own worth and dignity.** Incorporate healthy behaviors into your life. Strive to grow personally and professionally. Be responsible and accountable for your nursing practice (this includes your direct patient care and the overall accountability of the nursing profession). Broaden your knowledge and seek out learning experiences. Help advance the profession by contributing to practice, education, administration, and knowledge development (this improves patient care and your own worth and employability).

❑ **Participate in establishing, maintaining, and improving the health care environment.** Advocate for work conditions that are conducive to providing quality health care.

❑ **Get involved in professional organizations.** Help articulate nursing values, shape policies, and maintain and improve the integrity of the profession and its practice.

Page 28 shows a code of conduct that can help you establish ethical, trusting relationships with peers and colleagues.

Including Patient Partners While Following HIPAA Rules

The HIPAA privacy rules sometimes confuse nurses about who can be included in making decisions. It's important to remember, however, that you reduce errors and get the best results when patients involve important family and friends in health care

Code of Conduct

As a member of this team/group, I agree to work to make the following a part of my daily routine.

1. **To promote empowered partnerships by:**
   - Valuing your time and the contribution you make to the team/group.
   - Accepting the diversity in our styles—recognizing that you know yourself best and should be allowed to choose your own approaches.
   - Promising to be honest, and treating you with respect and courtesy.
   - Promoting independence and mutual growth.
   - Listening openly to new ideas and other perspectives.
   - Attempting to walk a mile in your shoes.
   - Committing to resolving conflict without resorting to using power.
   - Taking responsibility for my own emotional well being (if I feel bad about something, it's my responsibility to do something about it).
   - Ensuring that we both:
     - Stay focused on our joint purpose and responsibilities for achieving it.
     - Make decisions together as much as possible.
     - Realize that we're accountable for the outcomes (consequences) of our actions.
     - Have the right to say no, so long as it doesn't mean neglecting my responsibilities.
2. **To foster open communication and a positive work environment by:**
   - Using the concept of the "Golden Rule" ("Do unto others…").
   - Addressing specific issues and behaviors.
   - Acknowledging/apologizing if I've caused inconvenience or made a mistake.
   - Doing my "homework" before drawing conclusions.
   - Maintaining confidentiality when I'm used as a sounding board.
   - Using only ONE person as my sounding board before I decide to either give feedback or drop the issue.
   - Validating any rumors I hear.
   - Redirecting co-workers who are talking about someone to speak directly to the person.
   - Addressing unsafe or unethical behavior directly and according to policies.
   - Offering feedback as indicated:
     - Within 72 hours
     - Using "I" statements ("I feel . . ." rather than "You make me feel . . .")
     - Describing behaviors and giving specific examples
     - Limiting discussion to the event at hand and not discussing past history and telling you honestly and openly the impact of the behavior.
3. **To be approachable and open to feedback by:**
   - Taking responsibility for my actions and words.
   - Taking time to reflect on what was said, rather than blaming, defending, or rejecting.
   - Asking for clarification of the perceived behaviors.
   - Remembering that there's always a little bit of truth in every criticism.
   - Staying focused on what I can learn from the situation.

Source: © 2008 R. Alfaro-LeFevre. Available at www.AlfaroTeachSmart.com

decisions. Use your common sense. Follow HIPAA rules and privacy policies of where you work, but encourage patients to identify "personal partners" in their care. Be sure to get the names of personal partners on the chart, so that they can be involved as needed.

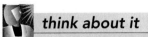

think about it

Patient-Centered Care—"Nothing About Me Without Me"*
Each patient and family holds the key to prevention of errors and optimum nursing care, and must be an integral part of all decision-making. When you provide information and encourage people to take an active role in their plan of care, you empower them to maximize health and open the door to patient satisfaction and health care efficiency.

Learn how to establish partnerships with mutual trust. Move from an *I'll-take-care-of-you* approach to one that sends the message, *I want you to know what to do when I'm not here.* Assume that patients know themselves well. Involve them by using comments like, "You know yourself best—tell me what you'd like to see happen," "What's most important to you?" and "I want you to be able to make informed choices—we share a common purpose and we're both responsible for what happens."

*This phrase was first used by an English midwife and has since been used by many authors.

CRITICAL THINKING EXERCISE I

NOTE: The point of the critical thinking exercises throughout this book is to help you to remember content and practice critical thinking skills, not to make you do time-consuming writing exercises. If you don't want to *write* the answers, think about mapping them, discussing them with someone else, verbalize them out loud to yourself, or tape-record them. If you don't need practice, skip the session entirely. The answers in the back of the book are example responses—they aren't the only answers. They are provided to help you to evaluate and correct your own thinking. If you aren't sure whether your response is acceptable, discuss it with a peer or ask your instructor.

What Is the Nursing Process and Why Learn About It?

To complete this session, read pages 5–29. Example responses start on page 241.

1. Using terms a layperson can understand, explain:
   a. The steps of the nursing process
   b. Five advantages of using the nursing process
   c. How the nursing process complements what other disciplines (eg, physicians and physical therapists) do
2. Give three reasons why using the nursing process is required.

(critical thinking continues on page 30)

CRITICAL THINKING EXERCISE I *(continued)*

3. Explain why the accuracy of each step of the nursing process depends on the accuracy of the preceding step.

4. What's wrong with this statement? *He's good at making diagnoses, but he needs to improve on his assessments.*

5. Imagine you work in a hospital. Consider the following patient satisfaction issues and think of three ways you could help nurses stay focused on the things that mean a lot to patients.

Patient Satisfaction: Top 10 Issues[12]

The 10 issues that most closely correlate with the likelihood that patients will recommend your hospital to others:

- Staff sensitivity to the inconvenience that health problems and hospitalizations cause
- Overall cheerfulness of the hospital
- Staff concern for patients' privacy
- Amount of attention paid to patients' special or personal needs
- Degree to which nurses took patients' health problems seriously
- Technical skill of nurses
- Nurses' attitudes toward patients calling them
- Degree to which the nurses kept patients adequately informed about tests, treatment, and equipment
- Friendliness of nurses
- Promptness in responding to the call button

Try This on Your Own

With a peer, in a group, or in a personal journal:

1. Discuss what the following "Think About It" items mean to you.

think about it

Nurses Are Stewards for Safe Passage. Just as a ship's steward protects passengers on a journey, your job as a nurse is to protect patients and help them navigate safe passage through the healthcare system. You hold patients' lives in your hands, but they are the ones who should be "at the helm, directing where they want to go." Involve patients and families early in decision-making. Ask questions like, "What are the main things you want to accomplish?" Help patients understand the concept of stewardship by saying something like, "I'm here to take care of you, but more importantly, I'm here to make sure you know how to take care of yourself when I'm not here". . . . "Let me know when you have questions or concerns". . . . "Stay involved in your care—you know yourself best and will do better if you let us know what you need and want."

Cutting Costs, Not Corners. Cutting costs doesn't mean "cutting corners." It means working to get *equal results within a budget.* For example, ask the pharma-

think about it *(continued)*

cist whether a generic antibiotic which is taken five times a day can be substituted for a more costly brand-name drug which is taken only three times a day. On the other hand, if you don't get the results you want because it's too inconvenient to take the generic drug five times a day, point out that it may be cheaper in the long run to use the more expensive brand drug. (Physician approval is required.)

Are You Culturally Competent? According to the Department of Health and Human Services, cultural competence is the ability to give effective care to people from different cultures.[15] This doesn't mean that you must know the beliefs of *every* culture—no one can know it all. It means that you need to learn about the values, beliefs, and customs of the populations you work with *most*. Get help when you find yourself caring for patients and families who are of a culture that you know little about. Remember that even when you *are* familiar with a certain groups' beliefs, you can't make assumptions. For example, most Amish people don't use electricity or technology. Yet, today, some Amish people have cell phones and leaf blowers. Work to develop your cultural competence: (1) Get in touch with your own values and beliefs. Understand how these affect your ability to give nursing care; (2) Work to understand, value, and incorporate your patients' cultural needs into the plan of care; (3) Don't make assumptions, as each person is unique within a cultural group. Specifically ask patients to tell you if they have any particular beliefs or traditions that need to be incorporated into the plan of care.

Fifty Years Ago—Porch Interviews and Two Bucks an Hour. On August 3, 1957, Dorothy Kavinsky, RN, of Hialeah, FL, interviewed for her first emergency room job. The interview occurred on the hospital porch and she was offered $2.36 an hour. We've come a long way![16]

2. Discuss how you feel about making mistakes. Identify ways you, your patients, and your peers can promote a culture of safety, rather than of blame.
3. Read and discuss the following online resources:
   - Brent, N. (n.d.) *Protect Yourself: Know your nurse practice act.* Available at the Nurse.com Web site: http://www.nurse.com/ce/syllabus.html?CCID=2813
   - Steefel, L. (2008). *ESL nursing students gain the courage to speak freely.* Available at the Nurse.com Web site: http://include.nurse.com/apps/pbcs.dll/article?AID=/20080128/NY02/80124012
   - Gordon, S. (2006). What do nurses really do? *Topics in Advanced Nursing eJournal, 6*(1). Available at the Medscape Web site: http://www.medscape.com/viewarticle/520714_3
   - U.S. Department of Health and Human Services. (2003). *HIPAA privacy rules: Frequently asked questions.* Available at the HHS Web site: http://www.hhs.gov/news/facts/privacy.html
4. Review the *Leading Health Indicators* addressed by *Healthy People 2010* in Box 1.6 (page 22). Decide where you, your peers, and your community stand in relation to efforts to improve health. Identify some things you could do to improve awareness of and actions for these efforts.

What's the Difference Between Nursing Process and Critical Thinking?

You may hear the term *nursing process* and *critical thinking* being used interchangeably, but there is a difference between these two terms: the nursing process *is a tool* and critical thinking is *how you use the tool.* Just like a car is a tool to take you where you want to go in your daily life, the nursing process gets you where you need to be with patient care. But you can't use a car or the nursing process without using your head. The more you use your brains, the better you can use any tool, whether it's a car or the nursing process.

Let's take a look at how to think critically—how to use your head. Remember that unlike the mindless thinking that happens when you do routine things like brushing your teeth, critical thinking is deliberate, purposeful, and informed. Consider the following description.

Critical Thinking Is Outcome-Focused Thinking That[6]:

- **Is guided by standards, policies and procedures, ethics codes, and laws** (individual state practice acts).
- **Is based on principles of nursing process, problem solving, and the scientific method** (requires forming opinions and making decisions based on evidence).
- **Carefully identifies the key problems, issues, and risks involved,** including patients, families, and major care providers in decision-making **early.**
- **Applies logic, intuition, and creativity** and is grounded in specific knowledge, skills, and experience.
- **Is driven by patient, family, and community needs,** as well as nurses' needs to give competent efficient care (eg, streamlining paperwork to free nurses for patient care).
- **Calls for strategies that make the most of human potential** and compensate for problems created by human nature (eg, finding ways to prevent errors, using information technology, and overcoming the powerful influence of personal views).
- **Is constantly re-evaluating, self-correcting, and striving to improve.**

R U L E

Critical thinking is contextual—it changes with circumstances (one size doesn't fit all). Look for changes *in the patient or situation* that require you to change your approach. For example, if you go from working in a hospital (where you're in charge and equipment and resources are plentiful) to working in home care (where you're a guest in someone else's home and have to improvise), you may have to re-think the whole process.

How to Become a Critical Thinker

Critical thinking is like any other skill: if you practice, it becomes more automatic. The exercises throughout this book are meant to help you develop, refine, and practice your ability to think critically in the context of nursing situations. As you complete each chapter, learning and applying the principles and rules of the nursing process, you begin to develop habits that help you be more automatic in your approaches to nursing situations. For now, study Boxes 1.8, 1.9, and 1.10 which list Critical Thinking Indicators (CTIs)—behaviors that evidence suggests promote critical thinking in nursing. Get a beginning idea of where you stand in relation to being a critical thinker—consider each indicator and rate your abilities using the following scale 0–10 scale:

0 = I'm not very good at demonstrating this indicator
10 = I almost always demonstrate this indicator.

---

box 1.8 Personal Critical Thinking Indicators (CTIs) (Behaviors Demonstrating CT Characteristics/Attitudes)

Personal CTIs are brief descriptions of behaviors that demonstrate characteristics that promote critical thinking. Indicators are listed in context of *clinical practice*.

❏ **Self-aware:** Clarifies biases, inclinations, strengths, and limitations; acknowledges when thinking may be influenced by emotions or self-interest.
❏ **Genuine:** Shows authentic self; demonstrates behaviors that indicate stated values.
❏ **Self-disciplined:** Stays on task as needed; manages time to focus on priorities.
❏ **Healthy:** Promotes a healthy lifestyle; uses healthy behaviors to manage stress.
❏ **Autonomous and responsible:** Shows independent thinking and actions; begins and completes tasks without prodding; expresses ownership of accountability.
❏ **Careful and prudent:** Seeks help when needed; suspends or revises judgment as indicated by new or incomplete data.
❏ **Confident and resilient:** Expresses faith in ability to reason and learn; overcomes disappointments.
❏ **Honest and upright:** Seeks the truth, even if it sheds unwanted light; upholds standards; admits flaws in thinking.
❏ **Curious and inquisitive:** Looks for reasons, explanations, and meaning; seeks new information to broaden understanding.
❏ **Alert to context:** Looks for changes in circumstances that warrant a need to modify thinking or approaches.
❏ **Analytical and insightful:** Identifies relationships; expresses deep understanding.
❏ **Logical and intuitive:** Draws reasonable conclusions (if this is so, then it follows that . . . because . . .); uses intuition as a guide to search for evidence; acts on intuition only with knowledge of risks involved.
❏ **Open and fair-minded:** Shows tolerance for different viewpoints; questions how own viewpoints are influencing thinking.
❏ **Sensitive to diversity:** Expresses appreciation of human differences related to values, culture, personality, or learning style preferences; adapts to preferences when feasible.
❏ **Creative:** Offers alternative solutions and approaches; comes up with useful ideas.
❏ **Realistic and practical:** Admits when things aren't feasible; looks for user-friendly solutions.
❏ **Reflective and self-corrective:** Carefully considers meaning of data and interpersonal interactions, asks for feedback; corrects own thinking, alert to potential errors by self and others, finds ways to avoid future mistakes.
❏ **Proactive:** Anticipates consequences, plans ahead, acts on opportunities.
❏ **Courageous:** Stands up for beliefs, advocates for others, doesn't hide from challenges.
❏ **Patient and persistent:** Waits for right moment; perseveres to achieve best results.

(box continues on page 34)

box 1.8 Personal Critical Thinking Indicators (CTIs) (Behaviors Demonstrating CT Characteristics/Attitudes) (continued)

❑ **Flexible:** Changes approaches as needed to get the best results.
❑ **Empathetic:** Listens well; shows ability to imagine others' feelings and difficulties.
❑ **Improvement-oriented (self, patients, systems):** *Self*—Identifies learning needs; finds ways to overcome limitations, seeks out new knowledge. *Patients*—Promotes health; maximizes function, comfort, and convenience. *Systems*—Identifies risks and problems with health care systems; promotes safety, quality, satisfaction, and cost containment.

Note: The preceding is the ideal—no one is perfect. Even the best thinkers' characteristics vary depending on circumstances such as comfort and familiarity with the people and situations at hand. What matters is *patterns* of behavior over time (is the behavior usually evident?). If you're a critical thinker, you can probably easily pick three or more of the above characteristics that you'd like to improve (critical thinkers are naturally focused on self-improvement).

box 1.9 Knowledge Critical Thinking Indicators (CTIs) (Requirements vary, depending on context [for example, specialty practice])

Clarifies:

❑ Nursing and medical terminology
❑ Nursing vs. medical and other models, roles, and responsibilities
❑ Signs and symptoms of common problems and complications
❑ Related anatomy, physiology, pathophysiology
❑ Normal and abnormal function (bio-psycho-social-cultural-spiritual)
❑ Factors that promote or inhibit normal function (bio-psycho-social-cultural-spiritual)
❑ Related pharmacology (actions, indications, side effects, nursing implications)
❑ Reasons behind interventions and diagnostic studies
❑ Normal and abnormal growth and development
❑ Nursing process, nursing theories, and research principles
❑ Applicable standards, laws, practice acts
❑ Policies and procedures and the reasons behind them
❑ Ethical and legal principles
❑ Spiritual, social, and cultural concepts
❑ Where information resources can be found
❑ How own thinking, personality, and learning style preferences may differ from others' preferences
❑ Personal values, beliefs, needs
❑ Organizational mission and values

Demonstrates:

❑ Ability to solve mathematical problems related to medication administration
❑ Focused nursing assessment skills (eg, breath sounds or IV site assessment)
❑ Related technical skills (eg, n/g tube or other equipment management)

---

box 1.10 Intellectual Skills Critical Thinking Indicators (CTIs)
(Behaviors Demonstrating Intellectual Competencies)

Nursing Process and Decision-Making Skills:

❑ Applies standards and principles when planning, giving, and adapting care
❑ Assesses systematically and comprehensively; uses a nursing framework to identify nursing concerns, uses a body systems framework to identify medical concerns
❑ Detects bias; determines credibility of information sources
❑ Distinguishes normal from abnormal; identifies risks for abnormal
❑ Determines significance of data; distinguishes relevant from irrelevant; clusters relevant data together
❑ Identifies assumptions and inconsistencies; checks accuracy and reliability; recognizes missing information; focuses assessment as indicated
❑ Concludes what's known and unknown; makes reasonable inferences (conclusions) and judgments—gives evidence to support them
❑ Considers multiple explanations and solutions
❑ Identifies both problems and their underlying cause(s) and related factors; includes patient and family perspectives
❑ Determines individualized outcomes; focuses on results
❑ Manages risks, predicts complications, promotes health, function, and well-being; anticipates consequences and implications—plans ahead accordingly

❑ Sets priorities and makes decisions in a timely way; includes key stakeholders in making decisions
❑ Weighs risks and benefits; individualizes interventions
❑ Reassesses to check responses and monitor results (outcomes)
❑ Communicates effectively orally and in writing
❑ Identifies ethical issues and takes appropriate action
❑ Identifies and uses technologic, information, and human resources

Additional Related Skills:

❑ Establishes empowered partnerships with patients, families, peers, and coworkers
❑ Teaches patients, self, and others
❑ Addresses conflicts fairly; fosters positive interpersonal relationships
❑ Facilitates and navigates change
❑ Organizes and manages time and environment
❑ Gives and takes constructive criticism
❑ Facilitates teamwork (focuses on common goals; helps and encourages others to contribute in their own way)
❑ Delegates appropriately; leads, inspires, and motivates others
❑ Demonstrates systems thinking (shows awareness of the interrelationships existing within and across health care systems)

Source: *Critical Thinking Indicators* © 2008 R. Alfaro-LeFevre. All rights reserved. No copying without written permission. Available: www.AlfaroTeachSmart.com

Using the Four-Circle CT Model

Another way to look at critical thinking is to use the four circles on the next page to get a "picture" of what it takes to think critically.

Going clockwise on the circles, here's what you need to do:

1. Develop CT attitudes, characteristics, and behaviors (top circle). When you develop CT characteristics like the ones in the box on page 33, the skills in the other circles come readily.

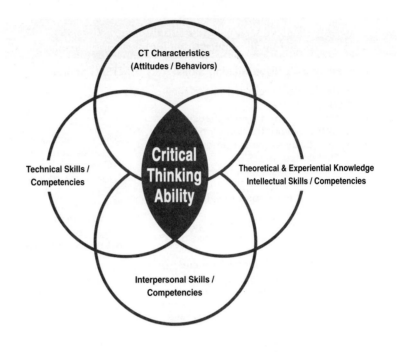

4-Circle CT Model
© 2002 R. Alfaro-LeFevre
www.AlfaroTeachSmart.com

2. **Acquire theoretical and experiential knowledge, as well as intellectual skills** (these skills are addressed in the Knowledge CTIs on page 34 and Intellectual CTIs on page 35).
3. **Gain interpersonal skills.** If you can't get along with others, you will be unlikely to think critically, because you will soon be out of the loop (people will avoid you). At the other end of the spectrum, if you're "too nice" to confront or give criticism, you contribute little to others' critical thinking and often lose brainpower to stress. Table 1-3 lists behaviors affecting interpersonal relationships.
4. **Practice technical skills.** Until technical skills (for example, IV skills or computer skills) are second nature, you have less brain power for critical thinking (due to the "brain drain" of mastering technical skills).

> ### R U L E
> **Develop your critical thinking skills by seeking out real and simulated experiences.** When you participate in patient care or work through simulated experiences, you learn deeply and become more proactive and able to plan ahead. Remember the proverb, *I hear, I forget . . . I see, I remember . . . I do, I understand* . . . Critical thinking skills are developed with practice and time.

table 1.3 Behaviors Affecting Interpersonal Relationships

Behaviors That Enhance Interpersonal Relationships	Behaviors That Inhibit Interpersonal Relationships
Conveying an attitude of openness, acceptance, and lack of prejudice.	Conveying an attitude of doubt, mistrust, or negative judgment.
Being honest.	Being deceptive.
Taking initiative and responsibility; responding to others' concerns.	Conveying an "it's not my job" attitude.
Being reliable.	Not meeting commitments, only partially meeting commitments, or not being punctual.
Demonstrating humility.	Demonstrating self-importance.
Showing respect for what others are, have been, or may become.	"Talking down" or assuming familiarity.
Accepting accountability.	Making excuses or placing blame where it doesn't belong.
Showing genuine interest.	Acting like you're only doing something because it's a job.
Conveying appreciation for others' time.	Assuming others have more time than we do.
Accepting expression of positive *and* negative feelings.	Showing anger when negative feelings are expressed.
Being frank and forthright.	Sending mixed messages, saying things just because we think it's what the other person seems to want to hear, or talking behind others' backs.
Admitting when we've been wrong.	Denying or ignoring when we've made an error.
Apologizing if we've caused distress or inconvenience.	Acting like nothing happened or making excuses.
Being willing to forgive and forget.	Holding grudges.
Showing a positive attitude.	Conveying an "it'll never work" attitude.
Conveying a sense of humor.	Acting like there's no room for anything but "serious business."
Allowing others control.	Trying to control others.
Giving credit where credit is due.	Ignoring achievements or taking credit that doesn't belong to us.

Willingness and Ability to Care

Using the nursing process means being willing and able to care for your patients. Caring is often an innate characteristic, but let's look at how it also requires commitment.

Willingness to Care

Being willing to care means making the choice to do what it takes to help others. This includes choosing to:

❏ Keep the focus on what's best for the consumer (patient, family, community)
❏ Respect the values, beliefs, and individuality of others
❏ Stay involved, even when problems become chronic or more complex
❏ Maintain a healthy lifestyle so you're able to help

Being willing to care also means making a commitment to make the following professional behaviors part of your everyday practice.

ANA Professional Practice Behaviors[13]

As a nurse, you must:

- Maintain knowledge, skills, and competence in current practices
- Evaluate the quality and effectiveness of your own performance and of nursing practice in relation to professional standards and rules and regulations
- Practice collegially, contributing to the professional development of peers and colleagues
- Collaborate with patients, families, peers, professionals, and others
- Integrate research findings into practice
- Use resources to improve safety, effectiveness, cost, and impact on planning and giving care.

Being Able to Care

Being able to care requires understanding ourselves and understanding others.

Understanding Ourselves

Because our tendencies, reactions, and habits tend to change as we grow and mature, gaining deep understanding of ourselves is a lifelong pursuit. When we learn about ourselves and recognize how our values and frame of reference influence our thinking and ability to understand others, we can take deliberate steps to be more objective and helpful.

Understanding Others

Understanding others takes active empathetic listening—being fully present and working to fully comprehend someone else's perceptions. It's like trying to "view the world through someone else's glasses" or "walk a mile in another's shoes." Read the following steps, and then think about how you can apply them to the case scenario that follows.

Listening Actively and Empathetically

1. Eliminate thoughts about how you, yourself, see the situation.
2. Listen carefully for *feelings*, trying to identify with how the other person perceives his situation. Don't allow yourself to think about how *you* feel or how you're going to respond; think only about the content of what you're hearing.
3. Reflect on what you heard; then name the feelings that were expressed.
4. Seek verification that you understood the message and the feelings correctly. Keep trying until you're sure you understand.
5. Detach, come back to your own frame of reference. Try to separate yourself from the emotions involved so that you can stay logical and objective.

CASE SCENARIO

Listening Empathetically Promotes Understanding the Real Issues and Therapeutic Communication

Today Pat is caring for Sharon, who just gave birth to healthy twin girls. Pat herself has always wanted children, but has been unable to conceive. Pat notes that Sharon seems very quiet. Recognizing the importance of being an active, empathetic listener, Pat has the following conversation with Sharon.

Pat: "You've been pretty quiet since I came on."

Sharon: "I can't help it. I'm supposed to be happy, but I'm sad. I wanted to have at least one boy."

Pat (makes a conscious effort to eliminate personal thoughts about the fact that this woman is crying over twin girls, when she, herself, has never been able to have *one* child—then rephrases what she heard): "You're supposed to be happy, but you feel sad?"

Sharon: "Yes."

Pat: (Uses silence to reflect on the feeling of sadness and encourage Sharon to continue)

Sharon: "The doctor told us one of the babies was a boy. I planned to name him after my father. My Dad is dying and I wanted to do this for him."

Pat (connects to what Sharon must be feeling): "That *would* be a disappointment."

Sharon (crying): "Yes. I had it all pictured in my mind."

Pat: (Stays quiet, conveys acceptance and understanding as Sharon cries)

Pat (detaches and becomes logical and objective): "Sharon, I know you feel sad right now. Hormones may be influencing how you feel. But, you have two beautiful little girls waiting to see you. Maybe we can figure out a girl's name that's a version of your father's. Shall I go get them?"

Sharon (smiling): "Yes. I only held them for a few minutes. I have to admit that it will be fun dressing two girls."

CRITICAL THINKING EXERCISE II

Critical Thinking and Willingness and Ability to Care

To complete this session, read pages 32–39. Only exercise number one has an example response (page 241).

1. Identify five critical thinking indicators you want to develop.
2. Complete the following sentence, using as many words as you choose: If I were to tell someone how I think, I would say that I . . .
3. In five sentences or less, explain the relationship between critical thinking and the nursing process.
4. In a personal journal, with a peer, or in a group:
   a) Discuss your personal experiences with the following caring behaviors.

Caring Behaviors

- Acknowledge that each person's experience is unique (don't assume you know—or make negative judgments about—others' feelings).
- Monitor patients closely and let them know you're doing it (eg, "I'll check on you every 15 minutes.")
- Keep people informed—listen actively and speak compassionately.
- Instill hope (creating a vision of what "can be").
- Offer companionship—just sit quietly.
- Avoid clichés (eg, "God gives you only what you can bear").
- Help people to stay in touch with positive aspects of their lives (eg, ask about friends, pets, special interests, or hobbies).
- Give patients and families resources to help themselves. For example, tell them about the *Top Ten Dos and Don'ts When Someone in Your Life Becomes Seriously Ill* at www.CarePages.com (click on Articles and Tips). CarePages are free personal Web sites that connect family and friends during illness or injury.

   b) Address how the following statements from ***Nursing: A Social Policy Statement***[14] relate to this chapter.
   - Health and illness are human experiences.
   - The presence of illness does not preclude health, nor does optimal health preclude illness.
   - An essential feature of contemporary nursing practice is the provision of a caring relationship that facilitates healing.
   - Humans manifest an essential unity of mind, body, and spirit.
   - Human experience is contextually and culturally defined.
   c) Explore the meaning of the "Voices" on the next page.
   d) Address the relationship between and among the key points on the map on the next page.

Try This on Your Own

1. **Improve your interpersonal skills.** Learn about your innate personality and how to get along with "difficult" people. Read *Don't Worry! Be Happy! Harmonize Diversity Through Personality Sensitivity,* available at http://www.nurse.com/ce/course.html?CCID=4217.

APPLYING NURSING PROCESS PRINCIPLES
AS DESCRIBED IN THIS BOOK

THINKING CRITICALLY ABOUT PATIENT CARE

☐ Communicate effectively (listen, speak, and chart carefully)
☐ Promote independence, function, comfort and well-being (as
   defined by patients themselves); guard patient privacy.
☐ Partner with patients, colleagues, and stakeholders to clarify
   expected outcomes and make care decisions
☐ Assess systematically—draw conclusions based on *facts*
☐ Address bio-psycho-social-cultural-spiritual needs
☐ Access information—apply knowledge and evidence
☐ Follow standards, policies, procedures, ethics codes, and laws
   (state practice acts).
☐ Remember that laws prohibit you from making medical diagnoses
   independently; but that *you* are *accountable* for reporting signs and
   symptoms and activating the chain of command as needed.
☐ Change your approach depending on the patient and situation
   (critical thinking is contextual and changes with circumstances)
☐ Perform interventions (assess, re-assess, revise, record)
☐ Monitor (evaluate) outcomes
☐ Keep patients safe (teach patients to speak up; report error-prone
   systems, follow safety procedures)
☐ Think ahead, think in action, think back (reflect on your thinking)
☐ Be accountable and responsible—improve care practices and
   your own knowledge and performance

voices

Who Guards the Patient?
"Safety lies at the crux of the care we deliver. And yet we all know that there are so
many factors that affect patient safety—from communication snafus through systems design problems through inadequate staffing . . . Nurses are in pivotal roles
within health care settings because they coordinate, implement, and evaluate the
patient care that is administered by the entire team on an ongoing basis."[17]

—*Rebecca B. Rice, RN, EdD, MPH*

Simply Being Nice and Making Work Fun Improves Outcomes
"[Studies show that] patients who come away from a positive encounter with a
nurse are more likely to follow prescribed directions, take medications, and seek
follow-up care . . . [however, if] a patient encounters a health care worker who's in a
negative emotional state, it becomes a springboard into other negative behaviors.
Down the road, their own outcomes suffer, and they just don't fare well. . . . Try to
make the work environment as fun as possible. If you see a staff member in a bad
mood, jump in and try to derail it before it becomes contagious."[18]

—*Howard Weiss, PhD*

(critical thinking continues on page 42)

CRITICAL THINKING EXERCISE II *(continued)*

2. Are you stressed out? Managing stress is an important part of staying healthy. Take the Life Stress Test at http://www.cliving.org/lifstrstst.htm. Think of things you can do to reduce your stress level.

3. Practice empathetic listening. Ask someone to tell you about an upsetting experience in his or her childhood and listen using the steps of empathetic listening listed on page 39. Discuss what can happen when you're too emotionally involved in patient situations. Identify ways you can manage your emotions to remain empathetic, but also objective and logical.

THIS CHAPTER AND NCLEX*

The following processes are integrated throughout:

1. Nursing process (five steps)
2. Caring

3. Teaching and learning
4. Communication and documentation

SUMMARY / KEY POINTS

- The nursing process—the first tool you need to learn to "think like a nurse"—is required by national practice standards, essential to thinking critically in the clinical setting, and a key part of NCLEX. It's a *cycle*—rather than a linear process—and it's purposeful, humanistic, systematic, organized, dynamic, and outcome-focused (results-oriented).

- The five steps—*Assessment, Diagnosis, Planning, Implementation,* and *Evaluation*—overlap and are interrelated. The accuracy of all of the steps depends on good communication skills and factual, relevant, and comprehensive assessment data.

- The nursing process complements what other health care professionals do by focusing on both the medical problems and on the *impact* of medical problems and treatment plans on patients' lives (human responses). The nursing process also aims to promote health by maximizing independence, sense of well-being, and ability to function, regardless of the presence of illness or disability.

- Using the nursing process requires you to apply national and state laws and local policies and procedures. It also requires following ethics codes and principles, and applying a code of conduct (see page 24).

- Being competent in using the nursing process requires a commitment to develop critical thinking behaviors (see CTIs listed on pages 33–35), strong interpersonal and technical skills, and being willing and able to care. The 4-circle CT model (page 36) gives you a picture of what it takes to think critically.

- Scan this chapter for important rules, maps, and diagrams highlighted throughout, then compare where you stand in relation to the expected learning outcomes on pages 3–4.

---

*Data from www.ncsbn.org/nclex.htm. See also "This Chapter and NCLEX" on pages 87, 137, 177, 202, and 221.

References

1. Caine, R., & Caine, G. (2002). *Making connections: Teaching and the human brain.* Reading, MA: Addison-Wesley.
2. On Purpose Associates. (n.d.). *Brain-based learning.* Retrieved February 7, 2008, from Funderstanding Web site: http://www.funderstanding.com/brain_based_learning.cfm
3. Hart, L. (2002). *Human brain, human learning* (3rd ed.). Covington, WA: Books for Educators, Inc.
4. American Nurses Association. (2004). *Nursing scope and standards of performance and standards of clinical practice.* Washington, DC: American Nurses Publishing.
5. Buppert, C. (2008). The legal distinction between the practice of medicine and the practice of nursing. *The Journal for Nurse Practitioners, 4*(1), 22–24.
6. Alfaro-LeFevre, R. (2008). *Critical thinking indicators: 2007–2008 evidence-based version.* Retrieved February 5, 2008, from http://www.alfaroteachsmart.com/cti.htm
7. Alfaro-LeFevre, R. (2009). *Critical thinking and clinical judgment: A practical approach to outcome-focused thinking* (4th ed.). Philadelphia: Saunders-Elsevier.
8. Carlson, K. (2008). *State regulations require more staff for some types of patients.* Retrieved February 5, 2008, from http://www.modbee.com/local/story/176897.html
9. Steefel, L. (2008). *ESL nursing students gain the courage to speak freely.* Retrieved February 5, 2008 from http://include.nurse.com/apps/pbcs.dll/article?AID=/20080128/NY02/80124012
10. Institute of Medicine. (2000). *To err is human: Building a safer health system.* Washington, DC: National Academies Press. Retrieved February 5, 2008 from The National Academies Press Web site: http://lab.nap.edu
11. American Nurses Association. (2001). *Code of ethics for nurses with interpretive statements.* Washington, DC: American Nurses Publishing.
12. McIntosh, T. (1997). Empathy: Why patients recommend hospitals. *Healthcare Benchmarks, 4,* 39.
13. American Nurses Association. (2004). *Nursing scope and standards of performance and standards of clinical practice.* Washington, DC: American Nurses Publishing.
14. American Nurses Association. (2003). *Nursing: A social policy statement* (2nd ed.). Washington, DC: American Nurses Publishing.
15. Department of Health and Human Services, Health Resources and Services Administration, Bureau of Health Professions (n.d.) *Other Definitions of Health Competence.* Retrieved February 5, 2008, from http://bhpr.hrsa.gov/diversity/cultcomp.htm
16. Hialeah nurse celebrates 50 years. (2008, January 28). *Nursing Spectrum* (Florida ed.), *18*(2), 13.
17. Rice, R. B. (2003). Patient safety: Who guards the patient? *Online Journal of Issues in Nursing, 8*(3), 1. Retrieved January 28, 2008, from www.nursingworld.org
18. Farella, C. (2000). Cooling the cauldron on your unit. *Nursing Spectrum, 10*(9). Retrieved February 7, 2008, from www.nurse.com

chapter 2

Assessment

what's in this chapter?

Stressing the points that *Assessment and Diagnosis* overlap significantly—and that the safety and efficiency of the entire plan depends on the accuracy and completeness of *Assessment*—this chapter examines how to do an assessment that's tailored to a specific patient situation (one size doesn't fit all). You study what an assessment that promotes critical thinking "looks like" and what behaviors (critical thinking indicators) help you to think critically during this phase. You learn that while in many cases you use standard or electronic tools to guide and record your assessments, YOU are the one who has to develop the knowledge and skills to make sure that the information *you record on those tools* is accurate and complete. To make clinical decisions, and to pass NCLEX and other competency tests, YOU are the one who has to develop habits that promote critical thinking during *Assessment*. This chapter helps you develop these habits, teaching you how to set priorities during assessment and when and how to do various types of assessments (data base assessments, focus assessments, and quick priority assessments). Finally, you get detailed guidelines for interviewing and examining patients and study how to complete six dynamic and interrelated phases of *Assessment:* (1) collecting data; (2) identifying cues and making inferences; (3) validating data; (4) clustering related data; (5) identifying patterns/testing first impressions; and (6) reporting and recording data.

ANA standards related to this chapter[1]

Standard 1   Assessment. The registered nurse collects comprehensive data pertinent to the patient's health situation.

critical thinking exercises

- **Critical Thinking Exercise III**   Developing Your Interview and Physical Assessment Skills
- **Critical Thinking Exercise IV**   Subjective and Objective Data; Cues and Inferences; Validating Data
- **Critical Thinking Exercise V**   Clustering Related Data
- **Critical Thinking Exercise VI**   Reporting and Recording Significant Data

expected learning outcomes

After studying this chapter, you should be able to:

■ Describe six characteristics of an assessment that promotes critical thinking, including why each one promotes critical thinking.

■ Clarify the relationships among the six phases of assessment (collecting data; identifying cues and making inferences; validating (verifying) data; clustering related data; identifying patterns/testing first impressions; reporting and recording data).

■ Discuss what can happen in the other steps of the nursing process if *Assessment* is incomplete or incorrect.

■ Explain why using *evidence-based standard tools* doesn't replace the need for you to develop *independent critical thinking* skills.

■ Compare and contrast the terms *data base* assessment, *focus* assessment, and *quick priority* assessment.

■ Apply ethical, cultural, and spiritual considerations when you perform an assessment.

■ Describe nurses' responsibilities in relation to assessing for disease, disability, and risk management.

■ Develop your interviewing skills, including knowing when and how to use open-ended questions, closed-ended questions, and exploratory statements.

■ Develop your physical assessments skills, including how to prioritize your assessment and gain information that clarifies information gained from your patient interview.

■ Identify *subjective* and *objective data* in a nursing assessment, explaining why both are needed.

(continued on next page)

Assessment: The First Step to Determining Health Status
Characteristics of an Assessment That Promotes Critical Thinking
Standard Assessment Tools and Evidence-Based Practice
Six Phases of Assessment

Collecting Data
What Resources Do You Use?
How to Ensure Comprehensive Data Collection

Data Base, Focus, and Quick Priority Assessments
Data Base (Start of Care) Assessment
Focus Assessment
Quick Priority Assessment (QPA)

Assessing Disease and Disability Management

Health Promotion: Screening for Risk Management and Early Diagnosis
Partnering With Patients to Make Informed Decisions

The Interview and Physical Assessment
Ethical, Cultural, and Spiritual Concerns

Developing Your Interviewing Skills

Guidelines: Promoting a Caring Interview
How to Establish Rapport
How to Listen
How to Ask Questions

expected learning outcomes (continued)

After studying this chapter, you should be able to:

- Identify patients' cues and make inferences (draw conclusions) based on evidence from patient assessment data.
- Explain why clustering data in more than one way (eg, both a body systems model and a nursing model) promotes critical thinking.
- Decide what information to report and record the next time you're in the clinical setting.
- Explain how to use the *Read Back Rule*, the *Repeat Back Rule*, and *SBAR* approach for communicating patient care.

Assessment: The First Step to Determining Health Status

Assessment—the first step to determining health status—is when you interview and examine the patient and gather data to find all the "necessary puzzle pieces" to get a picture of your patient's health status. Since the entire plan depends on the data you collect during this phase, you must ensure that your information is factual, comprehensive, and organized in a way that helps you get a sense of patterns of health or illness.

This chapter focuses on how *Assessment* leads to *Diagnosis.* Lets start by reviewing the following diagram from chapter one.

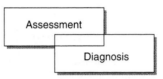

Remember that *Assessment* and *Diagnosis* overlap, and that you often move back and forth between these two steps. Sometimes, you even "work backwards." For example, you may be asked to screen patients for the diagnoses of *depression* or *coping problems*. In this case, you know the *diagnoses* that you're looking for (*depression* and *coping problems*)—you "work backwards" doing an *assessment* to decide whether or not the patient has depression or coping problems.

> ### RULE
> **The accuracy, efficiency, effectiveness, and safety of all the other steps of the nursing process—*Diagnosis, Planning, Implementation,* and *Evaluation*—depend on your ability to gather accurate, relevant, and comprehensive assessment data.** If your assessment is inaccurate, vague, or incomplete, you put your patient at risk for ineffective, inefficient, unsafe care.

Characteristics of an Assessment That Promotes Critical Thinking

To promote critical thinking, your assessment should have the following characteristics.

Purposeful. Your approach to assessment must change, depending on your purpose and the circumstances (context) of your patient's situation. For example: Do you aim to assess *all aspects* of care or *one specific problem?* Is your patient hospitalized or at home? Is the person an adult or a child? To think critically, clarify your purpose and consider your patients' circumstances.

Prioritized. You need to gain the most important information *first.* There's certain information you should gain *early* because it's likely to affect virtually every aspect of care, including how you proceed with your assessment. We discuss this in detail later when we discuss *Quick Priority Assessments.*

Focused and Relevant. You have to focus your assessment to gain the relevant facts you need to think critically.

Purposeful.

Prioritized.

Focused and Relevant.

Systematic.

Accurate and
Complete.

Recorded in a
Standard Way.

Systematic. Being systematic helps you to be comprehensive and to recognize if you have forgotten to look for—or omitted—something important.

Accurate and Complete. The most common error that happens in critical thinking is identifying problems or making judgments based on insufficient or incorrect data. Your information must be factual, and as complete as is warranted by your purpose. For example, an assessment that aims to get information about *one specific problem* is shorter than one that aims to get comprehensive data about *all aspects of care.*

Recorded in a Standard Way. Recording information in a standard way ensures that the *most important information* can easily be found by all members of the health care team. It also helps you form the habit of being systematic. As you record data over and over in a standard way, it becomes habitual.

Standard Assessment Tools and Evidence-Based Practice

Completing standard assessment tools at various points in care is required by standards and regulatory agencies. These tools are an example of *applying evidence-based practice* (EBP). EBP brings together *the best of what we know from research* and *the best of what we know from clinical experts.* Standard assessment tools—designed for specific purposes and situations—are considered *evidence-based* because they are developed based on expert opinion and research. Standard tools ensure that the most important information is recorded and communicated in the best way. Whether you're admitting a patient, transferring a patient, or simply recording daily assessments, one of the first questions you should ask is: Is there a standard form that I need to complete?

> **R U L E**
>
> **Just as pilots use Federal Aviation Administration–approved tools to reduce errors at various points during flight, you'll be required to use approved tools at specific points during patient care (eg, when you admit or transfer patients).** These tools help you be systematic and comprehensive. But they don't *think* for you. YOU are the one who has to do the critical thinking needed to ensure that the *information you record on the tools* is factual, relevant, and complete. YOU are the one who has to develop *assessment habits* that help you make clinical decisions. YOU are the one who has to have these habits "in your head" to be able to pass NCLEX and other competency tests.

Box 2.1 (page 49) describes critical thinking indicators (intellectual skills) needed in doing *Assessments.*

Six Phases of Assessment

The following six phases of *Assessment* can help you gain the facts you need for the next step, *Diagnosis.*

1. **Collecting Data:** You gather information about health status.
2. **Identifying Cues and Making Inferences:** You identify significant data and draw some beginning conclusions about what the data may indicate.

---

box 2.1 Major Intellectual Skills CTIs Related to *Assessment* (Behaviors Evidence Suggests Promote Critical Thinking)

The critical thinking nurse:

❏ Applies standards and principles
❏ Assesses systematically and comprehensively; uses a nursing framework to identify nursing concerns; uses a body systems framework to identify medical concerns
❏ Detects bias; determines credibility of information sources
❏ Distinguishes normal from abnormal; identifies risks for abnormal
❏ Determines significance of data; distinguishes relevant from irrelevant; clusters relevant data together
❏ Identifies assumptions and inconsistencies; checks accuracy and reliability; recognizes missing information; focuses assessment as indicated
❏ Communicates effectively orally and in writing
❏ Establishes empowered partnerships with patients, families, peers, and coworkers
❏ Sets priorities and makes decisions in a timely way; includes key stakeholders in making decisions
❏ Weighs risks and benefits; individualizes intervention
❏ Identifies ethical issues and takes appropriate action
❏ Identifies and uses technologic, information, and human resources
❏ Addresses conflicts fairly; fosters positive interpersonal relationships
❏ Facilitates and navigates change
❏ Organizes and manages time and environment
❏ Facilitates teamwork (focuses on common goals; helps and encourages others to contribute in their own way)
❏ Demonstrates systems thinking (shows awareness of the interrelationships existing within and across health care systems)

The knowledge indicators listed in the CTIs in Chapter 1 on page 34 and the CTIs listed on page 33 also apply.

Source: Alfaro-LeFevre, R. (2008). *Critical thinking indicators* (2007–2008 *Evidence-based version*). Retrieved from www.AlfaroTeachSmart.com

---

3. **Validating (Verifying) Data:** You double-check to make sure that your information is accurate and complete.
4. **Clustering Related Data:** You group related pieces of information together to help you to identify patterns of health or illness (eg, clustering data about nutrition together, the data about coping patterns together, and so forth).
5. **Identifying Patterns/Testing First Impressions:** You look for patterns and focus your assessment to gain more information to better understand the situations at hand. For example, you suspect that someone's data shows a pattern of poor nutrition and decide to find out what's contributing to this pattern (does the person have poor eating habits or could it be something else, such as not having enough money to eat well?).
6. **Reporting and Recording Data:** You report abnormal data (eg, a fever) and chart these on the patient's record according to policies and procedures.

Figure 2.1 shows how the six phases of *Assessment* lead to *Diagnosis.*

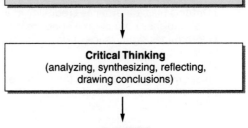

FIGURE 2.1 The above shows how the phases of *Assessment* set the stage for *Diagnosis*.

> **R U L E**
>
> **The six phases of *Assessment* are dynamic and interrelated.** For example the sixth phase—reporting and recording data—helps ensure that the first phase—collecting data—is accurate and complete (recording the data helps you recognize gaps in data collection). After *Assessment* becomes *habit,* the six phases are fluid and dynamic.

Let's look at the six phases of *Assessment,* starting with the first one, collecting data.

Collecting Data

Collecting data is an ongoing process. It begins when you first meet patients, and continues until they're discharged. This section addresses the resources and methods you use to gather information.

What Resources Do You Use?

The following bullets summarize the resources to consider when gathering data.

❏ Patients and significant others
❏ Nursing and medical records, including diagnostic and laboratory studies
❏ Consultations with other experts (eg, physicians, pharmacists, dieticians, clinical nurse specialists)
❏ Additional key stakeholders (eg, care givers, primary care providers, insurance companies)

While all of the preceding are important, remember the following rule:

> **RULE**
>
> **Even though data collection requires you to collect information from various resources, always consider your *direct assessment of the patient* to be your *primary source* of information.** Your direct assessment gives the most up-to-date information.

How to Ensure Comprehensive Data Collection

Comprehensive data collection often occurs in three phases:

1. **Before you see the person:** You find out what you can. This information may be limited (only name and age) or extensive (you may have medical records to review).
2. **When you see the person:** You interview the person and do a physical examination.
3. **After you see the person:** You review the resources you used and determine what *other resources* may offer additional information (eg, you may consult with a pharmacist to gain more information about a medication regimen).

Data Base, Focus, and Quick Priority Assessments

There are three major types of assessments, summarized below and addressed in detail in the following section.

1. **Data base (start of care) assessment:** Comprehensive information you gather on *initial contact* with the person to assess *all aspects* of health status. See example on pages 52–55 (Figure 2.2).
2. **Focus assessment:** Information you gather to determine the status of a *specific condition.* See Figure 2.3 (page 56) and Figure 2.4 (page 57).
3. **Quick Priority Assessments (QPA):** These are short, focused, prioritized assessments that you do to gain the most important information you need to keep in mind as you plan or give nursing care. See page 58 (Box 2.2).

> **RULE**
>
> **Depending on where you work, you may be required to enter data base, focus, and quick priority assessments into the computer.** Computer, print, and paper assessment forms help you be systematic and comprehensive. However, remember to think WITH the computer or form. Find ways to reflect on the big picture. Don't just dump data into computer data bases like the ones in Figures 2.5 and 2.6 (pages 59 and 60).

(text continues on page 57)

COMPLETE THIS SECTION FOR ALL PATIENTS
UNLESS SPECIFIC ASSESSMENT IS WARRANTED

Patient Name: _____

CULTURE/RELIGIOUS/SPIRITUAL	ACTION TAKEN
Religious Preference: ☐ None ☐ Catholic ☐ Protestant ☐ Jewish ☐ Other _____ Any special cultural, spiritual or religious needs while in the hospital? ☐ NO ☐ Yes Specify: _____	☐ Refer to Chaplain ☐ Other Referral

SOCIAL/DISCHARGE PLANNING	ACTION TAKEN
☐ Lives Alone ☐ Stairs ☐ Bathroom on same level as living quarters ☐ Lives with spouse/significant other/family/caretaker ☐ Lives in nursing home/assisted living ● ☐ Compromised in ADLs and/or lack of support network ● ☐ Special discharge needs ●_____ ☐ Insurance concerns ● ☐ Received supports prior to admission: ☐ unknown ☐ home care ☐ med equip ● ☐ Patient plans to be discharged to: _____ ☐ Discharge Transportation (Name) _____ (Phone#)_____ ☐ Unable to return to pervious living arrangement ● ☐ Financial concerns ● ☐ Evidence of physical/emotional abuse or neglect or domestic violence ● ☐ Current substance abuse ● ☐ No discharge planning needs identified	☐ Assist With ADLs ☐ Patient Education ● ☐ Refer to Case Manager Referral ● ☐ Refer to Social Work Referral

EDUCATION NEEDS ASSESSMENT

Learning Readiness: ☐ Willing to Learn ☐ Unable to Learn
Barriers to Learning: ☐ No Barriers ☐ Cognitive ☐ Cultural ☐ Educational ☐ Emotional
  ☐ Language ☐ Motivational ☐ Financial ☐ Physical ☐ Religious ☐ Refuses at this time
  ☐ Comments/Other _____

Plans to Overcome Barriers to Education: ☐ Family involvement ☐ Reinforcement ☐ Written Materials
  ☐ Audiovisual Aids ☐ Interpreter ☐ Other _____

Special Educational Needs: ☐ Disease Process ☐ Activity Level ☐ Diet ☐ Procedures ☐ Hygiene
  ☐ Medications (including Drug and Food Interactions) ☐ Medical Equipment/Assistive Devices
  ☐ Skin/Ostomy (Certified wound Ostomy Continence notified)
  ☐ Other _____

Teaching to be directed primarily to: ☐ Patient ☐ Family ☐ Other _____
Patient Folder Given? ☐ Yes ☐ No

Clinical Pathway Initiated? ☐ Yes ☐ See Flowsheet/Progress Note

Correct ID band in place ☐ Yes
  ☐ Patient Handbook/Patient's Right and Responsibilities reviewed.
  ☐ Patient/family oriented to room

Completed by RN: _____   Date:_____   Time:_____

Reviewed by RN: _____   Date:_____   Time:_____

FIGURE 2.2 Admission Tool.

Main Line Health

● *Jefferson Health System*

☐ Paoli Hospital ☐ Lankenau Hospital
☐ Bryn Mawr Hospital

INITIAL PATIENT ASSESSMENT

Complete shaded area **OR** ☐ See 24 Hour Flow Sheet ☐ See E.D. Triage Sheet
☐ See Critical Care Pathway

Date:	Time:	Height:	Weight:	Language spoken other than English:

Primary Care Physician: _____ Specialist: _____

Vital Signs Temp _____ P_____ RR_____ BP_____
O2 Sat _____ O2 _____ RA _____

Reason for procedure/hospitalization: _____

Procedure: _____

Allergies: Drug/Food/Latex/Tape/Dyes ☐ None Known

ALLERGIES	REACTION		ALLERGIES	REACTION		ALLERGIES	REACTION

ALL MEDICATIONS	☐ SENT HOME	☐ TO PHARMACY				
(Included over-the-counter drugs, vitamins, diet pills, and herbals currently being taken)	Dose	Route	Frequency	Last Taken	Reason for Taking/Comments
1.					
2.					
3.					
4.					
5.					
6.					
7.					
8.					
9.					
10.					
11.					

Recent Aspirin/Ibuprofen/Anti-inflammatory/Vitamin E/Blood Thinner: _____

PAST SURGICAL HISTORY

Past surgical History: _____

Previous anesthesia: ☐ General ☐ Spinal ☐ Other _____

Problems with Anesthesia? _____

Blood Donations-This Admission ☐ Autologous ☐ Direct Donor ☐ None

Figure 2.2 Continued.

Patient Name: _____ MR #: _____

HEALTH HISTORY   **Check Applicable Boxes Only**

NEUROLOGIC	CARDIOVASCULAR	RESPIRATORY	GASTROINTESTINAL
☐ CVA/TIA	☐ High Blood Pressure/	☐ Emphysema/Bronchitis	☐ Hiatal Hernia/Reflux
☐ Speech Difficulty	☐ Low Blood Pressure	☐ Asthma	☐ Hepatitis
☐ Swallowing/Choking	☐ Aneurysm	☐ Shortness of breath	☐ Ulcers
☐ Blackouts/Fainting/Vertigo	☐ Heart Attack	☐ TB	☐ Crohn's/Colitis
☐ Seizures	☐ Heart Failure	☐ Pneumonia	☐ Gall Bladder Disease
☐ Migraine/Headaches	☐ Murmur	☐ Seasonal/Environmental	☐ Irritable Bowels
☐ Numbness/Tingling	☐ Chest Pain/Angina	☐ Allergies	☐ Diverticular Disease
☐ Confusion	☐ Irregular Pulse	☐ Snoring/Apnea	☐ Ostomy _____
☐ Memory Changes	☐ Circulation Problem	☐ Breathing Devices: _____	☐ Recent change in bowel habits
☐ Head Injury	☐ Phlebitis/Clots		☐ Blood in stool
☐ Other _____	☐ Pacemaker/Defib.	☐ Other _____	☐ Last B.M. _____
☐ No identified problems	☐ High Cholesterol	No identified problems	☐ Other _____
	☐ Other _____		☐ No identified problems
	☐ No identified problems		

Comments: _____

MUSCULOSKELETAL	GENITOURINARY	PSYCHOSOCIAL	MISCELLANEOUS
☐ Arthritis	☐ Kidney Stones	☐ Alcohol use _____	☐ Vision Changes
☐ Muscle Weakness	☐ Prostate Problems	☐ Drug use _____	☐ Hearing Deficit
☐ Joint Replacement _____	☐ Ostomy	☐ Panic/Anxiety Attacks	☐ Glaucoma/Cataracts
☐ Spinal Problems	☐ Burning/Urgency Frequency	☐ Depression	☐ Blood/Bleeding Disorders
☐ Other _____	☐ Blood in Urine	☐ Physical/Psychological	☐ CA _____
☐ No identified problems	☐ Kidney Failure	☐ Abuse	☐ Skin Problems
METABOLIC	☐ Dialysis	☐ Tobacco use _____	☐ Hearing Deficit
☐ Diabetes Type: _____	☐ Breast Masses/	☐ Claustrophobia	☐ Infectious Disease/STD
☐ Thyroid	☐ Tenderness/Discharge	☐ ADD	☐ Head Circumference _____
☐ Hypoglycemia	☐ LMP _____	☐ Growth and Development	(if appropriate)
☐ Anemia	☐ Possibility of Pregnancy	not appropriate for age	☐ Immunizations up to date
☐ Other _____	☐ Breast Feeding	☐ Bereavement	(< > = 18 yrs)
☐ No identified problems	☐ Other _____	☐ Other _____	☐ Other _____
	☐ No identified problems	☐ No identified problems	☐ No identified problems

Comments: _____

Needs Assessment

☐ Orthodontic appliance	☐ Prosthesis	☐ Religious Items
☐ Dentures _____	☐ Glasses/Contacts	☐ Crutches/Walker/Cane/Wheelchair
☐ Hearing Aid	☐ Hairpiece	☐ Other _____

CURRENT PAIN		**CARE OR LEARNING NEED**

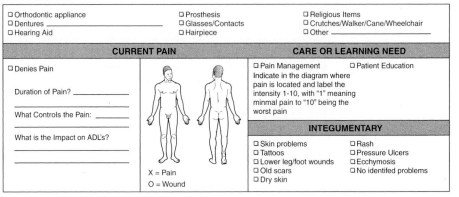

CURRENT PAIN

☐ Denies Pain

Duration of Pain? _____

What Controls the Pain: _____

What is the Impact on ADL's? _____
_____
_____

X = Pain
O = Wound

CARE OR LEARNING NEED

☐ Pain Management   ☐ Patient Education
Indicate in the diagram where pain is located and label the intensity 1-10, with "1" meaning minmal pain to "10" being the worst pain

INTEGUMENTARY

☐ Skin problems	☐ Rash
☐ Tattoos	☐ Pressure Ulcers
☐ Lower leg/foot wounds	☐ Ecchymosis
☐ Old scars	☐ No identifed problems
☐ Dry skin	

Advance Directives   ☐ NA (Patient < 18 years old)   ☐ Unable to Assess

Does the patient have an advance directive?	☐ Yes	☐ No	☐ Information Given	☐ Information Declined
If "Yes" copy in current chart? Obtain from previous chart	☐ Yes	☐ No	Follow-up action: ☐ Family to obtain copy for record ☐ Patient to formulate another advance directive (sample in "It's Up To You") ☐ Substance as stated by patient: _____	
If "No" does the patient wish to make an advance directive?	☐ Yes-Refer to Social Work	☐ No	☐ Patient declines stated context ☐ Patient/family declines to bring, and/or complete advance directive information	

FIGURE 2.2 Continued.

COMPLETE THIS SECTION FOR INPATIENTS ONLY
UNLESS SPECIFIC ASSESSMENT IS WARRANTED

Patient Name: _____ MR #: _____

NUTRITIONAL STATUS	☐ No Identified Problems	ACTION/TAKEN
If any of the following are present, send computer order to Nutrition Services ☐ Any Specific diet and/or restrictions ❶ ☐ Unintentional Weight Loss/Gain ? 10 lbs in the Last 6 Months ❶ ☐ Vomiting/Diarrhea for the Last 3 Days or Longer ❶ ☐ Poor Appetite for the Last 5 Days or Longer ❶ ☐ Swallowing Difficulties resulting in inadequate intake ❶ ☐ Newly Diagnosed Pt with Diabetes Need for Education ❶, ❷ ☐ Pressure Ulcer Stage II or greater ❶, ❸ ☐ Dialysis ❶ ☐ New to modified Diet and Needs Education ❶		❶ ☐ Nutrition Referral ❷ ☐ Diabetes Educator Referral ❸ ☐ Certified Wound Ostomy Continence Nurse Referral

RESPIRATORY ASSESSMENT	☐ No Identified Problems	ACTION/TAKEN
☐ Patient is pre-op for upper abdominal or thoracic surgery and has a history of Emphysema, Bronchitis, Asthma, or Pulmonary Fibrosis		☐ Respiratory Care Referred

FUNCTIONAL STATUS ASSESSMENT	☐ No Identified Problems			ACTION/TAKEN
	Independent	Some Assist	Total Assist	☐ Assist with ADL's
Feeding				
Bathing				
Dressing				
Toileting				
Transfer (bed to chair, to/from toilet)				
Walking/Use of Wheelchair				☐ Patient/Family Education

If any of the following are present, refer as follows:	ACTION/TAKEN
OCCUPATIONAL THERAPY ☐ No Needs Identified ☐ Condition Resulted in difficulty in use of one or both arms. ☐ Decreased Ability for Self-Care That Could Be Helped With Therapy. ☐ Physically Unable To Feed Self	☐ Physician Order Requested For: OCCUPATIONAL THERAPY

PHYSICAL THERAPY ☐ No Needs Identified
☐ Condition has Resulted in Walking, and Transfer That Could Be
  Resolved with Therapy.
☐ Condition has Resulted in Decreased Strength and/or Range of Motion
  of arms and legs.
☐ Condition has Resulted in Acute Increase in Muscle or Back Pain.
	PHYSICAL THERAPY

SPEECH THERAPY ☐ No Needs Identified ☐ Difficulty Swallowing or Signs of Choking While Drinking/Eating. ☐ Diagnosis of Stroke, Myasthenia Gravis and Multiple Intubations. ☐ Unable to Follow Simple Instructions for Daily Care and/or Unable to Communicate Wants and Needs.	SPEECH/LANGUAGE PATHOLOGY

FALL RISK ASSESSMENT* Low Risk 0–20 Moderate Risk 25–60 High Risk 65–100 *See Patient Safety: Fall Safety Program		
Fall Assessment Indicators	**Weight Score**	**Assessment Score**
Admission or transfer	5	
History of falls	20	
Recent change in functional mobility	20	
Alteration in elimination	20	
Diagnosis/Medication which effects cognition/mobility/balance	10	
Confusion/impairment of judgement/forgetful/agitated and or non-compliant	20	
Sensory/Visual/Perceptual impairment (unrelated to above)	5	
TOTAL SCORE	100	

FIGURE 2.2 Continued.

FOCUS ASSESSMENT: SKIN

Note to the patient: Please help us assess your problem by taking a few moments to complete the self-assessment below. To give you the best care possible, we need you to pay attention to your body and keep us informed. In accordance with national safety goals, we want **YOU** to be a key player in all your health care decisions. Please speak up if you have any concerns.

Are you experiencing any of the below? (Use back of page if you need more room.)

	Yes	No	Where?	Started When?	What Makes it Better?	What Makes It Worse?
Itching						
Tingling						
Pain						
Swelling						
Redness						
Rash						
Blisters						
Drainage						
Lumps/ Lesions/ Moles						
Circulation Problems						

Other Important Questions To Think About...

	Yes	No
Have you been exposed to heat, direct sunlight, or tanning beds?		
Do you have any other symptoms, like fatigue or fever?		
Have you been exposed to chicken pox, measles, or anything like that?		
Have you been wearing clothes that fit tightly anywhere on your body?		
Are you taking any medications that have skin side effects? (List meds below)		
Anything else you want us to know? (Write on back of page)		

☐ **Any Allergies (include medications)?**

☐ **Medications (Include herbal and over-the-counter meds):**

Mark Problems Below

FIGURE 2.3 Focus Assessment Tool.

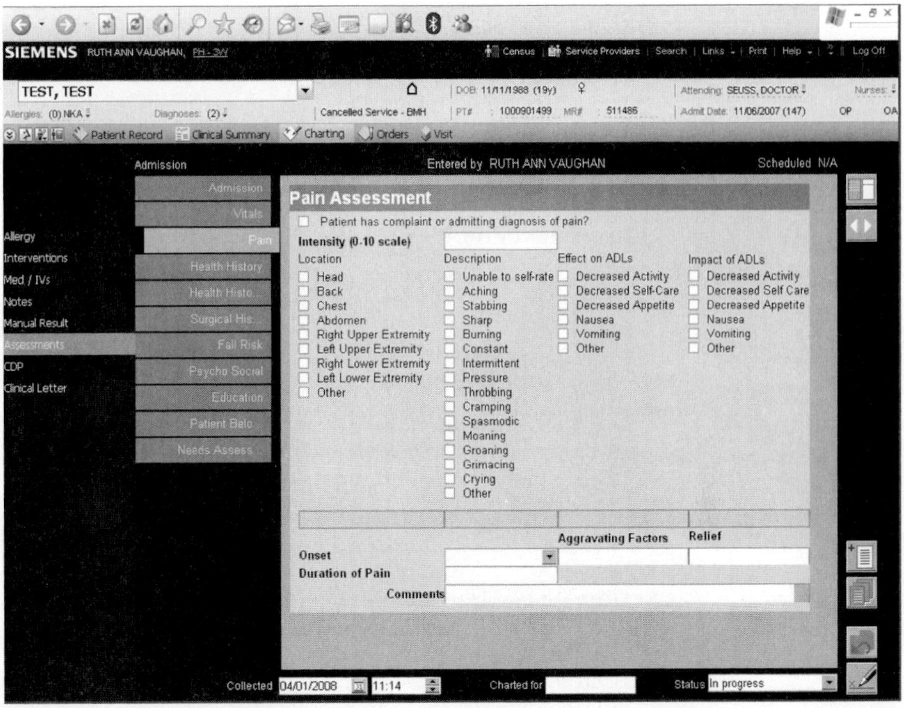

FIGURE 2.4 Computer screen showing focus assessment for pain. (Reprinted with permission from Paoli Memorial Hospital, Paoli, PA.)

Data Base (Start of Care) Assessment

Depending on the setting—for example, acute care versus long-term care—government and regulatory agencies mandate that nurses complete standard data base (start-of-care) assessment tools for each patient. These tools are designed to ensure that the major information that's required to plan and give care is easily found (this is often called the *minimum data set*—the minimum that *must* be collected for every patient—and may include information that must be recorded to get Medicare, Medicaid, and other third-party payer payments).

Focus Assessment

You may do a *focus assessment* as part of a comprehensive data base assessment or by itself to monitor specific aspects of care. For example, as part of a comprehensive admission assessment, you may do a focus assessment to determine the neurological status of someone with a head injury. Later, you're likely to continue neurological focus assessments every hour to check for changes in status.

The following are the types of questions you need to ask during initial and ongoing focus assessments.

box 2.2 Quick Priority Assessment (QPA)

DEFINITION: A QPA includes the things that you should find out *first* in all patient encounters. You often do the QPA categories in rapid succession, or at the same time (not necessarily one before the other). QPAs also include focus assessments you do when calling doctors or transferring care from one nurse to another (eg, the SBAR approach on page 61).

Assessment Priorities	Rationale
❑ Risks for infection, injury, or violence.	Keeping patients, yourself, and others safe is top priority. Address risks for patient infection or transmission of infection to others immediately (follow policies and procedures). Do the same for injury and violence risks.
❑ Problems (or risks for problems) with breathing, comfort, vital signs, or communication.	Problems and risks in these areas should be dealt with *early*. They also point to problems in *other areas* (eg, pain usually flags a problem that needs to be dealt with).
❑ Allergies ❑ Current medications and treatments ❑ Admitting Diagnosis / Chief Complaint ❑ Current and past medical problems ❑ Current and past nursing problems.	These flag known problems and risks and affect decisions about initiating certain treatments.

Examples of Initial Focus Assessment Questions

- What are your symptoms?
- Can you point with one finger to the areas that are bothering you?
- When did they start?
- What makes them better?
- What makes them worse?
- Are you taking any medications—prescribed, over-the-counter, or herbal remedies— that may be causing some of these symptoms?
- What else might be contributing to your symptoms?

Examples of Ongoing Focus Assessment Questions

- **What's the current status of the problem** (are there signs, symptoms, or risk factors for the problem)?
- **Compared with the baseline data** (data gathered before treatment began), does the information indicate that the problem is better, worse, or the same?
- **What factors are contributing to the problem,** and what has been done about these factors?
- **What's the patient's perspective** on the current status of the problem and how it's being managed?

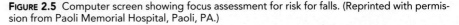

FIGURE 2.5 Computer screen showing focus assessment for risk for falls. (Reprinted with permission from Paoli Memorial Hospital, Paoli, PA.)

The following example focus assessment shows how to apply the preceding questions to assess for the problem of constipation.

Example Focus Assessment for Constipation

1. **What is the current pattern of bowel elimination?** Is there evidence of signs, symptoms, or risk factors for constipation?
2. **Compared to the baseline data, does the current data indicate that the constipation (or risk for constipation) has changed?** Are the signs, symptoms, and risk factors still present? Are there new ones?
3. **What factors are contributing to the constipation (eg, poor diet, lack of fluid intake, medication side effects, and immobility)?** How can we ensure enough roughage and fluid intake? Is there anything we can do about the immobility? What can be done about medication side effects (eg, can the drugs be changed? How can we be sure we stay on top of this problem?)?
4. **What's the patient's perspective on his current status and preventing and managing constipation?** Is he able to explain how to manage this problem? Is there a need for teaching?

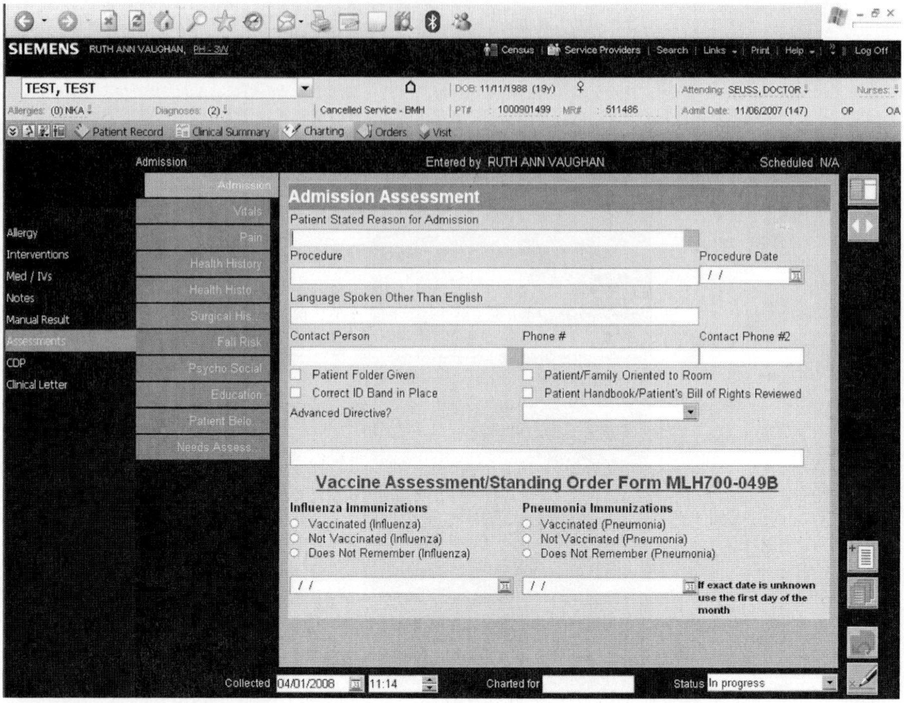

FIGURE **2.6** Computer screen showing first screen of an admission assessment. (Reprinted with permission from Paoli Memorial Hospital, Paoli, PA.)

Quick Priority Assessments (QPAs)

Knowing how to do QPAs is important for two reasons:

1. These assessments "flag" existing problems and risks.
2. The information you gain often affects every aspect of care, including how you proceed with your assessment. For example, if your patient shows signs of a communicable disease, you need to immediately consider what precautions to take, before you continue assessment.

R U L E

Quick Priority Assessments (QPAs) help you make the most of your time with patients and improves the quality, efficiency, and safety of nursing care. Box 2.2 (page 58) and the SBAR approach (next page) are examples of QPAs.

NOTE: Pronounced S-BAR and first used by the military to improve the effectiveness of communication between care givers, the SBAR approach is recommended by patient safety experts. SBAR forms vary depending on purpose and setting. Some places use SBAR for giving hand-off situations (when one nurse transfers patient care to another). Some places use SBAR forms like the one below for calling physicians about a problem.

→ Have the chart in hand before you make the phone call, and be sure you can readily communicate all of the following information.

S SITUATION: Have the chart in hand before you make the phone call, and be sure you can readily communicate all the following: Briefly state the issue or problem: what it is, when it happened (or how it started) and how severe it is. Give the signs and symptoms that cause you concern.

B BACKGROUND: Give the date of admission and current medical diagnoses. Determine the pertinent medical history and give a brief synopsis of the treatment to date (eg, medications; oxygen use; nasogastric tube; IVs, code status).

A ASSESSMENT: Give most recent vital signs and any changes in the following:

- ☐ Mental status – neuro signs
- ☐ Respirations
- ☐ Pulse – skin color
- ☐ Comfort – Pain

- ☐ GI status (nausea-vomiting-diarrhea, distention)
- ☐ Urine Output
- ☐ Bleeding-Drainage
- ☐ Other: _____

R RECOMMENDATION: State what you think should be done. For example:

- ☐ Come see the patient now
- ☐ Get a consultation
- ☐ Get additional studies (eg, CXR, ABG, EKG, CBC, other)
- ☐ Transfer the patient to ICU
- ☐ If the patient doesn't improve
- ☐ How frequent do you want vital signs.
- ☐ If there's no improvement, by when do you want us to call you?

*Data from: Haig, K, Sutton, S. and Whittington, J. (2006) SBAR: A Shared Mental Model for Improving Communication Between Clinicians. *Journal of Quality and Patient Safety*, 32(3), 167 – 175. Available: http://www.jcipatientsafety.org/fpfd/psp/SBAR.pdf

Source: R. Alfaro-LeFevre Handouts © 2007-2008 www.AlfaroTeachSmart.com

Assessing Disease and Disability Management

Many patients today live with chronic conditions—for example, diabetes, asthma, heart disease, cancer, or paralysis. You need to assess these conditions *early* for three main reasons:

1. You must be sure that the medical plan is current. You're responsible for ensuring that all medical problems are being managed by a qualified primary care provider. You don't plan nursing care unless the patient has an up-to-date medical evaluation.

2. **How you manage nursing care is influenced by the medical treatment plan** (eg, if you decide you need to encourage fluids in a patient with heart disease, you need to know if there are fluid restrictions).

3. **You need to find out how patients manage their diseases or disabilities.** Patients are the experts on how they manage their own care. If they're managing their diseases and disabilities well, follow their care management plan as much as possible (don't assume you have a better way). If they're managing these poorly, find out *why* so that the reasons can be addressed in the plan of care (eg, is there a lack of knowledge or is the problem a lack of resources?).

Health Promotion: Screening for Risk Management and Early Diagnosis

Increasingly today, your assessments will include screening for risk management and early diagnosis of common health problems.

Screening is often done at significant points during the life cycle. For example:

❑ Assessing infant development using standard scales
❑ Measuring height, weight, and vision in school-age children
❑ Assessing for problem drinking and depression beginning in adolescence
❑ Measuring cholesterol and fecal occult blood in adults

In many settings, standards require you to do focus assessments to address risks such as smoking. To meet the goals of *Healthy People 2010*—which aims to increase the length and quality of life of all people—you may be required to do specific health promotion counseling (eg, smoking cessation, weight control) during all important interactions.

Nurses also make a significant impact on patient outcomes by screening for many problems that were once considered only physician responsibilities. For example, nurses routinely screen for diabetes, depression, substance abuse, domestic abuse, violence, and vision and hearing problems.

Learn More About Health Screening and Prevention of Common Diseases. Access the *Healthy People 2010* documents online at http://www.healthypeople.gov/. Explore the **Agency For Healthcare Research and Quality** (AHRQ) Web site, (http://www.ahrq.gov/) where you can download the *Guide to Clinical Preventive Services* free from http://www.ahrq.gov/clinic/pocketgd.htm and find links to a wealth of resources—in English and Spanish—including clinical practice guidelines, research findings, public health preparedness, information technology, patient safety, and how to help patients be active healthcare consumers.

Partnering With Patients to Make Informed Decisions

A key part of assessment is partnering with patients to make informed decisions about what screening and prevention measures they should follow. This means moving from a *paternalistic* model ("we know what's best for you") to a *partnership* model ("we want you to be informed so that you can *choose the best for you*"). The following summarizes information from U.S. Preventive Services Task Force (USPSTF) related to discussing health screening with patients[2]:

The length of discussions about screening for health problems and use of medication to prevent diseases varies according to:

❏ The scientific evidence addressing how useful the service is
❏ The health, preferences, and concerns of each patient
❏ The decision-making style of each clinician
❏ Practical constraints, such as the amount of time available

The USPSTF points out that you can consider your patients decisions to be informed and mutually decided only if they:

❏ Understand the risks or seriousness of the disease or condition to be prevented
❏ Comprehend what the preventive service involves (including the risks, benefits, alternatives, and uncertainties)
❏ Have weighed their values about the potential benefits and harm associated with the service
❏ Have engaged in decision-making at a level at which they want and feel comfortable

The Interview and Physical Assessment

The nursing interview and physical assessment complement each other, as you can see in the following example.

E x a m p l e
You interview a woman who tells you, "My breathing doesn't feel right." You take a stethoscope and listen to her lungs. What you hear (whether the breath sounds are normal or abnormal) gives you additional information that complements and clarifies what you've been told.

Ethical, Cultural, and Spiritual Concerns

The success of your interview and examination is influenced by your awareness of ethical, cultural, and spiritual concerns. As a nurse, you must:

1. **Assess with respect for human dignity** and the uniqueness of the patient, unrestricted by considerations of social or economic status, personal attributes, or the nature of health problems.[3]

2. **Safeguard the client's right to privacy** by judiciously protecting information of a confidential nature. This is also law.

3. **Be honest.** Tell the person the truth about how you'll use the data (eg, "I have to write a paper examining someone's eating patterns. Would you be willing to tell me about your eating habits?").

4. **Respect cultural and religious beliefs** and be aware of physical tendencies related to culture. This includes being aware of:

   • **Biologic variations.** For example, differences among racial and ethnic groups (eg, skin color and texture, and susceptibility to diseases like hypertension or sickle-cell anemia).

   • **Comfortable communication patterns.** For example, how language and gestures are used, whether eye contact or touching is acceptable, and whether the person is threatened by being in close proximity to another.

   • **Family organization and practices.** We have diverse family units and practices. We must understand them to gain insight into factors that influence health status.

   • **Beliefs about whether people are able to control nature and influence their ability to be healthy** (eg, whether blood transfusions are allowed or whether rituals are required).

   • **The person's concept of "God" and beliefs about the relationship between spiritual beliefs and health status** (eg, "God gives you what you deserve.").

Developing Your Interviewing Skills

Your ability to *establish rapport, ask questions, listen, and observe* is central to building a therapeutic relationship. People seeking health care are in a vulnerable position. It's your job to help people feel like they're in good hands and that their main concerns will be addressed. The following guidelines can help you to establish trust, create a positive attitude, and reduce anxiety.

Guidelines: Promoting a Caring Interview

How to Establish Rapport

Before You Go Into the Interview

❑ **Get organized.** Be sure you have everything you need to have with you.

❑ **Don't rely on memory:** Have a printed or electronic assessment tool to guide the questions you'll ask (eg, use a standard tool).

❑ **Plan enough time:** The admission interview usually takes 30 to 60 minutes.

❑ **Ensure privacy:** Make sure you have a quiet, private setting, free from interruptions or distractions.

❑ **Get focused:** Clear your mind of other concerns (other duties, worries about yourself). Say to yourself, "Getting to know this person is the most important thing I have to do right now."

❏ **Visualize yourself as being confident, warm, and helpful:** This helps you to *be* confident, warm, and helpful—your genuine interest comes through.

When You Begin the Interview

❏ **Introduce yourself and give your name and position.** This sends the message that you accept responsibility and are willing to be accountable for your actions. This is especially important if you are a student.

❏ **Verify the person's name and ask what he or she would like to be called** (eg, "I have your name as Jack Riley. Is that correct? What would you like us to call you?"). Use the preferred name to help the person feel more relaxed and send the message that you recognize that this person is an individual who has likes and dislikes.

R U L E

In accordance with national patient safety goals, when you do an assessment or give nursing care, use at least two unique identifiers to be sure you have the right name and patient.[4] For example, ask the person his name and birth date and also check the ID bracelet to make sure it matches.

❏ **Briefly explain your purpose** (eg, "I'm here to do the admission interview to help us plan your nursing care.").

During the Interview

❏ **Give the person your full attention.** Avoid the impulse to become engrossed in your notes or in reading the assessment tool.

❏ **Avoid rushing.** It sends the message that you're not interested in what the person has to say.

❏ **Sit down.** This communicates that you're willing to take your time.

How to Listen

❏ **Listen actively and empathetically** (see page 39, in Chapter 1).

❏ **Use short, supplementary phrases that let the person know you understand** and encourage the person to continue. Some examples are, "I see," "Mm-hm," "Oh, no," "And . . . ," and "Then what?" A nod of the head and maintaining eye contact also lets the person know that you're listening.

❏ **Listen for feelings as well as words.** Someone who sighs, looks away, and says, "I'll be okay with this," might be telling you, "I doubt this will work."

❏ **Let the person know when you see body language** that sends a message that conflicts with what is being said (eg, "You say that you aren't having pain, but you look uncomfortable to me.").

❏ **Be patient If the person has a memory block.** This information may be remembered later when you ask related questions.

❏ **Avoid the impulse to interrupt.** If the interview is getting off track, allow people to finish sentences, then say, "We're getting off track. Can we get back to . . . ?"

❏ **Allow for pauses in conversation.** Silence gives both you and the person time to gather thoughts, and allows you to reflect on the accuracy of the information the patient has provided.

How to Ask Questions

❏ **Ask about the person's main problems first** (eg, "What are the main reasons you're here today?").

❏ **Focus your questions to gain specific information about signs and symptoms.** (eg, "Show me where the problem is." "Can you describe how this feels more specifically?" "When did this start?" "When does this seem to happen?" "Is there anything that makes it better?" "What makes it worse?")

❏ **Don't use leading questions** (questions that lead the person to a specific response; eg, "You don't drink alcohol, do you?" leads the person to a "no" answer).

❏ **Do use exploratory statements** (statements that begin with words like tell, describe, explain, and elaborate) to get the person to tell you more about specific conditions (eg, "Tell me more about your sleeping patterns."). Some authors use the term *leading statements* instead of *exploratory statements.* I use *exploratory statements* to avoid confusion with *leading questions,* which you *shouldn't* use.

❏ **Use communication techniques that enhance your ability to think critically and get the facts:**
   1. **Use phrases that help you see the other person's perspective** (eg, "From your point of view, what are the biggest problems?" or "What are the problems as you see them?").
   2. **Restate the person's own words.** This technique clarifies meaning and encourages the person to expand on what's been said (eg, "When you say . . . , what are you saying?" or "When you say . . . , does this mean . . . ?" or "Let me repeat what you said to make sure I understand.").
   3. **Ask open-ended questions** (questions requiring more than a one-word answer, such as "How are you feeling?" rather than "Are you feeling well?").
   4. **Avoid closed-ended questions** (those requiring a one-word answer) unless the person is too ill to elaborate or you're trying to clarify a response by getting a yes or no answer.

Table 2.1 gives examples of open-ended and closed-ended questions. Table 2.2 summarizes the advantages and disadvantages of using each of these types of questions.

How to Observe

❏ **Carefully assess areas connected to verbal complaints** (eg, if someone has abdominal discomfort, focus your assessment carefully on the abdomen).

❏ **Use your senses.** Do you see, hear, or smell anything unusual?

❏ **Note general appearance.** Does the person appear well-groomed, healthy, well-nourished?

table 2.1 Examples of Closed-Ended and Open-Ended Questions

Closed-Ended	Open-Ended
Are you happy about this?	How does this make you feel?
Do you get along with your husband?	How is your relationship with your husband?
Does this make you sick to your stomach?	How does this affect your stomach?

❏ **Observe body language.** Does the person appear comfortable? Nervous? Withdrawn? Apprehensive? What behaviors do you see?

❏ **Notice interaction patterns.** Be aware of the person's responses to your interviewing style (eg, sometimes cultural and personal differences create communication barriers).

table 2.2 Advantages and Disadvantages of Open-Ended and Closed-Ended Questions

Advantages	Disadvantages
Open-Ended Question	
Brings forth more information than a question that requires only a one-word response.	May allow the person to sidestep the question.
Gives people a chance to verbalize and involves them in dialogue.	Requires a more wordy response. This may be undesirable in an emergency situation or if the individual is confused, in pain, or having difficulty breathing.
Tends to bring forth a more honest reply.	Allows opportunity to ramble and get off track.
Usually less threatening and less likely to convey negative judgment.	
Often interpreted to imply sincere interest.	
Closed-Ended Question	
Helps clarify responses to open-ended questions.	May be more threatening.
Saves time in emergency situations.	Limits the amount of information offered.
Can be helpful in focusing the interview on specific data (eg, following a checklist that asks for history of specific illnesses, such as high blood pressure, heart attacks).	Does not encourage the person to express concerns from his or her point of view.
May be helpful for those who are confused, in pain, or having difficulty breathing.	Does not encourage active dialogue between the nurse and the person.

> **box 2.3** Common Communication Errors
>
> ❑ **Using first names without permission.** For some, being called by their first name by someone other than a close friend or family member is disrespectful.
> ❑ **Using endearing names.** Most people feel degraded when called "honey, deary, sweetie, pop, grandma" by anyone other than close family.
> ❑ **"Talking down."** For example, "So you've had a pain in your tummy?"
> ❑ **Using medical terminology with laypeople.** Many people don't know common medical terms such as void, vital signs, BM.
> ❑ **Using communication techniques you're comfortable with, without paying attention to the person's response.** For example, touching someone to offer support and not noticing that he withdraws, sending the message that he doesn't want to be touched.
> ❑ **Using passive, rather than active strategies in important situations** (see Rule on page 84).

How to Terminate the Interview

❑ **Give a warning** (eg, "We have 5 minutes to finish up . . . let's be sure we have covered the most important things you want us to know.")
❑ **Ask people to summarize their most important concerns,** then summarize the most important concerns as you see them (eg, "We've talked about a lot of things. To make sure I have it right, tell me the three most important things I can help you with.")
❑ **Ask, "what else?"** (eg, "Is there anything else you want me to know?")
❑ **Offer yourself as a resource** (eg, "I want to be kept informed on how you're doing. Let me know if something changes or if you have any questions.")
❑ **Explain care routines and provide information about who is accountable for nursing care decisions.** Consumers often are confused about who is responsible for what.
❑ **End on a positive note and encourage the person to become an active participant.** (eg, "We have a good start here. I want you to be actively involved in making decisions about your care.") Give information on SPEAK UP Initiatives (Box 1.3, page 19).

Box 2.3 lists common communication errors to avoid.

Developing Your Physical Assessment Skills

To develop your physical assessment skills, you need to work at being thorough, systematic, and skilled in the following techniques.

❑ **Inspection:** Observing carefully by using your fingers, eyes, ears, and sense of smell
❑ **Auscultation:** Listening with a stethoscope

❏ **Palpation:** Touching and pressing to test for pain and feel inner structures, such as the liver

❏ **Percussion:** Directly or indirectly tapping a body surface to determine reflexes (done with a percussion hammer) or to determine whether an area contains fluid (done by tapping fingers over surface)

How you organize your assessment is influenced by three things:

1. **The person's condition:** If the person is ill or has a specific complaint, begin by examining the problem areas before going on to other parts of the body (eg, if there's abdominal pain, examine the abdomen first; if someone is unconscious, assess neurological, respiratory, and cardiovascular status first).
2. **The standard tool that you're required to complete.** In many cases, these guide your approach.
3. **Your own preference.** You may choose a head-to-toe approach, beginning by assessing the head and neck, and continuing down the body to the thorax, abdomen, legs, and feet, in that order. Or you may choose a systems approach such as the one in Box 2.4 below.

The following guidelines help you to develop habits that promote a thorough and systematic physical assessment.

---

box 2.4 Systematic Head-to-Toe Physical Assessment

❏ **Neurologic status.** Check: mental status; orientation; pupillary reaction; vision and appearance of the eyes; gag reflex; ability to hear, taste, feel, and smell; gait; coordination; arm and leg reflexes; presence of pain or discomfort (eg, headache)
❏ **Respiratory status.** Check: throat, airway, breath sounds, rate and depth of breathing, cough, symmetry of chest expansion, presence of pain/discomfort (eg, chest pain)
❏ **Cardiac and circulatory status.** Check: apical heart rate, rhythm, heart sounds; quality of pulses (radial, brachial, carotid, femoral, dorsalis pedis); presence of peripheral edema; presence of pain/discomfort (eg, chest or extremity pain)
❏ **Skin status.** Check: color, temperature, skin turgor, edema, lesions, rashes, lumps, hair distribution. Specifically examine male and female breasts for lumps or nipple discharge. Check for itching/pain/discomfort.
❏ **Musculoskeletal status.** Check: muscle tone, strength, range of motion, presence of pain/discomfort (eg, aches, spasm)
❏ **Gastrointestinal status.** Check: condition of the lips, tongue, gums, teeth; bowel sounds; presence of abdominal distention; impaction; hemorrhoids; presence of pain/discomfort (eg, abdominal tenderness). If vomiting, check emesis for color and blood.
❏ **Genitourinary status.** Check color and amount of urine; presence of distended bladder; discharge (vaginal, urethral); condition of the vulva; testicular examination; presence of pain/discomfort

Guidelines: Performing a Physical Assessment

❏ **Promote communication.** Establish rapport, and use good interviewing techniques (rather than working in silence).

❏ **Provide privacy.** Uncover only the body parts being examined, keeping the rest of the body draped. Tell the person before touching a part of the body that she can't see (eg, "I'm going to feel this cyst on your back.").

❏ **Don't rely on memory.** Jot down notes to be sure of accuracy.

❏ **Choose a way to organize your assessment (eg, Box 2.4, previous page) and use it consistently, so that it becomes a habit.**

> ### R U L E
>
> **Pain and cough are the "fifth and sixth" vital signs.** When taking routine vitals signs—temperature, pulse, respirations, and blood pressure—ask about the "fifth vital sign" (whether the person has pain or discomfort) and assess closely to determine the cause. Cough is the sixth vital sign. While complete lung assessment is important, you can learn a lot from brief encounters. You can say something like, "Can you cough for me so I can hear how it sounds?" The person's ability (or inability) to comply with this request tells you a lot—for example, whether the person has pain with coughing, whether there's congestion, or whether the person's cough effort is strong enough to clear the lungs. This brief encounter can help you "flag" patients who need more in-depth assessment. (In some facilities, pulse oximetry is considered the sixth vital sign. Pulse oximetry is a non-invasive way to monitor the percentage of hemoglobin that is saturated with oxygen. The pulse oximeter consists of a probe attached to the patient's finger or ear lobe that is linked to an electronic unit).

Checking Diagnostic Studies

Your physical assessment is incomplete until you check results of diagnostic studies. These studies are like a "report card" on how the body is functioning—they provide key evidence that helps you to determine health status. The data you gathered during the interview and examination may be perfectly normal, but you could miss the serious problems if you don't check the lab studies (eg, kidney, liver, and hematological problems are often silent). Diagnostic studies may also confirm your suspicions (eg, you may suspect an infection and be able to confirm it by blood work).

> ### R U L E
>
> In accordance with national patient safety goals, follow policies and procedures for reporting (or taking orders for) critical lab values, including using the "Read Back" and "Repeat Back" rules.[4] Write down and read back verbal orders for lab studies. Write down and read back lab *results*. When you give lab results to physicians or others, have them repeat back the results.

CRITICAL THINKING EXERCISE III

Developing Your Interview and Physical Assessment Skills

To complete this session, read pages 64–70 and the example responses on page 241.

Part One: Developing Your Interviewing Skills

1. **Practice asking open-ended questions.** Restate each of the following questions as an open-ended question.
   a. "Are you feeling better?"
   b. "Did you like dinner?"
   c. "Are you happy here?"
   d. "Are you having pain?"
2. **Practice clarifying communication by using reflective statements** (restating what you hear) and making open-ended questions. For each of the following statements, write a reflective statement and an open-ended question that would help you to clarify what has been said.
   a. "I've been sick off and on for a month."
   b. "Nothing ever goes right for me."
   c. "I seem to have a pain in my side that comes and goes."
   d. "I've had this funny feeling for a week."
3. **Test your knowledge of communication techniques.** Read each of the following sentences and identify whether it is an open-ended statement (O), a closed-ended statement (C), a leading question (L), an exploratory statement (E), or a supplementary phrase or statement intended to help the person continue (S).
   a. "Are you afraid of dying?"
   b. "Tell me when this first started."
   c. "I see."
   d. "You're not still afraid to feed Hector, are you?"
   e. "How do you think you'll be doing this at home?"
   f. "Do you have a history of hypertension in your family?"
   g. "And . . . ?"
   h. "You do want your family to visit, don't you?"
   i. "How do you feel about being here?"
   j. "You don't need more practice, do you?"
   k. "Explain what you mean by 'a long time.' "
4. **Rephrase each leading question that you identified in number 3** to an open-ended question.

Part Two: Developing Your Physical Assessment Skills

1. **Because physical assessment and interviewing go hand-in-hand,** use the following situations to practice focusing your interview questions on areas of concern noted during the physical examination.

(critical thinking continues on page 72)

    a. You examine and find: The patient's hands and fingernails are filthy with ground-in dirt, although the rest of him is clean. What will you say or ask next?

    b. You examine and find: The patient has a lump on the back of his head. What will you say or ask next?

    c. You examine and find: The patient's respirations are 40. What will you say or ask next?

    d. You examine and find: The patient's right eye is red, teary, and inflamed. What will you say or ask next?

2. Now practice focusing your physical examination on areas of concern voiced by the patient.

    a. Patient states: "I have had a rash that comes and goes." What will you reply and examine?

    b. Patient states: "My stomach has been hurting me." What will you reply and examine?

    c. Patient states: "I find it burns when I urinate." What will you reply and examine?

    d. Patient states: "I feel like I'm heavier than usual, like I'm bloated with fluid." What will you reply and examine?

3. Your approach to the interview and physical assessment should be influenced by:

    a. Your own preference.

    b. The patient's condition.

    c. Both of the above.

    d. Neither of the above.

Try This on Your Own

1. Practice combining interviewing techniques with a physical examination. Do a mock interview and physical examination on a peer, friend, or family member using an assessment tool from a local clinical facility. Alternatively, use the assessment tool on pages 52–55. Be sure you can explain *why* the form requires you to collect each piece of data.

2. Practice doing a focus assessment. Ask someone you know who is taking medications to allow you to do an assessment of their medication regimen. Use the memory-jog TACIT addressed in the *Think About It* on page 73 to do the assessment.

3. With a partner or in a group, discuss how doing a quick priority assessment like the one in Box 2.2 (page 58) helps you prioritize your thinking during assessment.

4. Read the following article, then discuss the challenges of assessing culturally diverse patients.

Sensenig, J. (2007). Learning through teaching: Empowering students and culturally diverse patients at a community based nursing care center. *Journal of Nursing Education, 46*(8), 373–379.

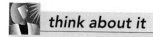

think about it

Medication side effects cause 90% of adverse drug events.[6] Prevent complications by using **TACIT** to remember what you need to assess when caring for patients taking medications or other treatments.

Therapeutic effect? (Is there a **t**herapeutic effect?)
Allergic or Adverse reactions? (Signs of **a**llergic or **a**dverse reactions?)
Contraindications? (Are there **c**ontraindications to giving this drug?)
Interactions? (Possible drug **I**nteractions?)
Toxicity/overdose? (Are there signs of **t**oxicity or **o**verdose?)

Source: Alfaro-LeFevre Clinical Cards © 2007 www.AlfaroTeachSmart.com. All rights reserved. No copying without permission.

Identifying Subjective and Objective Data

Considering both *subjective data* (what the person states) and *objective data* (what you observe) aids critical thinking because each complements and clarifies the other. For example, think about the following data.

❑ **Subjective data:** States, "I feel like my heart is racing."
❑ **Objective data:** Right radial pulse 150 beats per minute, regular, and strong

The preceding objective data support the subjective data—what you observe confirms what the person is stating.

Sometimes, what you *observe* and what the person *states* are different, as in the following data.

❑ **Subjective data:** States, "I feel fine."
❑ **Objective data:** Color pale, easily becomes short of breath

Above, what the *person states* isn't supported by what *you observe.* You need to investigate more to understand the full scope of the problems.

R U L E

Identifying both subjective and objective data promotes critical thinking because each of these complements and clarifies the other. Use the following to remember these two terms:

S—S: S subjective data = **S**tated
O—O: O objective data = **O**bserved

Use quotation marks and the patients' *own words* to give subjective data (eg, "pain comes and goes for no reason"). Use *specific, measurable terms* to give objective data (eg, *temperature of 100.6°F* is more specific and measurable than *temperature elevated*).

Examples of Subjective and Objective Data

Subjective Data	Objective Data
"I feel sick to my stomach."	Abdomen hard and distended
"My foot hurts."	Limps on left foot
"It burns when I urinate."	Urinated 150 cc clear urine

Identifying Cues and Making Inferences

The subjective and objective data you identify act as *cues*. Cues are data that prompt you to get a beginning impression of patterns of health or illness. For example, consider the following cues.

❑ **Subjective data:** "I just started taking penicillin for a tooth abscess."
❑ **Objective data:** Fine rash over trunk

The above gives you cues that may lead you to infer (suspect) that there's an allergic reaction to penicillin. How you interpret or perceive a cue—the conclusion you draw about the cue—is called an *inference*. In the preceding case, you make an inference about the rash: you decide the rash may indicate a penicillin allergy.

Your ability to identify cues and make correct inferences is influenced by your observational skills, your nursing knowledge, and your clinical expertise. Your values and beliefs also affect how you interpret some cues; make an effort to avoid making value judgments (eg, inferring that a person who bathes only once a week needs to be taught better hygiene, rather than wondering whether this could be a part of the person's culture).

To clarify your understanding of cues and inferences, study the following examples of cues and corresponding inferences.

Examples of Cues and Inferences

Cue	Corresponding Inference
"I have trouble moving my bowels."	May be constipated.
"I don't want to talk."	May be depressed or angry.
Blood pressure 60/50	Is in shock.
"I can't stand this pain any more."	Has severe pain.

Validating (Verifying) Data

Validating (verifying) that your information is factual and complete is a crucial step in critical thinking. It helps you to avoid making mistakes related to the following:

❑ Making assumptions
❑ Missing key information
❑ Misunderstanding situations

❏ Jumping to conclusions or focusing in the wrong direction
❏ Making errors in problem identification

For example, suppose you ask a woman whether she is pregnant, and she responds, "No." If you don't verify this by getting more information (eg, asking "When was your last period?" or finding out the results of a pregnancy test), you may operate under the assumption that the woman isn't pregnant when indeed she is, which can be dangerous (eg, drugs might be ordered that harm the fetus). The following guidelines help you know how to validate data.

Guidelines: Validating (Verifying) Data

❏ **Remember the following rule.**

> **R U L E**
>
> **More than one cue, more likely it's true—more than one source, more likely of course.** Critical thinking requires making judgments based on *evidence*. Look for *more than one cue* to support your conclusions. For example, if you suspect that your patient is at risk for skin breakdown, look for risk factors for *impaired skin integrity* (eg, assess feet and bony areas for dryness or redness; consider whether there are other risk factors present, such as immobility or advanced age). Also look for more than one source to verify your data. For example, if your patient's agitation causes you to suspect that there's a risk for violence, ask the family and check the chart for history of violence.

❏ **Data that can be measured accurately can be accepted as being valid** (eg, height, weight, diagnostic study results). However, keep in mind that there's always the possibility of a lab error or other factors that may alter the accuracy of studies (eg, a fasting blood sugar test that's done even though the person ate an hour earlier).
❏ **Data that someone else observes (indirect data) may or may not be true.** Verify information by directly observing and interviewing the patient *yourself.*
❏ **The following techniques help you validate questionable data.**
  • Double-check information that's extremely abnormal or inconsistent with patient cues (eg, use two scales to check an infant who appears much heavier or lighter than the scale states; repeat an extremely high or low laboratory result).
  • Double-check that your equipment is working correctly.
  • Recheck your own data (eg, take a patient's blood pressure in the opposite arm or 10 minutes later).
  • Look for factors that may alter accuracy (eg, check whether someone who has an elevated temperature and no other symptoms has just had a hot cup of tea).
  • Ask someone else, preferably an expert, to collect the same data (eg, ask a more experienced nurse to recheck a blood pressure when you're not sure).
  • Compare subjective and objective data to see if what the person *states* is consistent with what you *observe* (eg, compare actual pulse rate with perceptions of "racing heart").

• Verify your inferences with the patient (eg, "You look uncomfortable.").
• Compare your impressions with those of other key members of the health care team (eg, "He seems anxious.").

CRITICAL THINKING EXERCISE IV

Subjective and Objective Data; Cues and Inferences; Validating Data

To complete this session, read pages 73–76. Example responses are on page 242.

Part I. Subjective and Objective Data

1. List the *subjective data* noted in the following case history that follows (what does Mr. Michaels *state?*).

Case History

Mr. Michaels gives his age as being 51 years old. He was admitted yesterday with chest pain. His physician has ordered the following studies: electrocardiogram, chest x-ray examination, and complete blood studies including a blood sugar test. Results of these studies were just posted on the chart. When you talk with Mr. Michaels, he states, "I feel much better today—no more pain. It is a relief to get rid of that discomfort." You think he appears a little tired or weary; he seems to be talking slowly and sighs more often than you think is normal. He denies being weary. His vital signs are as follows:

T: 98.6 P: 74 (regular) R: 22 BP: 140/90

2. List the *objective data* noted in the preceding case history (what information is *observed?*).

Part II. Cues and Inferences

1. List the cues in the case history in Part I.
2. List the inferences that you might make about the cues you identified.

Part III. Validating Data

1. From the cues and inferences that you identified in Part II, indicate in three separate columns those that you feel are *certainly valid, probably valid,* and *only possibly valid.*
2. For the data listed in the *possibly valid* and *probably valid columns,* identify some methods of clarifying whether they are indeed true (eg, what other questions might you ask?).

Try This on Your Own

In a clinical conference or with another student, choose data from a real patient and identify cues. Then discuss the inferences that you might make from the cues. Discuss the validity of the cues and inferences and how you might clarify or validate your inferences.

Clustering Related Data

Just as putting similar puzzle pieces together helps you get a beginning idea of what the puzzle will look like when it's finished, clustering related health data together helps you get a beginning picture of various aspects of health status.

Assessment tools guide you to cluster data together (eg, information about nutrition is mostly in one place, information about activity is mostly in one place, and so on). However, no tool does *all the clustering* you need to do to understand each and every problem. You have to *think* about the relationships among data on the tool. For example, the data clustered under *nutrition* also relates to data under *skin status* (poor nutrition is a risk factor for skin problems). The following section helps you to learn principles of clustering data that are central for you to be able to think critically.

Clustering Data According to Purpose

Many nurses want *one way* to cluster data to meet all purposes. However, remember the truth of the clichés "one size doesn't fit all" and "more than one way is a must today." If you cluster data only one way, you get a narrow view and may miss important problems. You have to be sure that you cluster your data according to your purpose. For example, clustering data according to *Gordon's Functional Health Patterns* (Box 2.5) helps you identify nursing concerns, but it isn't very helpful when deciding how to set priorities—*Maslow's Hierarchy of Human Needs* (also in Box 2.5) is better for this purpose.

---

box 2.5 Clustering Data According to Purpose

Note: Clustering data according to *Functional Health Patterns (Gordon)* helps you identify nursing diagnoses and problems. Clustering data according to *Human Needs (Maslow)* helps you set priorities.

Functional Health Patterns (Gordon)

❏ **Health-Perception–Health-Management:** Perception of general health status and well-being. Adherence to preventive health practices.
❏ **Nutritional–Metabolic:** Patterns of food and fluid intake, fluid and electrolyte balance, general ability to heal.
❏ **Elimination:** Patterns of excretory function (bowel, bladder, and skin), and client's perception.
❏ **Activity–Exercise:** Pattern of exercise, activity, leisure, recreation, and activities of daily living; factors that interfere with desired or expected individual pattern.
❏ **Cognitive–Perceptual:** Adequacy of sensory modes, such as vision, hearing, taste, touch, smell, pain perception, cognitive functional abilities.
❏ **Sleep–Rest:** Patterns of sleep and rest/relaxation periods during 24-hour day, as well as quality and quantity.

(box continues on page 78)

---

box 2.5 Clustering Data According to Purpose (continued)

❏ **Self-Perception–Self-Concept:** Attitudes about self, perception of abilities, body image, identity, general sense of worth, and emotional patterns.
❏ **Role–Relationship:** Perception of major roles and responsibilities in current life situation.
❏ **Sexuality–Reproductive:** Perceived satisfaction or dissatisfaction with sexuality. Reproductive stage and pattern.
❏ **Coping–Stress-Tolerance:** General coping pattern, stress tolerance, support systems, and perceived ability to control and manage situations.
❏ **Value–Belief:** Values, goals, or beliefs that guide choices or decisions.

Human Needs (Maslow)

❏ **Physiologic (survival) needs (Priority #1):** Food, fluids, oxygen, elimination, warmth, physical comfort.
❏ **Safety and security needs (Priority #2):** Things necessary for physical safety (eg, a cane) and psychological security (eg, a child's favorite toy).
❏ **Love and belonging needs (Priority #3):** Family and significant others.
❏ **Self-esteem needs (Priority #4):** Things that make people feel good about themselves and confident in their abilities (eg, being well-groomed, having accomplishments recognized).
❏ **Self-actualization needs (Priority #5):** Need to grow, change, and accomplish goals.

R U L E

Cluster Data According to Your Purpose:

1. **To identify nursing diagnoses and problems,** use a nursing model (eg, Gordon's Functional Health Patterns in Box 2.5 preceding page).
2. **To identify signs and symptoms of possible medical problems,** use a medical model (eg, body systems, Box 2.6 below).
3. **To set priorities, use a model designed for that purpose.** For example use, *Maslow's Human Needs* or the *ABC's Approach* (Airway, Breathing, Cardiac, and Circulatory status).
4. **Clustering data one way, then clustering it another way helps you think critically** because each way of clustering reveals different patterns.

---

box 2.6 Clustering Data According to Body Systems

Clustering in this way helps you identify data that should be referred to the physician.

1. Cluster together a brief client profile (vital statistics), including the following: name, age, reason the individual is seeking health care, vital signs, any known medical problems or diagnoses, allergies, or problems with diet.
2. Cluster together any data you suspect may be abnormal for any of the following systems:
   ❏ Respiratory system   ❏ Gastrointestinal system
   ❏ Cardiovascular system   ❏ Musculoskeletal system
   ❏ Nervous system   ❏ Genitourinary system
   ❏ Integumentary system (skin)

The following diagram shows the relationship between clustering data and identifying health problems.

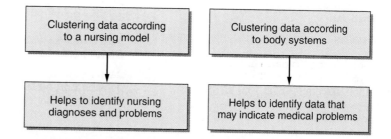

To recognize both medical and nursing problems, cluster your data two ways: use a body systems and a nursing model. If you cluster data according to body systems *only,* you're likely to miss key information that helps you to identify *nursing problems.* If you cluster data according to a nursing model *only,* you may miss information that helps you identify *medical problems.*

Box 2.7 shows the same data organized in several different ways.

Find Out More About Nursing models. You can learn about *King's Systems Interaction Model, Neuman's Systems Model, Roy's Adaptation Model, Orem's Self-Care Model, Watson's Human Science and Care Model,* and others by exploring the links at http://healthsci.clayton.edu/eichelberger/nursing.htm.

---

box 2.7 Examples of the Same Patient Data Organized According to Human Needs, Functional Health Patterns, and Body Systems

Data

1. 21-year-old male
2. Married, no children*
3. Occupation: Firefighter*
4. Ht: 6'1"; Wt: 170 lb
5. T: 98; P: 60; R: 16
6. BP: 110/60
7. Unconscious from head injury
8. Spontaneous respirations
9. Lungs clear
10. History of seizures
11. Foley draining clear urine
12. Wife states he's always constipated
13. Tube feeding via nasogastric tube every 4 hours
14. Extremities rigid
15. Has reddened areas on both elbows

16. Allergic to penicillin
17. Wife states she feels as though she is falling apart*
18. Wife states that before the accident, he took pride in being physically fit*
19. Wife states that they were considering converting to Catholicism before the accident*

Data Organization by Maslow's Human Needs

❑ Physiologic: 1, 4, 5, 6, 7, 8, 9, 10, 11, 12, 13, 14, 15, 16, 18
❑ Safety and security: 7, 10, 13, 17, 19
❑ Love and belonging: 2, 17, 19
❑ Self-esteem: 2, 3, 18
❑ Self-actualization: 3

(box continues on page 80)

box 2.7 Examples of the Same Patient Data Organized According to Human Needs, Functional Health Patterns, and Body Systems (continued)

Data Organization by Gordon's Functional Health Patterns

❑ Health-perception–health-management pattern: 10, 18
❑ Nutritional–metabolic pattern: 4, 5, 6, 8, 9, 11, 13, 15, 16
❑ Elimination pattern: 11, 12, 13, 15
❑ Activity–exercise pattern: 5, 8, 9, 14
❑ Cognitive–perceptual pattern: 7
❑ Sleep–rest pattern: 7
❑ Self-perception–self-concept pattern: 18
❑ Role–relationship pattern: 1, 2, 3
❑ Sexuality–reproductive pattern: 2

❑ Coping–stress-tolerance pattern: 17
❑ Value–belief pattern: 19

Data Organization by Body Systems to Determine What Should Be Referred to the Physician

❑ Vital statistics (client profile): 1, 4, 5, 6, 7, 10, 16
❑ Respiratory system: 8, 9
❑ Cardiovascular system: 5, 6, 9
❑ Nervous system: 7, 10
❑ Musculoskeletal system: 14
❑ Gastrointestinal system: 12, 13
❑ Genitourinary system: 11
❑ Integumentary system: 15

*These data are more likely to be clustered according to a nursing model only and therefore are not assigned a category under the body systems organization.

CRITICAL THINKING EXERCISE V

Clustering Related Data

To complete this session, read pages 77–80. Example responses can be found on page 242.

1. Why is it important to organize data according to both a body systems framework and a nursing model?
2. Get a piece of paper and cluster the following data according to body systems and according to any holistic nursing model you choose.

Case History Data

1. Age: 36
2. Married, has three small children
3. Occupation: Landscape architect and homemaker
4. Religion: Episcopalian
5. Medical diagnosis: Pneumonia
6. T: 100; P: 100; R: 28; BP: 104/68
7. States she is concerned about how her husband is caring for the children, that it is "tough on him."
8. States she feels weak and tired all the time, but can't seem to rest because she keeps coughing all the time.
9. Appetite poor. Has eaten less than half of regular meals. Is forcing fluids well (1000 mL per shift).
10. States she smokes a pack of cigarettes a day.
11. States she always has been in good health and never had to be hospitalized (even gave birth at home).

12. States that all of the tests that have to be done make her nervous; she is worried about getting AIDS from needle sticks.

13. Lungs have bilateral rhonchi; she coughs up thick, yellow mucus.

14. Chest x-ray examinations show improvement over the past 2 days.

15. White blood cell count is elevated at 16,000.

3. When you organized the previous data, you may have found that some categories had no data listed. If this happens to you in the clinical area, what should you do?

Identifying Patterns/Testing First Impressions

After you cluster your data into related groups, you begin to get initial impressions of patterns of human functioning. But you must test these impressions and decide if the patterns really are as they appear. Testing first impressions involves:

❏ deciding what's relevant
❏ making tentative decisions about what the data suggest
❏ focusing your assessment to gain more in-depth information to better understand the situations at hand.

Like the puzzle analogy, you put some of the puzzle pieces together and you think you know what the picture looks like. But sometimes those *last few pieces* surprise you with details that change the whole picture. Think about the following example in which a nurse clustered the following data together.

❏ **Objective data:** 72-year-old male; blind; bruises over right arm and on forehead
❏ **Subjective data:** "I bump into things a lot. I use my cane to find my way."

The above suggests that there's a pattern of frequent injury related to blindness. However, there isn't enough information. You need to examine the data, decide what's relevant and irrelevant, and look for reasons why he has bruises. For example, think about the following relevant and irrelevant data in relation to this blind man's injuries.

❏ **Relevant:** elderly, blind, says he bumps into things, uses a cane, has bruises on right arm and forehead
❏ **Irrelevant:** male

The above supports the conclusion that the injuries are related to blindness. But you need to ask more questions, such as "Does he live alone, or is someone else responsible for his care?" and "Are the injuries really caused by blindness?" Perhaps he's falling down because of weakness or dizziness. After all, if he's using the cane correctly, do you think he'd bump himself all the time? These questions that come to mind when identifying patterns guide you to collect additional information to *test initial impressions* and describe the problems more clearly. For example, with the man just described, you could use probing questions to clarify how and why he keeps hurting himself. You may find that his injuries are related to fainting, poor cane use, abuse, or anticoagulant medications.

To focus your assessment on testing first impressions and gaining key data about patterns of health or illness, keep the following critical thinking principles in mind.

1. **Determine what's relevant and irrelevant:** Ask yourself what relevant information might be missing.
2. **Remember cause and effect:** Find out *why* or *how the pattern came to be* (look for contributing factors). Remember that there's usually more than one contributing factor (health problems are complex situations).

Reporting and Recording

The final phase of *Assessment* is reporting and recording. This section focuses mainly on charting during *an initial data base assessment.* Additional guidelines for charting during *Implementation* are on page 108.

Reporting Abnormal Findings

Reporting anything you suspect might be abnormal does three things:

1. It promotes early diagnosis and treatment, even if you don't have the knowledge to diagnose the problems yourself.
2. It keeps others who are also accountable for your patient's care informed.
3. It helps you to learn. You get help in determining whether the information is significant.

Recording anything you suspect is abnormal helps you and other caregivers to identify downward trends in patient status. Remember the importance of *Thinking Back* (reflecting on thinking) addressed in the rule on page 12. *Reflect* on what you chart, asking yourself questions like, *What could I have missed here?*

Deciding What's Abnormal

There are many things to consider when deciding what's abnormal (eg, age, disease process, culture, stress tolerance). If you're a student or a novice, be sure that you work with more experienced nurses (mentors, preceptors, instructors). Ask them to review your assessment data to be sure you're not missing something.

To decide if your patient has abnormal findings, compare your patient's data with accepted standards for normalcy. If the findings aren't *within normal limits,* consider it to be *abnormal.* For example, if you're caring for an adult and find a resting pulse of 110 beats per minute, you'd suspect this is abnormal because normal limits for an adult resting pulse is 60 to 100 beats per minute.

Remember that normal limits may vary from person to person and from situation to situation. For example, a pulse of 110 beats per minute may be normal for a child or for someone who's anxious, but abnormal for a sleeping adult who usually has a resting pulse of 60 beats per minute. Always ask yourself, How normal is this for someone of this age, this culture, with this lifestyle, these problems, or in this situation?

Box 2.8 shows questions to ask to determine normal versus abnormal.

box 2.8 Determining Normal versus Abnormal

Ask the Person

❏ Would you say this is normal or abnormal for you?
❏ What would you describe as normal for you?

Ask Yourself

❏ What's accepted as normal for someone who's this person's age? Physical stature? Culture? Developmental status?
❏ What's accepted as normal for someone who has:
    This disease process?
    This medication regimen?
    This person's beliefs or cultural background?
    This occupation, this socioeconomic level, this lifestyle?
❏ If I compare the data I've collected with the data gathered on admission (baseline data) or the data gathered in the past 24 to 48 hours, are there changes that reflect increasing problems?
❏ Are there too many slightly abnormal factors that, when put together, suggest an overall picture of abnormal?
❏ Is what the individual accepts as normal detrimental to his or her health?

R U L E

Follow policies and procedures for *Activating the Chain of Command.* When you suspect that patients need more qualified assessment or treatment than you're able to do, follow policies and procedures for getting help. Be persistent—stay with the problems until your patients get the qualified help they need. Record all attempts to contact physicians about changes in patients' conditions. Include the name of the physician notified, a brief summary of the reason for the call, and the physician's response. If you leave a message with an answering service, record the name of the person you spoke with and the date and time of the phone call.

Guidelines: Reporting and Recording

General Guidelines

❏ **In accordance with National Patient Safety Goals, follow policies and procedures for:** (1) communicating patient status from one care giver to another and (2) charting on the patient's record.[7] For example, patient safety experts recommend using the SBAR approach on page 58 when phoning physicians, during change-of-shift reports, and when transferring patients from one place to another (called "handing-off" patients).
❏ Report and record abnormal data (eg, a fever), as well as responses to current treatments. *See also page 200 in Chapter 5, Implementation.*
❏ If something on the data base form isn't applicable to your patient's situation, put "N/A" (stands for "not applicable"). Don't leave it blank.

Guidelines: Verbal and Phone Communications

❏ Identify yourself by name and position. If you're a student, you may not be allowed to take verbal or phone orders.

❏ State the patient's name, diagnosis, and location. Then ask, "Do you know whom I'm talking about?" This gives the person time to focus on that particular patient. It also helps you know how much background information you need to give.

> ### R U L E
>
> Use the "Read Back" and "Repeat Back" rules in *all* important communications.[7] When you get verbal orders—or take down laboratory values—write down what you hear (or enter it into the computer), then *read it back* ("I put that you want him started on amoxicillin 500 mg qid"). *Repeat back* key information ("You're not allergic to anything."). Ask others to repeat what you have said ("Please repeat what I said so that I know we have it right."). Passive strategies like *head-nodding* or *listening without saying anything* contribute to communication errors.

Guidelines: Recording the Nursing Data Base

❏ **Guard the privacy of all records—it's law.**

❏ **Complete the data base as soon as you can.** Charting when you're memory is fresh promotes accuracy and helps you identify things you may have forgotten to do. Late charting leads to omissions and errors. In court, juries may interpret late charting to be substandard care. If you have to leave the unit before completing the data base, make sure that you chart the most important information (eg, vital signs, allergies, and medications) before you leave.

> ### R U L E
>
> Policies and procedures for recording the nursing data base vary from one place to another, but follow them closely—they're designed to guide you to complete a data base that provides legal documentation of accepted standards of care (this documentation also affects whether or not hospitals get reimbursed for the cost of patient care).[8,9,10]

❏ Remember that documentation standards are rapidly changing to reflect evidence-based care and improve care quality.

> ### R U L E
>
> In many cases, standards dictate that certain information must be recorded within a specific time frame after initial contact with patients. You'll be required to record diagnoses present on admission—and that key evidence-based interventions were initiated within specific time frames (for example, patients with certain infections must be given an antibiotic within a certain time frame from admission). Be sure that you follow these standards closely, as they aim to ensure timely, evidence-based care that improves care quality and are key to getting Medicare, Medicaid, and other insurance reimbursements.[11]

❏ **Check "do not use" lists** to be sure you don't use abbreviations that are potentially dangerous. You can find links to "do not use" lists at the Institute for Safe Medication Practices (ISMP) Web site (www.ismp.org) and the Joint Commission Web site (www.jointcommission.org).

E x a m p l e
Right: States "I quit going to therapy."
Wrong: Not compliant.

❏ **Avoid terms that have a negative connotation** (eg, "drunk," "disagreeable"). In court, they may convey a negative attitude on your part.
❏ **Keep it short, record the facts, and be specific.**

E x a m p l e
Right: Breath sounds diminished at lower left base. Complains of "piercing pain" with inspiration at the lower left base. Respirations 32, pulse 110, BP 130/90.
Wrong: Seems to have breathing problems and complains of chest pain.

❏ **If you make an inference, support it with evidence.**

E x a m p l e
Right: Seems upset. States he's "fine" and that he's "not upset," but he doesn't make eye contact, uses only one-word answers, and states he doesn't "feel like talking."
Wrong: Seems upset.

❏ **If you make a mistake, follow policies and procedures for correcting it.** With written charts, *never cover up the original words.* It may imply intent to cover up the facts, which is considered malpractice. Instead, draw a line through the original words, write "error," make the correction and put your initials.
❏ **If you gain information from significant others,** list the name and the relationship of the person to the patient (eg, "Wife states he's allergic to morphine.").

Guidelines: Charting on Electronic Records

❏ Know your state's rules and regulations and your facility's policies and procedures for patient data, confidentiality, and disclosure.
❏ Follow electronic charting policies and procedures carefully (including procedures for error correction).
❏ Never tell anyone your password. Change it often to avoid anyone guessing (most facilities automatically change it every 45–90 days).
❏ Tell your immediate supervisor if you suspect someone is using your code.
❏ Don't leave patient information displayed on the computer screen; log off the computer when you're not using it; retrieve printouts immediately.
❏ Make sure that backup files are kept as indicated.
❏ Find a way to *reflect* on your charting. Don't just dump data in. Double-check for accuracy, look for trends, and *think* about what you could be missing.

> **Learn more about communication and keeping patients safe.** Explore the common types of adverse events, causes of adverse events, patient safety practices, and national and international patient safety goals at http://www.jointcommission.org/PatientSafety/PSP/
>
> **Learn more about what—and what not—to chart.** Access *Charting The Course for Nursing: Who Benefits When Charting is Complete*, a free online video, from www.nursingcenter.com/AJNdocumentation.

CRITICAL THINKING EXERCISE VI

Reporting and Recording Significant Data

To complete this session, read pages 81–86. Example responses are on page 242.

1. **Practice identifying what's normal and abnormal.** Study the following data. In the space to the left, put "N" next to the normal data, "A" next to the abnormal data.
   a. States he usually has a bowel movement every other day.
   b. Temperature of 101°F.
   c. Pulse rate of 72 and regular (adult).
   d. Pulse rate of 150 (adult).
   e. Has hives over entire body.
   f. Infant cries as mother leaves the room.
   g. Patient complains of pain with urination.
   h. Grandmother suddenly does not recognize favorite grandchild.
   i. Grandmother says, "I can see okay as long as I wear my glasses."
   j. Infant cries, pulls at ears, and cannot be consoled by his mother.
2. **Learn how to ask relevant questions.** Having a holistic assessment tool that's tailor-made to gain specific information in specific situations (eg, in labor and delivery) is the key to getting relevant, complete data. Asking yourself *why each piece of information that the tool guides you to collect is required* helps you develop the critical thinking skill of *asking relevant questions.* Go through Figure 2.2, beginning on page 52, and decide why each piece of data is required. (No example response listed for this one.)

Try This on Your Own

1. **No matter what type of charting you use, you need to know** *basic principles* **to chart effectively.** Read and discuss the following articles.
   • Monarch, K. (2007). Documentation, part 1: Principles for self-protection. *American Journal of Nursing, 107*(7), 58–60.
   • Ferrell, K. (2007). Documentation, part 2: The best evidence of care. *American Journal of Nursing, 107*(7), 61–64.
2. **Learn more about patient safety, communication practices, and charting that helps your patients and protects you from lawsuits.** Visit the Internet resources listed in the box above.
3. **With a peer or in a group,** discuss the implications of the *Voices* on page 87.

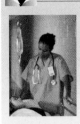

voices

Stepping into Peoples' Lives

As a nurse, you will step into people's lives . . . carry immense responsibility . . . see people at their worst, see people at their best . . . never be bored, always be frustrated . . . experience devastating failures, experience resounding triumphs . . . cry a lot, laugh a lot . . . see life begin and end . . . and KNOW WHAT IT IS TO BE HUMAN AND HUMANE[12]

—*Melodie Chenevert, RN, BSN, MN, MA*

Families' Most Important Needs

A recent study shows that the following are families' most important needs: to feel there's hope and that hospital staff care about patients; to have the waiting room near the patient; to be called at home about the patient's condition; know specific facts about the patient's prognosis; to have questions answered honestly; receive information about the patient once per day; to get explanations in understandable terms; to see the patient frequently.[13]

—*Researchers Shirley Fry, MSN, RN, and Nancy Warren, PhD, RN*

Spiritual Needs Matter

Spirituality encompasses the whole of a person's being. Although many people do not subscribe to a recognized, organized system of beliefs—an established religion—virtually all humans are spiritual beings and uphold certain individual principles. These principles shape their view of themselves, the world, and God or a higher power.[14]

—*Susan Richardson, RN, MS, CS*

It Depends

I know my students are thinking critically when I ask them a question and they answer "It depends"[15]

—*Toni C. Wortham, RN, BSN, MSN*

THIS CHAPTER AND NCLEX*

❑ Initial = Assessment. When you see the word *initial,* the correct response is likely to refer to what needs to be *assessed.*

❑ If the question gives assessment data, decide whether you have *enough information* to make the diagnosis or to intervene. If you do not, the correct answer probably addresses what *else* needs to be assessed.

❑ When asked to prioritize, apply Maslow's Hierarchy of Needs (see Box 2.5 on page 77)

❑ Always look for *abnormal data* in the assessment information, as it influences decision-making.

❑ See also "This Chapter and NCLEX" on pages 42, 137, 177, 202, and 221.

*The author acknowledges the help of Deanne Blach (www.deanneblach.com) and Judith Miller (www.judymillernclexreview.com) in developing NCLEX tips.

SUMMARY / KEY POINTS

- The accuracy, efficiency, effectiveness, and safety of all the other steps of the nursing process depend on your ability to gather accurate, relevant, and complete assessment data.
- *Assessment* and *Diagnosis* overlap—you often move back and forth between these two steps, even "work backwards" (you know the diagnoses and you assess their status).
- To promote critical thinking, your assessments should be purposeful, prioritized, focused, relevant, systematic, accurate, complete, and recorded in a standard way.
- Box 2.1 (page 49) describes critical thinking indicators (intellectual skills) needed to complete Assessment.
- The diagram on page 50 shows how the six dynamic and interrelated phases of Assessment lead to *Diagnosis*.
- Ensuring comprehensive data collection means gathering data *before you see the person, when you see the person,* and *after you see the person;* consider *your direct patient assessment* to be your primary source of information.
- This chapter discusses three types of assessment—Data Base, Focus, and Quick Priority Assessments.
- Assessing how patients manage their diseases and disabilities is an important part of *Assessment;* health promotion and screening for prevention and early diagnosis is also important.
- Partnering with patients means moving from a paternalistic model ("we know what's best for you") to a partnership model ("we want you to be informed so that you can choose the best for you").

- The interview and physical assessment complement one another; you gain *subjective data* from what patients tell you and *objective data* from your physical assessment.
- Standards mandate that you apply ethics principles and assess patients' cultural, spiritual, and communication needs.
- Your ability to establish rapport, ask questions, listen, and observe is central to building a therapeutic relationship.
- Physical assessment skills include learning inspection, auscultation, palpation, and percussion. Your physical assessment is incomplete until you check results of diagnostic studies.
- Your ability to identify cues and make correct inferences is influenced by your observational skills, your nursing knowledge, and your clinical expertise.
- Validating (verifying) that your information is factual and complete is a crucial step in critical thinking.
- To avoid missing nursing or medical problems, use both a body systems framework and a holistic nursing model (eg, Functional Health Patterns) to cluster data.
- Identifying patterns and testing first impressions help you be comprehensive and avoid jumping to conclusions.
- Report and record abnormal data in a timely way; it ensures early detection of patient problems and helps you to learn (because you find out what data are abnormal enough to indicate a problem).
- Scan this chapter for important rules, maps, and diagrams highlighted throughout; then compare where you stand in relation to the expected learning outcomes on page 45–46.

References

1. American Nurses Association. (2004). *Nursing scope and standards of performance and standards of clinical practice.* Washington, DC: American Nurses Publishing
2. U.S. Preventive Services Task Force. (2007). *Guide to clinical preventive services: Recommendations of the U.S. Preventive Services Task Force.* Retrieved March 15, 2007, from http://www.ahrq.gov/clinic/pocketgd.htm
3. American Nurses Association. (2004). *Nursing scope and standards of performance and standards of clinical practice.* Washington, DC: American Nurses Publishing.
4. The Joint Commission. (2008). *2008 national patient safety goals.* Retrieved March 18, 2008, from http://www.jointcommission.org/PatientSafety/National PatientSafetyGoals/08_hap_npsgs.htm
5. The Joint Commission. (2008). *2008 national patient safety goals.* Retrieved March 21, 2008, from http://www.jointcommission.org/PatientSafety/National PatientSafetyGoals/08_hap_npsgs.htm
6. Elixhauser, A., & Owens, P. (2007, April). Adverse drug events in U.S. hospitals, 2004. *Healthcare Cost and Utilization Project, Agency for Healthcare Research and Quality (HCUP-AHRQ) Statistical Brief #29.* Retrieved March 19, 2008, from www.hcup-us.ahrq.gov/reports/statbriefs/sb29.jsp
7. Haig, K., Sutton, S., & Whittington, J. (2006). SBAR: A shared mental model for improving communication between clinicians. *Journal on Quality and Patient Safety, 32*(3), 167–175.
8. The Joint Commission. (2008). *2008 national patient safety goals.* Retrieved March 21, 2008, from http://www.jointcommission.org/PatientSafety/National PatientSafetyGoals/08_hap_npsgs.htm
9. Monarch, K. (2007), Documentation, part 1: Principles for self-protection. *American Journal of Nursing, 107*(7), 58–60.
10. Ferrell, K. (2007). Documentation, part 2: The best evidence of care. *American Journal of Nursing, 107*(7), 61–64.
11. Centers for Medicare and Medicaid Services. (2008). *The Centers for Medicare and Medicaid Services (CMS) announces payment reforms for inpatient hospital services in 2008.* Retrieved April 22, 2008, from http://www.cms.hhs.gov/apps/media/press/release.asp?Counter=2335&intNumPerPage=10&checkDate=&checkKey=&srchType=1&numDays=3500&srchOpt=0&srchData=&keywordType=All&chkNewsType=1%2C+2%2C+3%2C+4%2C+5&intPage=&showAll=&pYear=&year=&desc=&cboOrder=date
12. Chenevert, M. (2006). *A student's road survival kit* (5th ed.). St. Louis, MO: Mosby-Elsevier.
13. Fry, S., & Warren, N. (2007). Perceived needs of critical care family members: A phenomenological discourse. *Critical Care Nursing Quarterly, 30*(2), 181–188.
14. Richardson, S. (2001). Making a spiritual assessment. *Nursing Spectrum* (Florida ed.), *11*(5), 11.
15. Wortham, T. (verbal communication, May 8, 2008)

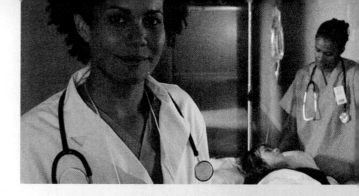

chapter 3

Diagnosis

what's in this chapter?

In this chapter, you learn about *Diagnosis*—the pivotal second step of the nursing process: if you diagnose the problems and risks *correctly,* you can start a plan to manage them; if you diagnose them *incorrectly,* your plan may actually make things *worse.* Here, you learn the legal implications of the term *diagnosis.* Focusing on the importance of identifying human responses to diseases, treatments, and changes in daily life, you explore how nurses' responsibilities related to *diagnosis* are growing—what your responsibilities are—and how to accurately diagnose and record health problems. You examine the impact of chronic diseases and disabilities on people's lives, and learn the implications of moving from the *Diagnose and Treat* (DT) approach to the more proactive *Predict, Prevent, Manage, and Promote* (PPMP) approach. You learn the importance of predicting and preventing potential complications. Finally, you examine how to: (1) include patients as partners in the diagnostic process; (2) be a safe, effective diagnostician; and (3) map diagnoses to promote critical thinking.

ANA standards related to this chapter[1]

Standard 2   Diagnosis. The registered nurse analyzes the assessment data to determine the diagnoses or issues.

critical thinking exercises

■ **Critical Thinking Exercise VII**   Nurses' Responsibilities as Diagnosticians; Key Terms Related to Diagnosis; Differentiating Between Nursing Diagnoses and Other Problems

■ **Critical Thinking Exercise VIII**   Recognizing, Mapping, and Stating Nursing Diagnoses

■ **Critical Thinking Exercise IX**   Predicting Potential Complications/Identifying Problems Requiring a Multidisciplinary Approach, Pulling It All Together

expected learning outcomes

After studying this chapter, you should be able to:

- Give three reasons why *Diagnosis* is a pivotal point in the nursing process.
- Explain why ANA standards state that nurses determine both diagnoses and issues.
- Compare and contrast the *Diagnose and Treat* model with the *Predict, Prevent, Manage, and Promote* model.
- Address the pros and cons of using critical paths and computer-assisted diagnosis.
- Discuss the legal implications of the term diagnosis.
- Make decisions about what standard terms to use in various clinical settings.
- Make decisions about your responsibilities related to identifying actual and potential nursing problems and actual and potential medical problems.
- Explain the possible consequences of diagnostic errors.
- Identify resources that can assist you to make diagnoses.
- Draw diagrams or maps that show a diagnosis and all contributing factors.
- Give summary diagnostic statements using the PES (PRS) system.
- Apply basic principles of diagnostic reasoning—including taking specific steps to avoid diagnostic errors—to make diagnoses in the clinical setting.
- Decide where you stand in relation to critical thinking indicators related to *Diagnosis*.

From Assessment to Diagnosis:
A Pivotal Point

Diagnosis: What ANA Standards Say

Nurses' Growing Responsibilities as Diagnosticians

Diagnose and Treat (DT) Versus Predict, Prevent, Manage, and Promote (PPMP)

Multidisciplinary Practice

Disease and Disability Management

Point-of-Care Testing

Critical Pathways (Care Maps)
Advantages of Critical Paths
Disadvantages of Critical Paths

Informatics and Computer-Assisted Diagnosis
Using Standard or Recognized Terms
How to Use Standard Languages
Computer-Assisted Diagnosis
Limitations of Computer-Assisted Diagnosis

Becoming a Competent Diagnostician

Key Terms Related to Diagnosis

Recognizing Risk Factors: The Key to Proactive Approaches

Critical Thinking Indicators (CTIs) Related to Diagnosis

(continued on next page)

From *Assessment* to *Diagnosis:* A Pivotal Point

The following diagram shows how the key phases of *Assessment* lead to a pivotal point in the nursing process: *Diagnosis.*

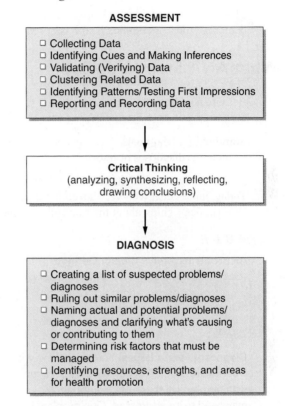

ASSESSMENT

- ☐ Collecting Data
- ☐ Identifying Cues and Making Inferences
- ☐ Validating (Verifying) Data
- ☐ Clustering Related Data
- ☐ Identifying Patterns/Testing First Impressions
- ☐ Reporting and Recording Data

Critical Thinking
(analyzing, synthesizing, reflecting, drawing conclusions)

DIAGNOSIS

- ☐ Creating a list of suspected problems/ diagnoses
- ☐ Ruling out similar problems/diagnoses
- ☐ Naming actual and potential problems/ diagnoses and clarifying what's causing or contributing to them
- ☐ Determining risk factors that must be managed
- ☐ Identifying resources, strengths, and areas for health promotion

Diagnosis is a pivotal point for the following reasons.

1. **The purpose of Diagnosis is to clarify the exact nature of the problems and risk factors you need to address to achieve the overall expected outcomes of care.** If you don't completely understand the problems and what factors are contributing to them, you're not going to know what to do about them.
2. **The conclusions you make during this phase affect the entire plan of care.** If your conclusions are correct, your plan is likely to be on target. If they aren't—for example if you're operating on *assumptions* rather than on sound reasoning that's based on evidence—your plan is likely to be flawed, maybe even dangerous.

> **R U L E**
>
> ***Diagnosis*—At Least 50% of Your Challenge.** Diagnosis—clearly and specifically identifying problems and risk factors that must be managed—requires in-depth critical thinking and is at least 50% of the challenge of developing the plan of care. The accuracy

and relevancy of the entire plan depends on your ability to clarify the problems and what factors are causing or contributing to them. If you make errors in this phase, your whole plan may be useless, even dangerous.

This chapter is designed to help you become a competent, efficient diagnostician in the context of today's complex health care setting.

Diagnosis: What ANA Standards Say

Because applying standards is essential to critical thinking, let's begin by looking at how the wording of *ANA Standard II* has changed to include the word *issues,* as follows:

Standard II: Diagnosis. The registered nurse analyzes the assessment data to determine the diagnoses or issues.[2]

Adding *issues* to Standard II reflects the realities of today's health care setting: Today, nurses deal with very specific problems (eg, diagnoses) and ill-defined problems (issues). Think about the rule and example that follows.

R U L E

All Problems Aren't Clearly Defined. The rapid pace and complexity of health care today requires you to deal with both *specific* and *ill-defined* problems. With a specific problem, major causative factors are clear. With ill-defined problems (issues), there are many causative or contributing factors present, and they're changing.

E x a m p l e

Diagnoses versus Issues. You're working with someone with the diagnosis of *Self-Care Deficit (Dressing).* As you help him get dressed, he mentions that he doesn't get along with his physical therapist. You begin the process of exploring interpersonal issues that may need to be addressed. One problem is very specific, while the other is muddy, with a lot of unknowns. Due to time constraints, you may only be able to talk briefly about the interpersonal issues, getting a beginning idea of whether this is something that needs to be addressed on the plan of care. In this case, it's appropriate to say something like, "I'm concerned that there are some interpersonal issues here we all need to explore."

The Terms Diagnoses, Disorders, Problems, and Issues Are Often Used Interchangeably

We'll use *diagnoses* when referring to *very specific problems* that are clearly defined and require detailed or long-term solutions. We'll use *disorders, problems,* or *issues* when the problem is less clear or when there's a simple, quick solution.

Nurses' Growing Responsibilities as Diagnosticians

Before you learn how to make diagnoses, it's important for you to realize that nurses' roles as diagnosticians are changing.

Laws and standards continue to change to reflect how nursing practice is growing. Depending on qualifications and practice setting, nurses have a wide range of responsibilities related to diagnosis and treatment of health problems. Physicians diagnose and treat medical problems from the perspective of medical science. As a nurse, you diagnose and treat medical problems from the perspective of *nursing science.* This means that you focus on *human responses.* You monitor patient responses to medical treatments and also the *impact* of medical problems and changes in daily life on the individual's sense of well-being. For example, many people who have problems with incontinence suffer feelings of isolation because they're concerned about leakage and odor.

Because of the increased use of technology in the diagnosis and treatment of patient problems, the boundaries between nursing and physician responsibilities are sometimes blurred. It is, however, important for you to understand some basic responsibilities that are central to your role as a nurse.

As a beginning nurse, you're responsible for:

❑ **Recognizing signs and symptoms** of common health problems and those that may indicate the need for more expert diagnosis (eg, if your patient has unexplained weight loss, it needs to be evaluated by a physician as it may indicate medical problems such as cancer or diabetes).

❑ **Predicting problems in those at risk** and taking steps to manage risks and prevent complications (eg, if you identify that someone is at risk for falls, you must begin a plan to prevent falls).

❑ **Identifying human responses** (how problems, signs and symptoms, and treatment regimens *impact on patients' lives*) and promoting optimum function, independence, and quality of life.

❑ **Initiating actions and referrals in a timely way to ensure appropriate, qualified treatment** (eg, if your patient is hemorrhaging, notify the doctor immediately and start interventions aimed at correcting the problem—for example, putting the head of the bed down or applying pressure to the site that's bleeding).

R U L E

Unless you're an Advanced Practice Nurse (APN)*, state laws prohibit you from making medical diagnoses independently. You are, however, **accountable** for giving high priority to assessing for—and reporting—signs and symptoms that may indicate the need for attention from a professional more qualified than you are.[3] For example, if your patient has signs and symptoms of a myocardial infarction (eg, chest pain and shortness of breath), you're accountable for: (1) suspecting that this could be the problem; (2) recognizing that it is a high priority; (3) doing what you can to address the problem (eg, raise the head of the bed); and (4) reporting it immediately. **This is called "Activating the Chain of Command"** (follow policies and procedures for getting help; be persistent—stay with the problems until your patient gets qualified help they need).

---

*For more information, see Appendix A (Advanced Practice Nurses' Roles).

Let's look at five main factors that impact on your diagnostic role today. These factors are summarized here and addressed in more depth in the next section.

1. The shift from *Diagnose and Treat (DT)* to *Predict, Prevent, Manage, and Promote (PPMP).*
2. More emphasis on the importance of multidisciplinary practice and disease management (the use of nurses to help people manage chronic diseases by themselves at home).
3. The development and refinement of critical pathways (also called critical paths, clinical pathways, or care maps).
4. Informatics (the use of computers to process and manage information) and computer-assisted diagnosis and decision support.
5. More awareness that the scope of nursing practice has a flexible boundary that responds to the changing needs of society.[4]

Diagnose and Treat (DT) Versus Predict, Prevent, Manage, and Promote (PPMP)

As addressed briefly in Chapter 1, the DT approach implies that we wait for evidence of problems before beginning treatment. The PPMP approach focuses on early intervention to prevent and manage problems and their potential complications. It is based on research or clinical evidence. We now know the typical course of most health problems, and we also know how to *alter* the course through early intervention.

The PPMP approach requires you to do three things:

1. **In the presence of known problems,** predict the most common and most dangerous complications and take immediate action to: a) prevent them, and b) manage them in case they can't be prevented.

E x a m p l e
As a beginning nurse working in the emergency department, you admit a woman you suspect is having a heart attack. You report this problem immediately so that steps can be taken to control the problem and its potential complications (eg, an IV is inserted so that medications can be given to improve blood flow to the heart and prevent arrhythmias, if needed).

2. **Whether problems are present or not,** you look for evidence of risk factors (things that we know may cause problems, such as risky sexual behaviors). If you identify risk factors, you aim to reduce or control them, thereby preventing the problems themselves.

E x a m p l e
You do an assessment and decide a teenage boy is in excellent health. However, you recognize that he has risky sexual behaviors. Recognizing that these behaviors puts the young man at risk for contracting HIV and other sexually transmitted diseases, you focus on addressing the risky behaviors (eg, you contact a peer counselor to discuss the need for safe sex).

3. In all situations, you coach and counsel patients to use behaviors that promote optimum function, independence, and sense of well-being.

E x a m p l e
You're caring for someone who is asthmatic and has just had a colonoscopy. As you give discharge instructions, you address the importance of exercising. You point out that a daily walking program strengthens muscles, prevents osteoporosis, improves endurance, is key to weight control, and promotes lung and cardiovascular function (all are especially important for asthmatics).

Using the PPMP model requires knowledge of health promotion behaviors and also disease process, treatment, and prognosis (the usual course and outcome of injury or disease). Keep in mind that the term *predict* in PPMP doesn't mean that a complication *will* happen. For example, it's an assumption to think like this: *My patient has this problem, so I can predict that he'll also have these complications.* The PPMP approach means you *anticipate* the possibility of complications and plan ways to detect, prevent, and manage them early.

Multidisciplinary Practice

The importance of collaborative and multidisciplinary approaches significantly impacts on your role as a diagnostician. As a nurse, you must be keenly aware that you don't work in isolation. Many problems require more than nursing resources to be resolved in a timely manner. As you'll see later in this chapter, you must know when you're "out of your league," so to speak. You are the one on the "front line." You often will be the one who recognizes that making referrals to other experts (eg, physical therapists and nutritionists) are the key to establishing a plan that avoids delays in recovery and gets results efficiently.

Disease and Disability Management

As the population ages, more nurses are involved in disease management, which involves helping patients with self-management of chronic diseases and disabilities at home (see Box 3.1). In disease and disability management, nurses are responsible for teaching patients how to manage signs and symptoms themselves, giving guidelines for when to call the doctor. They help patients adapt to limitations of disabilities and help them find resources to maximize their quality of life. Nurses, in partnerships with physicians, provide the bulk of care by applying their knowledge and using evidence-based guidelines. Nurses are key players in reducing costs and improving quality of life by working with chronically ill patients to improve adherence to treatment plans, diets, and medications.

Point-of-Care Testing

Another result of moving to the PPMP approach is that there is an increase in the use of point-of-care testing—diagnostic testing done by nurses at home or at the bedside—to improve efficiency and ensure early detection of problems. Examples of point-of-care

> **box 3.1** Health Promotion and Chronic Disease and Disability Prevention*
>
> Chronic diseases have a long course of illness. They rarely resolve spontaneously and they're generally not cured by medication or prevented by vaccine. Chronic diseases—such as heart disease, cancer, and diabetes—account for 7 of every 10 deaths and affect the quality of life of 90 million Americans. Chronic disabling conditions cause major limitations in activity for 1 out of every 10 Americans (25 million people). Prolonged courses of illness and disability often result in extended pain and suffering, as well as in decreased quality of life. Although chronic diseases are among the most common and costly health problems, they are also among the most preventable. Adopting healthy behaviors such as eating nutritious foods, being physically active, and avoiding tobacco use can prevent or control the devastating effects of these diseases. The U.S. can't reduce its enormous health care costs, much less its priority health problems, without addressing the prevention of chronic disease and disability in a more aggressive manner.

*Adapted from: http://www.doh.state.fl.us/Family/chronicdisease/

tests are blood glucose measurement and testing stool for blood. In specialty units (eg, intensive care), nurses may be accountable for complex point-of-care tests. Be sure you check with policies and procedures to know what tests you are responsible for doing and which ones are done by the laboratory. Be sure that you're prepared for point-of-care testing by practicing performing the tests if you're not doing them on a frequent basis (in some cases, you will need to pass competency tests to prove competence).

Critical Pathways (Care Maps)

Through research and interdisciplinary clinical studies, most facilities continue to develop and refine critical pathways. Critical pathways—also called clinical pathways and care maps—are standard plans that predict the day-by-day care required to achieve outcomes for specific problems within a certain time frame (pages 173–176 shows an example). There are advantages and disadvantages to using critical paths.

Advantages of Critical Paths

Advantages of critical paths include:

1. Give outcome-focused, evidenced-based approaches.
2. Alert you to frequently encountered problems and predicted care for specific situations (eg, repair of a fractured hip).
3. Help you learn the usual treatment course for common problems through repeated experience in using the paths with different patients.

Disadvantages of Critical Paths

There are some disadvantages in using critical paths:

1. You may be so influenced by knowing major diagnoses and predicted care in advance that it's easy to become complacent, thinking, I already know the problems, so I don't have to worry too much about assessment.

2. It's not unusual for patients to be experiencing other important problems that aren't covered by the path.

When using critical pathways, keep an open mind and think independently. Always determine your patient's specific needs rather than assume she "fits" the typical critical path.

Informatics and Computer-Assisted Diagnosis

Informatics—the use of computers to manage information and support decisions—is an important, growing field. Depending on purpose, informatics programs are designed differently. For example, some software are designed for billing purposes, and some are designed to support clinical decision-making. It's important to remember the following points.

❏ Although well-established, the field of informatics is still evolving and continues to change.
❏ In many cases, beginning definitions and theoretical structures have been proposed, but it will be some time before stable definitions, concepts, and systems are achieved.
❏ Computer programs aren't a "one-size-fits-all" proposition. You need to use a critical mind to decide what computer tools are useful in context of each particular situation.

Using Standard or Recognized Terms

Table 3.1 (next page) shows key organizations working to standardize terms to facilitate the use of computers for decision support, documentation, and research.

ANA practice standards state that you must use standard or recognized terminologies.[5] Understand that using standard or recognized terminologies doesn't mean you will use *only* the terms addressed by each organization in Table 3.1. Terms are usually tailored to each unit or health care organization.

> **R U L E**
>
> **How to Decide What Terms To Use.** When you begin to work in a new setting, review the *Do Not Use List,* ask whether there is a list of recommended terms, and take note of the terms used in standards, policies, protocols, procedures, and computer programs (these are the terms you must use).

Although not all facilities use standard terms from languages such as NANDA (North American Nursing Diagnosis Association) International, NIC (Nursing Interventions Classification), NOC (Nursing-Sensitive Outcomes Classification), keep in mind the following key points.

❏ **Developing nursing languages is important work**—as terms are developed, the concepts are also carefully studied, broadening nursing's knowledge base and proving nursing's worth by identifying exactly what problems nurses diagnose, what interventions nurses must use, and what outcomes nurses can influence.

table 3.1 Examples of Groups Developing Standard Languages (Vocabularies)

Group Name	Focus	Purpose
North American Nursing Diagnosis Association-International (NANDA-I)	Diagnoses	Increase the visibility of nursing's contribution to patient care by continuing to develop, refine, and classify phenomena of concern to nurses (see Nursing Diagnosis Quick Reference section). **Web site:** http://www.nanda.org
Nursing Interventions Classification (NIC)	Interventions	Identify, label, validate, and classify actions nurses perform, including direct and indirect care interventions (interventions done directly with patients, for example, teaching, and those done indirectly, for example, obtaining laboratory studies). **Web site:** http://www.nursing.uiowa.edu
Nursing-Sensitive Outcomes Classification (NOC)	Outcomes	Identify, label, validate, and classify nursing-sensitive patient outcomes and indicators to evaluate the validity and usefulness of the classification, and define and test measurement procedures for the outcomes and indicators. **Web site:** http://www.nursing.uiowa.edu
Home Health Care Classification (HHCC)	Diagnoses, Interventions, and Outcomes	Provide a structure for documenting and classifying home health and ambulatory care. Consists of two interrelated taxonomies: HHCC of Nursing Diagnoses and HHCC of Nursing Interventions. **Web site:** http://www.sabacare.com
International Classification for Nursing Practice (ICNP®)	Diagnoses, Interventions, and Outcomes	Capture nursing's contributions to health and provide a framework into which existing vocabularies and classifications can be cross-mapped, enabling comparison of nursing data from various countries throughout the world. **Web site:** http://www.icn.ch/icnp.htm
SNOMED CT (Systematized Nomenclature of Medicine—Clinical Terms)	Comprehensive clinical terminology	Integrate, link, and map terms from various disciplines such as medicine, nursing, and occupational therapy. **Web site:** http://www.nlm.nih.gov/research/umls/Snomed/snomed_main.html

❏ **Most of this work of language development is done at a national or international level by highly educated nurses** who have broad knowledge of nursing problems, theories, and approaches, and who also understand the many challenging aspects of building a taxonomy (classification) of terms.

❏ **Not all terms are clinically useful** (eg, some are too broad or cumbersome). It takes years of hard work and development before "the cream (the most useful terms) floats to the top." Some organizations, for example the Association of Perioperative Registered Nurses (AORN) and the Association of Rehabilitation Nurses (ARN), have done excellent work in narrowing down the terms that are most useful for their practice (see Box 3.2).

---

box 3.2 Examples of Nursing Diagnoses Commonly Used in Two Different Settings

Rehabilitation Nursing*

Activity Intolerance
Bathing or Hygiene Self-Care
  Deficit
Body Image Disturbance
Caregiver Role Strain
Colonic Constipation
Dressing and Grooming Self-Care
  Deficit
Feeding Self-Care Deficit
Impaired Physical Mobility
Impaired Swallowing
Impaired Thought Processes
Impaired Verbal Communication
Ineffective Individual Coping
Ineffective Family Coping
Knowledge Deficit
Pain
Pressure Ulcer
Reflex Incontinence
Risk for Injury
Risk for Disuse Syndrome
Toileting Self-Care Deficit
Urinary Retention

Perioperative Nursing†

Risk for Perioperative Positioning
  Injury‡
Risk for Infection‡
Altered Protection
Pain
Risk for Peripheral Neurovascular
  Dysfunction
Risk for Aspiration
Risk for Impaired Skin Integrity
Risk for Altered Body Temperature
Risk for Injury
Risk for Fluid Volume Deficit
Fluid Volume Deficit
Fluid Volume Excess
Anxiety
Fear
Hypothermia
Impaired Skin Integrity
Impaired Tissue Integrity
Inability to Sustain Spontaneous
  Respirations
Knowledge Deficit

---

*Data from: Association of Rehabilitation Nurses. Rehabilitation Nursing Foundation's Nursing Diagnosis Publications Task Force. (1995). *21 Rehabilitation nursing diagnoses.* Glenview, IL: Author. See also: Association of Rehabilitation Nurses, (2007) Evidence-Based Rehabilitation Nursing: Common Challenges and Interventions. Glenview, Illinois: Author *Evidence-Based Rehabilitation Nursing: Common Challenges and Interventions.* This book addresses 13 patient problems commonly encountered in rehabilitation nursing (Pain, Falls, Pressure Ulcers, Bowel, Bladder, Mobility, Cognition, Safety Awareness, Knowledge Deficit, Behavior Management, Depression, Self-Care Deficit, and Swallowing).

†Data From: Beyea, S. (Ed.). (2002). *The perioperative nursing data set* (2nd ed.). Denver, CO: Association of periOperative Registered Nurses.

‡Identified as critical nursing diagnoses. All others listed are primary nursing diagnoses. List is incomplete. See Beyea (2002) listed above for complete list.

How to Use Standard Languages

Rather than spending a lot of time trying to determine linkages among standard terms from taxonomies such as NANDA, NIC, and NOC (work that challenges experts and is still evolving), do the following.

1. Be sure you understand *conceptually* the relationships among the terms *diagnosis, intervention,* and *outcome* (see Box 3.3 on the next page).

box 3.3 Relationships Among Diagnosis, Interventions, and Outcomes

Term	Basic Concept	Example
Diagnosis	Actual and potential problems	Risk for Injury related to dizziness
Intervention	Specific treatments or actions needed to prevent, resolve, or manage actual and potential problems.	Stress the importance of not walking alone. Have someone close by, carefully monitoring for dizziness when patient is walking. Teach family to do the same.
Outcome	Specific data that will be observed in the patient to show that he or she has benefited from care (outcomes may relate to problems or intervention): 1) **Problem outcomes** state what will be observed in the patient when the problems are managed. 2) **Intervention outcomes** state what will be observed in the patient to show that intervention produced the desired results.	**Example Problem Outcome:** Patient is free from injury and management of risk factors is recorded on the plan of care (eg, walked with assistance only). **Example Intervention Outcomes:** ❑ Patient agrees to call for help before walking. ❑ Patient always has assistance when walking.

2. **Determine resources** that best guide you to assess, diagnose, and manage the commonly encountered problems in the setting in which you practice (eg, medical–surgical textbooks, maternal–child textbooks, care planning books, and so forth).

3. **When you're in a new setting,** check with your instructor or supervisor to find out whether there are standard terms that must be used (usually these are the terms that are used in policies, procedures, care-planning guides, and decision-support software).

4. **Before you take any tests**—especially before taking national licensing or certification tests—find out what terminology will be used. To get up-to-date information and resources for NCLEX go to: www.ncsbn.org.

R U L E

Become familiar with priority diagnoses (those that are clearly nursing's responsibility in each particular clinical setting). When you're in a new setting, ask your supervisor or instructor for a list of commonly encountered diagnoses (eg, Box 3.2). Assess every patient you have for the presence of any of the commonly encountered diagnoses; then continue looking for other problems. Assessing every patient for commonly encountered diagnoses *first,* helps you learn the priority diagnoses that you should know "in your head."

The Quick Reference to Nursing Diagnoses (pages 223–240) gives information on the frequently encountered NANDA diagnoses.

Computer-Assisted Diagnosis

Electronic support systems are valuable tools that can spot trends, facilitate problem identification, and help you learn; but you must use them with an active, critical mind, asking yourself questions like, How does this compare with my patient's situation, down to the last detail? and What could I be missing? Many patients today have multiple diagnoses which interact in ways that make "normal" or predicted approaches given by a computer program useless (eg, a program may call for the patient to exercise three times a day, but the patient has a heart problem that restricts activity; some patients react differently due to medications).

Think about the following benefits and limitations of computer-assisted diagnosis.

Benefits of Computer-Assisted Diagnosis

Computers:

❏ Store large amounts of data, keeping them all available for recall as needed.
❏ Process large amounts of data faster than humans can.
❏ Perform at a consistent level (not affected by human factors like fatigue, environmental distractions, boredom, or complacency).
❏ Prompt you to enter data, improving accuracy and completeness of documentation and diagnosis.
❏ Spot trends and flag potential problems or mistakes, such as drug interactions or incorrect dosages.
❏ Facilitate diagnostic reasoning by suggesting possible diagnoses, depending on matching assessment data.

Limitations of Computer-Assisted Diagnosis

Computers:

❏ Assume that information you enter into them is true.
❏ Can't think for you. Learn to think *with* the computer—analyze and interpret computer-generated information in context of individual situations.
❏ May not be up-to-date with minute-to-minute changes in patient status.
❏ Don't relieve you of the responsibility of recognizing when what the computer says doesn't *apply* to the current situation (or is completely wrong).

> **RULE**
>
> **Developing Sound Diagnostic Reasoning Habits Is Like Learning Mathematical Principles.** Before you can safely use computers to diagnose problems, you must internalize principles of *Assessment* and *Diagnosis*. If you don't form thinking habits based on the principles and rules in this chapter and the previous one, it's as if you worked in a bank without ever having learned simple rules of addition, subtraction, multiplication, and division.

Becoming a Competent Diagnostician

To be a competent diagnostician, act in your patients' best interest, and protect yourself from legal problems, you must understand key terms related to *Diagnosis*. Study the following terms, which are listed in the order in which you need to learn them (you need to know the first term to understand the second, and so on).

Key Terms Related to Diagnosis

Competency. Having the knowledge and skills to identify problems and risks and to perform actions safely and efficiently in various situations.

E x a m p l e
After the first semester of nursing, the student demonstrated competency in giving medications. **Discussion:** You're considered competent to perform an action or diagnose health problems after you've completed appropriate courses and passed tests (clinical and theoretical) demonstrating competency.

Qualified. Being competent and having the authority to perform an action or give a professional opinion.

E x a m p l e
Although you know you're competent to give intravenous (IV) medications in one hospital, when you go to another hospital, you check policies to determine whether you still have the authority to do so before you can consider yourself qualified to give IV medications. **Discussion:** Authority to do assessments, perform nursing actions, and give professional advice is derived from the following: laws, licensure, and certification; national, state, and community standards; facility standards, policies, procedures, and protocols; and other health care professionals (eg, instructors, supervisors, APNs, physicians).

Nursing Domain. Activities and actions a nurse is legally qualified to do. Also refers to diagnoses a nurse is qualified to make.

E x a m p l e
Inserting a nasogastric tube prescribed by a physician is in the nursing domain as long as the nurse is qualified to do so. **Discussion:** The nursing domain includes actions that nurses do independently (eg, monitoring function of a nasogastric tube) and activities that nurses do when delegated by a physician or APN (eg, inserting a nasogastric tube). As you progress with your education and clinical experience, your nursing domain will include a wider range of activities. You're responsible for maintaining competency within your practice domain.

Medical Domain. Activities and actions a physician is legally qualified to do. Depending on state regulations, APNs are also legally qualified to do some things in the medical domain.

E x a m p l e
Performing surgery is in the medical domain as long as it's allowed by law and the physician is qualified to do so. **Discussion:** When nurses take on responsibility for actions that previously belonged only to the medical domain, the actions must be approved by state rules and regulations. Boards of nursing usually issue position statements that describe what nurses can or can't do related to a specific problem or procedure.

Accountable. Being responsible and answerable for something.

E x a m p l e
If you do an assessment and you miss key problems, you're *accountable* for what happens (eg, if you miss an area of skin redness and the area becomes ulcerated because of lack of treatment, you're accountable).

Definitive Interventions. The *most specific* actions or treatments required to prevent, resolve, or manage a health problem.

E x a m p l e
If a patient has bacterial pneumonia, you might encourage fluids, assist with coughing, and administer oxygen. However, if you don't have the definitive intervention of giving an antibiotic that's effective against the specific bacteria, you're highly unlikely to get a cure.

Outcome. The result of prescribed interventions. Usually refers to the *desired* result of interventions (that the problem is prevented, resolved, or managed); includes a specific time frame for when the outcome is expected to be achieved.

E x a m p l e
"By 3 days after total knee replacement surgery, the person will show no signs of infection, will be able to walk with a walker, and be ready to be discharged to a rehabilitation facility."

Signs. Objective (observable) data known to suggest a health problem (rashes and fever are signs).
Symptoms. Subjective (reported) data known to suggest a health problem (pain and fatigue are symptoms).
Cues. Signs and symptoms that prompt you to suspect the presence of a health problem (rashes, fever, pain, and fatigue) or a desire to improve health ("I want to improve my eating habits.").
Diagnose. To make a judgment and specifically name the actual and potential health problems or risk factors present, based on evidence from assessment data.

E x a m p l e
After performing an assessment, the nurse diagnosed Risk for Aspiration related to decreased level of consciousness and poor cough reflex.

Diagnosis. In addition to referring to the second step of the nursing process, *diagnosis* means two things:

1. The *process* of diagnosing (eg, "We learn diagnosis in the first semester.")
2. The *result* of the diagnostic process (eg, "What's the diagnosis?")

E x a m p l e
After carefully analyzing and interpreting the patient's data, the doctor made the diagnosis of *inferior myocardial infarction*.

> **R U L E**
>
> **Legal Implications of Using the Term Diagnosis.** The term *diagnosis* implies that there's a situation or problem requiring appropriate, qualified treatment. This means if you diagnose a problem, you must decide whether you're qualified to treat it and willing to accept responsibility for treating it. If you're not, you're responsible for getting qualified help.

Definitive Diagnosis. The most specific, most correct diagnosis.

E x a m p l e
If you suspect a medical problem may be present, you consult a physician so that a *definitive diagnosis* can be made. **Discussion:** Being *very specific* about the diagnosis is essential to being able to determine definitive treatment. Would you be satisfied with a diagnosis of "lung disease," or would you want a definitive diagnosis like pneumonia, lung cancer, or asthma?

Rule Out. To decide that a certain problem is *not* present.
Discussion: Ruling out is a key part of diagnosis. When you make a definitive diagnosis, you rule out several other problems that your patient's signs and symptoms may represent.

E x a m p l e
The nurse made the diagnosis of *Activity Intolerance related to sedentary lifestyle*, after the doctor ruled out that cardiac or respiratory problems were contributing to the problem.

Life Processes. Events or changes that occur during one's lifetime (growing up, aging, maturing, becoming a parent, moving, separations, losses).
Discussion: Nurses are very involved in helping patients and families with transitions that occur across the lifespan.
Nursing Diagnosis. A clinical judgment about an individual, family, or community response to actual or potential health problems and life processes. Nursing diagnoses provide the basis for selection of nursing interventions to achieve outcomes for which nurses are accountable.[6] **Discussion:** Nursing diagnoses often are called *human responses* because we, as nurses, focus on how people *respond* to changes in health or life circumstances—for example, how they're responding to illness or to becoming a parent. This definition is evolving, to include a broader range of problems.[7] Each specialty organization often develops its own definition. Sometimes this term is used in a "generic" way, considering *any nursing opinion* to be a nursing diagnosis.

E x a m p l e
Risk for Injury related to poor balance.
Table 3.2 compares the terms nursing diagnosis and medical diagnosis.

Defining Characteristics. A cluster of signs, symptoms, and related factors usually seen with a specific nursing diagnosis (see Defining Characteristics heading throughout the Quick Reference to Nursing Diagnoses section, pages 223–240).

table 3.2 Comparison of Nursing Diagnoses and Medical Diagnoses

Nursing Diagnoses	Medical Diagnoses
Main Focus 1. The *impact* of disease, trauma, or life changes upon patients and families (human responses) 2. Problems with functioning independently (activities of daily living) 3. Quality of life issues (eg, pain, ability to do desired activities)	*Main Focus* 1. Diseases, trauma, pathophysiology 2. Complex behavioral and brain disorders 3. Quality of life issues (eg, pain, ability to do desired activities, but to a lesser extent than nursing—they often refer these types of problems to other disciplines)
Primary Manager of Problem Nurse (may use other resources such as physical therapy or physician expertise, but the nurse accepts primary responsibility for monitoring status and allocating resources)	*Primary Manager of Problem* Physician or advanced practice nurse (APN)
Definitive Diagnosis Authority to make the definitive diagnosis within the nursing domain.	*Definitive Diagnosis* Nurse is required to seek physician or APN for definitive diagnosis.
Nursing Responsibilities 1. Identification of signs, symptoms, and risk factors 2. Early detection of actual and potential problems 3. Initiation of a comprehensive plan to prevent, correct, or control the problems (nurse is the primary manager of the problems) 4. Monitoring patient responses to nursing care	*Nursing Responsibilities* 1. Identification of risk factors, anticipating potential complications 2. Monitoring to detect and report early signs or symptoms of potential complications or change in status 3. Initiating actions within the nursing domain to prevent or minimize the problems and their potential complications 4. Implementing medical orders (physician or APN is primary manager of the problems) and monitoring responses to treatment.

Medical Diagnosis. Problems with anatomy or physiology (eg, diseases or trauma) that require definitive diagnosis by a qualified physician, APN, or physician's assistant. Also includes complex brain and behavioral disorders. Often validated by medical diagnostic studies.

E x a m p l e
Acute myocardial infarction (MI)

Potential Complications. Problems that may occur because of current diagnoses, treatment, invasive monitoring, or diagnostic studies.

E x a m p l e
See the potential complications listed on the inside back cover and facing page.
Discussion: You're responsible for monitoring to detect early signs and symptoms of potential complications.

Multidisciplinary Problem. A problem requiring treatment by more than one discipline—for example, nursing, medicine, physical therapy, and occupational therapy.

E x a m p l e
Care management of someone with a fractured hip. **Discussion:** All disciplines are accountable for independent and physician-prescribed actions within their domain of practice. Figure 3.1 (below) shows key questions to ask to determine whether the problem you identified is a nursing diagnosis or a medical or multidisciplinary problem.

Related Factor. Something known to be associated with a specific health problem (eg, history of frequent falls is a related factor for *Risk for Injury*).
Risk Factor or Etiology. Something known to cause, or contribute to, a diagnosis (eg, decreased vision is a related factor for *Risk for Injury*).
Discussion: The terms related factors, risk factors, and etiology often are used interchangeably.
Risk (Potential) Diagnosis. A health problem that may develop if preventive actions are not taken.

E x a m p l e
Risk for Injury related to poor balance and history of frequent falls. **Discussion:** Table 3.3 (next page) compares nursing responsibilities for actual, potential, and possible diagnoses/problems.

Syndrome Diagnoses. A diagnosis that has a cluster of other diagnoses (see example in Box 3.4).
Wellness Diagnosis. Human responses to levels of wellness in an individual, family, or community that have a readiness for enhancement.[8] **Discussion:** NANDA uses *readiness for enhanced* as a prefix for wellness diagnoses.

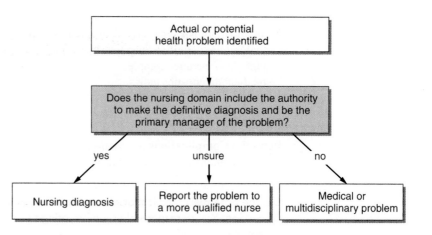

FIGURE 3.1 Key question to determine whether you've identified a nursing diagnosis or multidisciplinary problem.

table 3.3 Nursing Responsibilities for Actual, Risk (Potential), and Possible Diagnoses/Problems

Diagnosis/Problem	Nursing Responsibilities
❏ Actual Diagnosis/Problem: The person's data show signs and symptoms or defining characteristics of the diagnosis. **Example:** *Ineffective Breathing Pattern related to pain and thick mucus* as evidenced by coughing up thick mucus, statements of pain with deep inspiration, and poor chest expansion	❏ Compare patient's signs and symptoms with the signs and symptoms of the diagnoses you suspect; determine cause or related factors. Decide whether to treat independently or refer the problem.
❏ **Risk (Potential) Diagnosis/Problem:** The person's data show the related (risk) factors of the diagnosis/problem but **no** signs, symptoms, or defining characteristics. **Example:** *Risk for Ineffective Breathing Pattern related to pain*	❏ Control risk factors and monitor for onset of signs and symptoms (this indicates that the diagnosis/problem has become an *actual* diagnosis/problem, requiring treatment).
❏ **Possible Diagnosis/Problem:** You suspect a diagnosis/problem is present, but the person's data need more clarifying before you can decide whether the diagnosis/problem is present. **Example:** *Possible Ineffective Breathing Pattern*	❏ Collect more data to clarify whether or not the diagnosis/problem is present or whether there are related (risk) factors present.

E x a m p l e

Readiness for Enhanced Parenting. In acute care settings, the plan of care addresses only actual and risk (potential) diagnoses, which are considered the most important immediate concerns. In the community and in home care, more opportunities are present to focus on wellness diagnoses.

---

box 3.4 Cluster of Diagnoses Seen With Disuse Syndrome*

❏ Impaired Physical Mobility
❏ Risk for Constipation
❏ Risk for Impaired Respiratory Function
❏ Risk for Infection
❏ Risk for Activity Intolerance
❏ Risk for Injury
❏ Risk for Impaired Thought Processes
❏ Risk for Body Image Disturbance
❏ Risk for Powerlessness
❏ Risk for Impaired Tissue Integrity

*This diagnosis is commonly seen in bedridden nursing home residents.

Recognizing Risk Factors: The Key to Proactive Approaches

As we shift to the proactive PPMP model, the importance of recognizing and managing risk factors becomes clear. Often, there are no actual problems, but there *are* risk factors that indicate a need for close monitoring (and in some cases, treatment). For instance, suppose you're caring for a pregnant woman who is a smoker. Knowing that smoking contributes to low birth weight in infants and also puts the mother at risk for other problems such as blood clot formation, hypertension, and lung disease, you know to monitor this woman more closely and to continue to work with the woman to stop smoking.

Make the shift from having only a problem-solving mentality to having a proactive, preventive way of thinking. Move from asking only *Have I missed any problems?* to also asking *Have I missed any risk factors that need attention?*

Critical Thinking Indicators (CTIs) Related to Diagnosis

Before we go on to address how to apply critical thinking to make diagnoses, let's take a look at the major CTIs that relate to *Diagnosis.* Reflect on where you stand in relation to the CTIs in Box 3.5. Remember that the knowledge CTIs listed on page 34 and CTIs on page 35 in Chapter 1 also apply.

---

box 3.5 Major Critical Thinking Indicators (*CTIs*) Related to Intellectual Skills Required for *Diagnosis*

Nursing Process and Decision-Making:

❑ Applies standards and principles when planning, giving, and adapting care
❑ Assesses systematically and comprehensively; uses a nursing framework to identify nursing concerns, uses a body systems framework to identify medical concerns
❑ Detects bias; determines credibility of information sources
❑ Distinguishes normal from abnormal; identifies risks for abnormal
❑ Determines significance of data; distinguishes relevant from irrelevant; clusters relevant data together
❑ Identifies assumptions and inconsistencies; checks accuracy and reliability; recognizes missing information; focuses assessment as indicated
❑ Concludes what's known and unknown; makes reasonable inferences (conclusions) and judgments—gives evidence to support them
❑ Considers multiple explanations and solutions
❑ Identifies both problems and their underlying cause(s) and related factors; includes patient and family perspectives
❑ Manages risks; predicts complications; promotes health, function, and well-being; anticipates consequences and implications—plans ahead accordingly
❑ Sets priorities and makes decisions in a timely way; includes key stakeholders in making decisions
❑ Communicates effectively orally and in writing
❑ Identifies ethical issues and takes appropriate action
❑ Identifies and uses technologic, information, and human resources

Additional Related Skills:

❑ Establishes empowered partnerships with patients, families, peers, and co-workers
❑ Teaches patients, self, and others

(box continues on next page)

box 3.5 Major Critical Thinking Indicators (*CTIs*) Related to Intellectual Skills Required for *Diagnosis* (continued)

❑ Addresses conflicts fairly; fosters positive interpersonal relationships
❑ Facilitates and navigates change
❑ Organizes and manages time and environment
❑ Facilitates teamwork (focuses on common goals; helps and encourages others to contribute in their own way)
❑ Demonstrates systems thinking (shows awareness of the interrelationships existing within and across health care systems)

Source: *Critical Thinking Indicators (2007–2008 Evidence-Based Version).* © 2008 R. Alfaro-LeFevre. All rights reserved. Do not copy without written permission. Available: www.AlfaroTeachSmart.com

CRITICAL THINKING EXERCISE VII

Nurses' Responsibilities as Diagnosticians; Key Terms Related to Diagnosis; Differentiating Between Nursing Diagnoses and Other Problems

To complete this session, read pages 93–111. Example responses can be found on page 242.

1. **Short answer:**
   a. How do you know if an action is within your domain of practice?
   b. List two key nursing responsibilities related to nursing diagnoses and two related to medical diagnoses.

2. **Check your knowledge of key terms.** For each definition (numbers 1–20), write the letter of the word that best matches the definition. Use each letter only once.

   a. diagnose
   b. diagnosis
   c. medical domain
   d. wellness diagnosis
   e. definitive diagnosis
   f. risk diagnosis
   g. accountable
   h. competency
   i. being qualified
   j. life process

   k. nursing domain
   l. outcome
   m. legal implications of diagnosis
   n. medical diagnosis
   o. nursing diagnosis
   p. definitive interventions
   q. risk (related) factor
   r. signs
   s. symptoms
   t. rule out

   ____ **1.** Something known to contribute to (or be associated with) a specific problem
   ____ **2.** A health problem for which someone is at risk
   ____ **3.** The judgment that's made after drawing conclusions about assessment data; also may refer to the skill of analyzing data to make a judgment
   ____ **4.** To make a judgment and identity and name risk factors, problems, or strengths based on evidence from an assessment
   ____ **5.** Being responsible and answerable for something
   ____ **6.** Range of activities and actions that a physician is legally qualified to initiate or prescribe
   ____ **7.** Range of activities and actions that a nurse is legally qualified to initiate or prescribe

(critical thinking continues on page 112)

___ **8.** Implies that there's a situation or problem that requires appropriate qualified treatment

___ **9.** Usually refers to the desired or expected result of interventions (ie, the problem is prevented, resolved, or controlled)

___**10.** Usually referred to as human responses; these provide the basis for selection of nursing interventions to achieve outcomes for which nurses are accountable

___**11.** A clinical judgment about an individual, family, or community in transition from a specific level of wellness to a higher level of wellness

___**12.** Events or changes that occur during one's lifetime (eg, becoming a parent, aging, separations, losses)

___**13.** The most specific diagnosis

___**14.** The most specific actions required to prevent, resolve, or control a problem

___**15.** A problem requiring definitive diagnosis and treatment by a qualified physician; APNs also may treat some of these problems

___**16.** Having the knowledge and skill to perform an activity or give opinions

___**17.** Having the competency and authority to perform an activity

___**18.** Objective (reported) data known to be associated with a diagnosis

___**19.** To decide that a problem isn't present

___**20.** Subjective (reported) data associated with a diagnosis

3. **Differentiating between nursing and medical diagnoses.**

  a. Write "N" in front of the phrases that describe characteristics of nursing diagnoses. Leave blank the ones that do not.

___ **1.** Deals mostly with problems with anatomy and physiology

___ **2.** Includes health problems as identified from patients' unique human perspectives.

___ **3.** Definitive diagnosis is often validated by medical diagnostic studies.

___ **4.** Deals mostly with actual or potential problems with human responses to disease or life changes

___ **5.** Signs and symptoms don't improve after nurse-prescribed interventions are performed.

___ **6.** Signs and symptoms improve after nurse-prescribed interventions are performed.

  b. For each of the following problems, write "N" in front of those that are nursing diagnoses.

___ **1.** Hemorrhage related to clotting problems

___ **2.** Ineffective Airway Clearance related to copious secretions

___ **3.** Risk for Injury related to generalized weakness

___ **4.** Intravenous therapy

___ **5.** Ineffective coping related to lack of resources

___ **6.** Impaired Skin Integrity (right toe blister) related to pressure point from cast

___ **7.** Potential cardiac arrhythmias related to low potassium level

___ **8.** Diabetes

___ **9.** Risk for Aspiration related to difficulty managing copious secretions

___**10.** Potential Malnutrition related to prescribed NPO (nothing by mouth)

___**11.** Imbalanced Nutrition: Less than Body Requirements related to poor appetite

___**12.** Impaired Physical Mobility related to prescribed bed rest

___**13.** Pneumothorax (collapsed lung)

___**14.** Potential thrombus formation related to venous shunt placement

4. Compare and Contrast: List one way the DT and the PPMP models are the same and one way that they're different.

Try This on Your Own

1. **Learn more about helping patients self-manage chronic diseases and disabilities.** Read and discuss the following article, which addresses how the use of evidence-based principles of learning can contribute to the empowerment of patients as they adopt self-management skills aligned with healthy behaviors. You can also take a continuing-education test for this article.

   Suter, P., & Suter, N. (2008). Timeless principles of learning: A solid foundation for enhancing chronic disease self-management. *Home Healthcare Nurse. 26*(2), 82–88.

2. **Learn about the importance of establishing and sustaining healthy work environments.** Review and discuss the Healthy Work Environment Standards at http://www.aacn.org/AACN/hwe.nsf/vwdoc/HWEHomePage

3. **In some cases, errors in diagnosis result in misuse of restraints and seclusion.** With a partner or in a group, go to the following Web site and discuss some of the true case histories posted there: http://groups.msn.com/SIDEEFFECTS/restraint.msnw

4. **With a partner or in a group,** discuss the *Think About It* and the *Voices* after this exercise.

think about it

No Patient Is a Critical Path. Critical paths are developed for specific *problems*, not specific *people*.

voices

Predicting, Preventing, and Managing Violence

The most significant factor that helps to predict, prevent, and manage violence is asking about history of previous violent episodes. With angry or high-risk patients, ask questions like, "Have you ever felt out of control or been violent in the past?" . . . "What do you do when you feel like you're getting out of control?" . . . "What can we do when you're feeling like this?"

—*Nico Oud, RN, MNSc, Dipl.N.Adm (personal communication, 2008)*

Learning How to Make Definitive Diagnoses

In both nursing and medicine, learning how to make a definitive diagnosis—how to determine the most specific, correct diagnosis—is a challenge for teachers to teach and students to learn. There are two reasons for this:

1. As often in cases with many complex skills gained through experience over time, expert clinicians forget how hard it was to learn "the basics," thereby making it hard to teach novices.
2. Novices are overwhelmed by worrying about what they don't know.

Think of it this way: For most of you, using computers is second nature. You have done it for so long that you forget how daunting and tedious computer skills can be at first. Only when you have to teach a novice do you remember how hard it was at the start. You find yourself doing a lot of backtracking and saying things like, "Well, usually you do . . . ," ". . . except for . . . ," "Yes, I know I said that, but not in this case . . . ," "You'd better write this down."

This section is designed to help you learn the basics of becoming a competent diagnostician and also to give you tools and strategies that help you move more quickly from being a tentative beginner to a more confident student in the skill of diagnosis.

Let's start by looking at principles and rules that are fundamental to making diagnoses.

Fundamental Principles and Rules of Diagnostic Reasoning

❏ As shown in the diagram at the beginning of this chapter, at the big-picture level, **making diagnoses involves** the following.
  1. Creating a list of possible problems/diagnoses
  2. Ruling out similar problems/diagnoses
  3. Naming actual and potential problems and clarifying what's causing or contributing to them
  4. Determining risk factors that must be managed
  5. Identifying resources, strengths, and areas for health promotion

Rationale: Making diagnoses requires you to consider several possibilities, not just one. Listing *all the possible problems* gives you a visual aid that you can reflect on. Ruling out *other similar diagnoses* helps ensure that you don't mislabel the problem. Identifying both the problem and its cause(s) shows that you have a complete understanding of the problem. It also helps you decide what to do about the problem. For example, you may have two people who have Immobility. One has Immobility because of paralysis after a spinal cord injury, and the other has it because of medically prescribed bed rest—two very different problems. Identifying and managing risk factors is proactive—it prevents problems before they happen. Taking advantage of resources and strengths to manage or improve health is cost-effective, helps boost patient self-esteem, and reframes situations to focus on the positive (it's easy to get bogged down with problems and forget the good things that are happening).

❑ **Know your qualifications and limitations.** Get help when needed. **Rationale:** People have the right to be assessed by a qualified health care professional. Although you may feel that you have the knowledge to do an assessment and diagnose the problems, you must determine—for your patient's health and your own legal protection—whether you have the authority to do so.

❑ **Keep an open mind.** Avoid tendencies to be overly influenced by past experiences or by information you gain from patient charts or others (eg, you may assess someone whose chart reports a history of chronic arthritic back pain and fail to consider that an increase in back pain could signify something else, like a kidney problem). **Rationale:** Keeping an open mind prevents you from "tunnel vision," a common critical thinking error.

❑ **Making diagnoses involves comparing your patient's cues (signs and symptoms) with the "textbook picture" of the diagnoses you suspect. Rationale:** You make a *definitive diagnosis* when your patient's data closely match the "textbook picture" of the diagnosis you suspect.

❑ **Name the problems by using the labels that most closely match assessment cues.** For example, if you suspect *Anxiety* or *Fear,* compare the cues with the defining characteristics of Anxiety and Fear. If the cues are most similar to Anxiety, name the problem Anxiety. If the cues are most similar to the defining characteristics of Fear, label the problem Fear. **Rationale:** *Diagnosis* is based on recognizing when patient cues match the signs and symptoms or defining characteristics of a specific diagnosis.

❑ **When you suspect a specific problem, look for other signs, symptoms, and risk factors commonly associated with the problem.** For example, if you suspect infection because of localized pain and swelling, look for *other* signs of infection (fever, redness, heat, drainage). **Rationale:** *Diagnosis* is based on evidence: the more evidence (cues) you have, the more likely you are to be correct.

R U L E

Remember, "More than one cue, more likely it's true. More than one source, more likely, of course."

❑ **When you make a diagnosis, back it up with evidence.** Be ready to give the cues (signs, symptoms, risk factors) that led you to make the diagnosis. **Rationale:** Cues (signs, symptoms, risk factors) are like "key puzzle pieces"; if you don't have them, you can't complete the puzzle and label the problem. For example, your patient may have a productive cough and fever, causing you to suspect pneumonia. The doctor needs evidence from a chest x-ray examination, sputum culture, and white blood cell count to complete the puzzle and make the diagnosis.

❑ **Include problems from patients' perspectives.** Ask them to tell you their three biggest problems. **Rationale:** Patients know themselves best, and must be included in the diagnostic process. Things that the patient sees as problems should be given a high priority.

❑ **Patients often complain of two or more related problems.** The first step is to identify the primary problem by looking at *relationships* between and among the problems.

For example, someone may complain of both *anxiety* and *insomnia.* The person may be most upset about the insomnia. It's your job to determine the primary problem, which quite likely is *anxiety.* **Rationale:** Often one problem creates another (in this case the *anxiety* may be causing *insomnia*).

❏ **Although intuition is a valuable tool for problem identification, never make diagnoses on intuition alone:** look for evidence to verify your intuition. See Box 3.6 below. **Rationale:** Diagnosis is based on evidence.

❏ **Look for flaws in your thinking: (1) What other problems could the cues represent?** For example, if someone tells you he's been having increasing episodes of left shoulder pain due to an old injury, consider the possibility that this pain also could represent a cardiac problem. **(2) What could be influencing the status of the problems you suspect?** For example, you may have ruled out the possibility of infection because there is no fever, but when you check all the data, you realize that an anti-inflammatory drug has been taken, reducing body temperature. **Rationale:** We're all vulnerable to misinterpretation. Looking for flaws in thinking is a critical thinking principle that helps reduce diagnostic errors.

❏ **If you miss a problem, mislabel a problem, or identify a problem that isn't there, you made a diagnostic error,** which may result in inappropriate, dangerous treatment. **Rationale:** An error in diagnosis is likely to cause an error in treatment. Box 3.7 lists common causes and possible consequences of diagnostic errors. Box 3.8 gives a checklist to help you avoid diagnostic errors.

❏ **Diagnosis is incomplete until you identify not only the problems, but also strengths, resources, and areas for improving health** (Box 3.9, page 118). **Rationale:** Identifying strengths is the key to efficiency (you draw on these strengths when planning care). At all patient encounters, in accordance with *Healthy People 2010,* nurses should actively consider areas for health promotion. What better way is there to reduce the need for nursing care than to motivate people to improve their health on their own? Successful nurses are good teachers.

❏ **Share your diagnoses with patients and ask them whether they understand what the diagnoses mean** (as appropriate, ask whether they agree with your opinion).

---

box 3.6 How to Use Intuition Safely

1. Recognize that although you have no evidence that a problem exists, your intuition is sending up a red flag that says, "There is a problem here; watch this patient closely," or "This patient needs help." Assess closely for existing signs and symptoms that validate the presence of the problem that you suspect. (You should say to the patient, physician, or another nurse, "My intuition tells me that . . ." or "I have the feeling that. . . .")

2. If you know that something is wrong but can't put your finger on any specific problem, increase the frequency and intensity of nursing assessment to monitor closely for early detection of signs and symptoms.

3. Before you act on intuition alone, weigh the risks of the possibility of your actions causing harm (either aggravating the situation or creating new problems) against the risk of not acting at all (other than to monitor more closely).

box 3.7 Diagnostic Errors

Causes of Diagnostic Errors

❑ Overvaluing the probability of one explanation or failing to consider all of the data because of a *narrow* focus.
  Example: Deciding that anxiety is related to psychological stress rather than considering whether there might be some physical problem, such as poor oxygenation, causing the anxiety.
❑ Continuing to *analyze* when you should be *acting* to get help.
  Example: Continuing to see if repositioning and emotional support help a breathing problem, even though they make no difference.
❑ Failing to recognize personal biases or assumptions.
  Example: Assuming that someone who doesn't bathe daily has a poor self-image.
❑ Making a diagnosis that's too general (not being specific enough in choosing a diagnostic label to name the problem).
  Example: Using *Impaired Urinary Elimination* instead of *Stress Incontinence related to weakness of bladder sphincter muscles.*
❑ Failing to include the correct diagnosis in the initial list of possible problems.
  Example: Listing the problems of *Noncompliance* but not including the possible problems of *Ineffective Coping or Ineffective Management of Therapeutic Regimen.*
❑ Rushing to get done, either when collecting or analyzing data.
  Example: Rushing through assessment or choosing any diagnosis that's close so you get to report on time, rather than communicating that you ran out of time to the next nurse.

Risks of Diagnostic Errors

When you miss a problem, mislabel a problem, or fail to fully understand a problem, you run the risk of any of the following:

❑ Initiating interventions that actually aggravate the problems.
❑ Omitting interventions that are essential to solving the problems.
❑ Allowing problems to exist or progress without even detecting that they are there.
❑ Initiating interventions that are harmless but wasteful of everyone's time and energy.
❑ Influencing others that problems exist as described incorrectly.
❑ Harming patients and placing yourself in danger of legal liability.

box 3.8 Avoiding Diagnostic Errors

Do you:

❑ Take the time to be sure your data are accurate and complete?
❑ Compare your patients' signs and symptoms with the "textbook picture" of the diagnoses you suspect?
❑ Recognize your biases and avoid value judgments?
❑ Consider other problems that the cues might signify?
❑ Look for flaws in your thinking?
❑ Identify the cause(s) of the problem(s)?
❑ Include what the patient sees as problems?
❑ Choose the most specific diagnostic label(s) that best describes the problem(s)?
❑ Inform the patient (and significant others) of what you see as problems?
❑ Ask someone to double-check you when you're unsure?
❑ Validate the diagnosis with the client?

box 3.9 Identifying Resources and Strengths

1. **Ask the person (and significant others)** the main questions:
   - ❏ Can you tell me some things about yourself that you view as strengths, as healthy aspects?
   - ❏ Can you think of any things that aren't really problems but you'd like to improve?
   - ❏ Who would you say are your best resources that can help you?

   Rationale: Answers to these questions help everyone to recognize assets and areas that could be improved.
2. **Cluster together data** that indicate normal or positive functioning. Label these areas as strengths and share them with the person and significant others. For example, you might say, "You've made the decision to seek help, which is a healthy thing to do." **Rationale:** This strategy helps both you and the person requiring care to focus on strengths as well as problems.
3. **List the strengths** that will assist you in preventing, resolving, or controlling the identified problems. **Rationale:** These are the strengths that you use to develop an efficient care plan.

Examples

❏ **Physical strengths:** In good health; exercises daily and has excellent cardiac and respiratory reserve; eats a balanced diet; demonstrates physical adaptation; upper torso and arms are powerful (compensating for paraplegia).

❏ **Psychological and personal strengths:** Demonstrates effective coping; copes with chronic pain by using guided imagery and by judicious use of pain medications; motivated; wants to be independent and healthy; knowledgeable; relates understanding of health care management and available resources; demonstrates good problem-solving skills; able to adjust daughter's therapy schedule for optimum results and convenience; has strong support systems.

Rationale: Patients have the right to be informed of diagnoses and must be partners in developing the plan of care.

Pages 119–120 show the first two pages of a tool to guide diagnostic reasoning (the complete tool can be downloaded from www.AlfaroTeachSmart.com). Using a tool like this consistently can help you develop good diagnostic reasoning.

Patients as Partners in Diagnosis

To reduce errors and improve results, patients and families must be active partners in care; this includes being actively involved in making diagnoses. Too often patients come into the health care system "unfocused"—they haven't given much thought to deciding what their major problems are. To improve efficiency and results, many places now give their patients written forms to help them identify their major concerns before meeting with the doctor or nurse. Developing tools that help patients assess their own problems and what's causing them saves time and improves accuracy. The patient self-assessment tool on pages 121–122 and the focus assessment tool in Chapter 2 on page 56 are examples of these types of tools.

COMPREHENSIVE ANALYSIS TOOL
A Guide For Diagnostic Reasoning

NOTE: This tool is designed for *beginning students* caring for *adult patients.* It's NOT intended to replace standard assessment tools. Rather, it helps you to do in depth analysis to *draw conclusions* about the data recorded on them. While this guide prompts you to approach diagnosis systematically, it doesn't replace the need for independent judgment or ability to apply basic principles of diagnostic reasoning. Using this tool consistently will help you develop habits that prioritize your approach to diagnosis.

Keeping a nursing focus – to maximize patient self-mangement, bio-psychosocial function, and quality of life – this tool guides you through the process of thinking about nursing concerns. It incorporates principles from *Gordon's Functional Health Patterns and Maslow's Human Needs*, and considers *Healthy People 2010* recommendations (for example, screening for depression). It also prompts you to check for disease often included in disease management programs. To help you prioritize, it lists questions according to things you need to think about early (for example, whether signs and symptoms are caused by a communicable disease).

This tool patient self-assessment tools are available for download free *for personal or student use only* at: www.AlfaroTeachSmart.com (click on *Publications*, then *Handouts*).

1. List admitting diagnoses and current major problems according to patient, family, and medical records.

2. Rule out presence of infection or communicable disease (check for fever, fatigue, pain, redness, heat, swelling, drainage, exposure to communicable disease or toxic substance; travel to foreign country).

3. Rule out whether patient signs and symptoms are actually medication problems. Consider all drugs taken (including over-the-counter and herbal remedies). Use **SODA** to jog your mind:

   ☐ **S**ide effects?

   ☐ **O**ver dosage?

   ☐ **D**rug interactions?

   ☐ **A**llergy or **A**dverse reactions?

4. Rule out whether the patient's signs and symptoms are actually allergic responses or due to history of surgery or trauma. Check for patient history of the following:

☐ Arthritis or Back Pain	☐ Depression/mental	☐ Thyroid Disease
☐ Asthma or other Lung Disease	health problems	☐ Vascular/Circulation
☐ Bleeding problems	☐ Diabetes	Problems
☐ Cancer (Breast, Prostate, Other)	☐ Hypertension	☐ Wound Healing Problems
☐ Congestive Heart Failure/	☐ Infection/HIV	☐ Surgery/trauma
Heart Disease	☐ Obesity	☐ Skin problems
☐ Neurological problems	☐ Kidney Disease	☐ Other diseases/problems:

5. Has there been significant weight loss or gain? (Consider as far back as 6 weeks. Remember that unexplained weight loss may indicate serious medical problems like cancer, or diabetes; unexplained weight gain may indicate serious kidney, heart, or thyroid disease).

COMPREHENSIVE ANALYSIS TOOL
A Guide For Diagnostic Reasoning

6. Determine smoking pattern and possible role in current problems:

Yes ☐ Quit Smoking ☐ Never Smoked Packs per day _____

7. For pre-menopausal women (age <55 years), rule out possibility of pregnancy (many drugs, diagnostic studies, or treatments affect the fetus).

8. Rule out whether there are problems (or risk factors for problems) with any of the following.

		(Circle those that apply)		
☐ Breathing or coughing, or oxygenation?	Yes	No	AR[1]	Pos[2]
☐ Blood pressure, pulse, bleeding, circulation?	Yes	No	AR	Pos
☐ Pain, stiffness or discomfort?	Yes	No	AR	Pos
☐ Body temperature or sweating?	Yes	No	AR	Pos
☐ Ability to think or perceive environment?	Yes	No	AR	Pos
☐ Communication (seeing, hearing, or speaking)?	Yes	No	AR	Pos
☐ Eating, digestion, or nutrition?	Yes	No	AR	Pos
☐ Bowel elimination?	Yes	No	AR	Pos
☐ Dehydration, edema or electrolyte imbalance?	Yes	No	AR	Pos
☐ Movement, range of motion, or activity intolerance?	Yes	No	AR	Pos
☐ Rashes, skin problems, ulcers, or tissue perfusion?	Yes	No	AR	Pos
☐ Sleeping?	Yes	No	AR	Pos
☐ Infection (vulnerable or contagious to others)?	Yes	No	AR	Pos
☐ Safety (risk for injury or falls; weakness or seizures)?	Yes	No	AR	Pos
☐ Anxiety, coping or managing stress?	Yes	No	AR	Pos
☐ Drug or alcohol dependence?	Yes	No	AR	Pos
☐ Growth and developmental challenges?	Yes	No	AR	Pos
☐ Life style changes (eg, divorce, moving, new parent)?	Yes	No	AR	Pos
☐ Roles, relationships, sexuality, or self-esteem?	Yes	No	AR	Pos
☐ Patient or family education needs?	Yes	No	AR	Pos
☐ Difficulties at home or work?	Yes	No	AR	Pos
☐ Ability to do desired, as well as necessary activities?	Yes	No	AR	Pos
☐ Personal, religious, spiritual, cultural beliefs?	Yes	No	AR	Pos
☐ Ethical issues?	Yes	No	AR	Pos
☐ Socio-economic issues?	Yes	No	AR	Pos

> **HOW TO PRIORITIZE: Problems usually present in a cluster** (patients rarely have only one problem). Before going on to the next page, study the above and consider *relationships* among the problems. For example, if pain is contributing to depression or movement problems, **pain** is a major problem. If you're unsure whether a problem is present, ***collect more data.***

AR[1] = At Risk for problem (no signs and symptoms present, but risk factors are evident).

Pos[2] = Possible problem (insufficient data, but you suspect a problem).

COMPREHENSIVE PATIENT SELF-ASSESSMENT TOOL

Note to Our Patient Partners: Because YOU are the one who knows yourself best, we want you to be informed, involved participants in your care. Studies show that people who are actively involved in making decisions about their care are likely to have the best results. In all aspects of your care, remember the following Speak Up steps, from the Joint Commission:

□ **S**peak up if you have questions or concerns. If you don't understand, ask again. It's your body and you have a right to know.*

□ **P**ay attention to the care you are receiving. Make sure you're getting the right treatments and medications by the right health care professionals. Don't assume anything.

□ **E**ducate yourself about your diagnosis, your testing procedures, and your treatment plan.

□ **A**sk a trusted family member or friend to be your advocate.

□ **K**now what medications you take and why you take them. Medication errors are the most common health care errors.

□ **U**se hospitals, clinics, surgery centers, or other types of health care organizations that have undergone rigorous on-site evaluations against established state-of-the-art quality and safety standards, such as that provided by the Joint Commision.

□ **P**articipate in all decisions about your treatment. You are the center of the health care team.

1. Get focused and help us prioritize. Tell us your 3 biggest problems or concerns.

2. Please list any current medical problems.

3. List any surgery you have had, including date when surgery was done.

4. (For women) when was your last menstrual period?

5. Do you smoke?   □ Yes   □ Quit Smoking   □ Never Smoked   Packs per day _____

If you smoke, we strongly recommend that you stop. Please ask for our information on smoking cessation. You CAN do it, with help!

*Speak Up approach is courtesy of the Joint Commission, http://www.jointcommission.org/

First two pages of tool. Download complete tool from www.AlfaroTeachSmart.com

6. Do you drink alcohol? ☐ Yes ☐ No   If yes, how much per week?

7. List allergies and medications (include over-the-counter and herbal drugs).

Allergies:

Drug	Dose	Taken how often?	Last dose?	Prescribing doctor?

8. Could any of your symptoms be medication related? Remember SODA:

☐ **S**ide effects?

☐ **O**ver dosage?

☐ **D**rug interactions?

☐ **A**llergy or **A**dverse reactions?

9. What screening tests have you had done (eg, colonoscopy, mammography)?

10. Put an X on the box, if you have a family history of any of the following:

☐ Cancer ☐ Glaucoma

☐ Heart disease ☐ Mental health problems

☐ Diabetes ☐ Other

☐ Hypertension

11. Children/Pregnancies:

Number of living children you have: ____ Number deceased: ____

For women, number of pregnancies you have had: ____

> R U L E
>
> **Partner With Patients to Identify Problems.** Help patients prioritize their problems by asking things like, "What are your three biggest problems?" Verify your opinions by asking patients whether they understand and agree. For example, "It seems like you are drinking to cope with your pain . . . do you think that's possible?" **Rationale:** Identifying problems should always begin by asking patients first.

Clarifying Causes and Contributing (Risk) Factors

Problem Identification is incomplete until you understand what's *causing* or *contributing to* the problems. Keeping in mind the importance of focusing on the whole person, not just the disease(s), the following are some steps to take to identify contributing factors.

1. Ask patients and families questions like the following:
 • What do you think is causing or contributing to the problem(s)?
 • How do your symptoms impact on your ability to do daily activities?
 • How has your life changed?
 • How are you coping with these changes?
 • What resources (personal, community) might be able to help you?
2. Determine whether there are factors related to developmental age, disease, treatment, or changes in lifestyle that may be contributing to the problem(s).
3. Find out if there are cultural, socioeconomic, ethnic, or spiritual factors that may be contributing to the problem(s).
4. Check your other resources for data collection (eg, medical records, other health care professionals, literature review) to identify other factors that might be causing or contributing to the problem(s)?

> R U L E
>
> **Until you clarify all the factors that are causing (or contributing to) the problems you identify, *Diagnosis* is incomplete.** You must determine *all the contributing factors* to be able to decide: a) the most important factors that must be managed; and b) what has to be done to manage the problem. Figure 3.2 (next page) shows a map demonstrating how the problem of *Impaired Skin Integrity* may have many contributing factors. Page 125 gives a worksheet to help you be systematic when determining factors contributing to a problem.

> R U L E
>
> **Always ask yourself whether it's possible that the signs and symptoms you identify could represent a medical problem that needs in-depth assessment by a more qualified professional.** For example, if you're caring for someone with chronic constipation,

be sure that this problem has been evaluated by a physician. Figure 3.3 (page 127) shows how a nurse determines the cause of constipation compared with how a physician determines the cause of constipation. Notice that the medical evaluation examines whether the constipation is a sign of undiagnosed cancer.

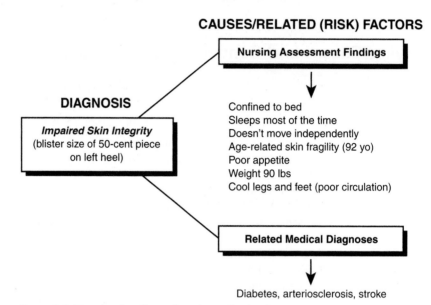

CAUSES/RELATED (RISK) FACTORS

DIAGNOSIS

Nursing Assessment Findings

Impaired Skin Integrity (blister size of 50-cent piece on left heel)

Confined to bed
Sleeps most of the time
Doesn't move independently
Age-related skin fragility (92 yo)
Poor appetite
Weight 90 lbs
Cool legs and feet (poor circulation)

Related Medical Diagnoses

Diabetes, arteriosclerosis, stroke

FIGURE 3.2 Map showing diagnosis and contributing factors.

Identifying Nursing Diagnoses

The Quick Reference to Nursing Diagnoses section beginning on page 223 gives the following information for commonly encountered diagnoses.

❏ **Title (Label) and Definition:** A concise description of the problem.
❏ **Defining Characteristics:** The cluster of signs and symptoms often associated with the diagnosis.
❏ **Related (Risk) Factors:** Factors that can cause or contribute to the problem.

NANDA International officially updates its information every 2 years. Some of the diagnoses have been studied extensively (eg, *Risk for Injury*) and others have not (eg, Personal Identity Disturbance). The quick reference guide beginning on page 223 gives commonly encountered nursing diagnoses. The following guidelines can help you identify nursing diagnoses.

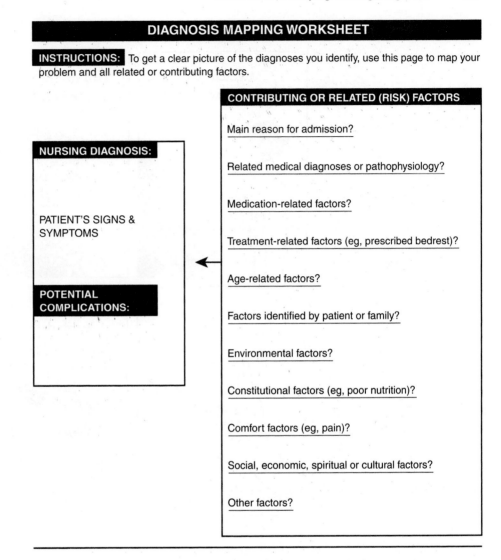

DIAGNOSIS MAPPING WORKSHEET

INSTRUCTIONS: To get a clear picture of the diagnoses you identify, use this page to map your problem and all related or contributing factors.

NURSING DIAGNOSIS:

PATIENT'S SIGNS & SYMPTOMS

POTENTIAL COMPLICATIONS:

CONTRIBUTING OR RELATED (RISK) FACTORS

Main reason for admission?

Related medical diagnoses or pathophysiology?

Medication-related factors?

Treatment-related factors (eg, prescribed bedrest)?

Age-related factors?

Factors identified by patient or family?

Environmental factors?

Constitutional factors (eg, poor nutrition)?

Comfort factors (eg, pain)?

Social, economic, spiritual or cultural factors?

Other factors?

Guidelines: Identifying Nursing Diagnoses

To identify <u>actual</u> nursing diagnoses, compare your patient's signs and symptoms with the defining characteristics of the diagnoses you suspect. The nursing diagnosis that has defining characteristics that most closely match your patient's data is the definitive nursing diagnosis. For example, if you suspect *Anxiety* or *Fear,* compare defining

H.M.O. (HELP ME OUT)®

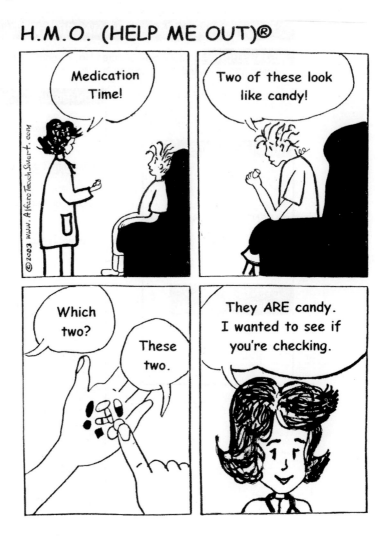

characteristics for both diagnoses with your patient's signs and symptoms. Then choose the diagnosis that most closely matches your patient's signs and symptoms.

To identify <u>risk (potential)</u> nursing diagnoses, compare your patient's risk factors with the related (risk) factors listed under the diagnoses you suspect. Use the nursing diagnosis label that has related (risk) factors that most closely match *your patient's* risk factors. For example, if your patient's risk factors match the related (risk) factors listed under *Acute Pain* more closely than Chronic Pain, then use *Acute Pain.*

To identify syndrome diagnoses, compare your patient's signs and symptoms with the related factors and defining characteristics of the syndrome diagnosis you suspect (see *Disuse Syndrome* versus *Rape Trauma Syndrome*).

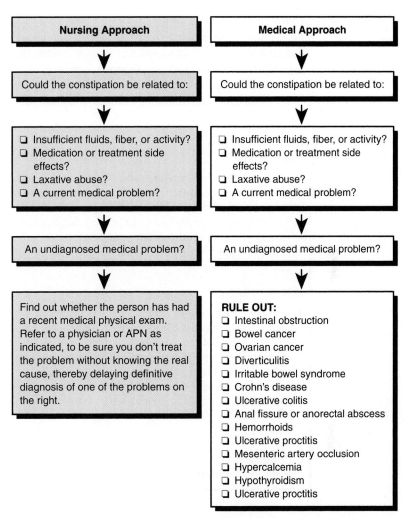

Figure 3.3 Nursing versus medical approach to determining cause of constipation.

To identify wellness diagnoses, compare patient statements for desired improved health with the defining characteristics of the wellness diagnosis you believe is appropriate. Use the phrase *Readiness for Enhanced* before the diagnostic label. For example, *Readiness for Enhanced Parenting.*

Mapping Diagnoses

Now that we know more about how the brain handles information, we have begun to do more mapping and diagramming of problems and diagnoses. Statements tend to constrain the brain (we sometimes spend more time thinking about the *rules* of statements than we do thinking about the *data*). Mapping and diagramming promote freedom and allow you to draw a picture of how you see the relationships among key aspects of a given problem (eg, Figure 3.2, page 124). Identifying relationships is a key critical thinking principle that's essential for making correct diagnoses.*

Think about the following changes in thinking about how diagnoses should be recorded.

Old Thinking

1. Students must learn to write two-part statements that state the problem and its cause, using "related to" to link the problem and its cause. For example: Impaired Skin Integrity (Left Heel Blister) related to pressure on left heel.
2. Students must identify causes of nursing diagnoses that can be remedied by independent nursing actions only.
3. Students must focus *only* on identifying problems that are managed independently by nurses.

Current Thinking

1. While two-part summary statements are helpful, they may limit critical thinking in early stages: Problems often have several causes and contributing factors. Some students may be able to express their thinking better by mapping or diagramming the diagnostic process. If mapping is used, students must know how to document the diagnoses in accordance with workplace policies.
2. Students need to learn to think in depth and identify ALL factors contributing to a problem (eg, page 125). When they consider all factors, they can decide what they will do independently and to what they will need to refer to ensure management of *all factors*.
3. Students must focus as much on identifying signs and symptoms that may indicate potential medical problems and complications, as they do on identifying problems that belong only to nursing.

Writing Diagnostic Summary Statements Using the PES or PRS Format

As explained earlier, using very specific rules for stating diagnoses can limit critical thinking in the early stages of problem analysis. However, there are times when writing a diagnostic statement after in-depth analysis fosters critical thinking, because it forces you to summarize the *most important* elements. This section explains how to write summary statements by using the PES (Problem, Etiology, Signs and Symptoms) method, also called the PRS (Problem, Related Factors, and Signs and Symptoms) method.

---

*For detailed guidelines on using mapping, see "Nuts and Bolts of Mapping" at www.AlfaroTeachSmart.com

To use the PES (or PRS) method:

1. State the problem.
2. Use "related to" to link the problem and its etiology—the cause or related (risk) factors.
3. Give the signs and symptoms that show evidence that the diagnosis is present, using the words "as evidenced by."

E x a m p l e

1. Actual Nursing Diagnosis (Three-Part Summary Statement)

Problem:	Impaired Communication
	related to
Related Factors:	language barrier
	as evidenced by
Signs and Symptoms:	speaking and understanding only Spanish

2. Risk (Potential) Nursing Diagnosis (Two-Part Summary Statement):

Problem:	Risk for Impaired Skin Integrity
	related to
Related Factors:	excessive sweating, and confinement to bed

R U L E

When writing diagnostic summary statements, be as explicit as you can: Add "secondary to" after the PES (or PRS) format to address key related problems (eg, left hip *decubitus ulcer* related to immobility and loss of sensation *secondary to* spinal cord injury).

The following gives a checklist to be sure you include the most important information in your summary statements for nursing diagnoses.

Checklist for Writing Diagnostic Statements:

Is the statement:

- Based on evidence from the nursing assessment?
- Specific and clear?
- Written with accepted terminology?
- Descriptive of both the problem and its cause?
- Written in a way that there's a high probability that others with the same knowledge and experience agree with the diagnosis?
- Reflective of a problem that you are authorized to manage?

Did you:

- Use "related to" to link the problem and it's cause
- Add "as evidenced by" when indicated?

think about it

Confirmation Bias: A Common Diagnostic Mistake
Be aware of confirmation bias (the human tendency to see only evidence that supports your initial beliefs). For example, a colleague of mine who is an APN works in an emergency department. A staff nurse reported that she had just admitted a patient with appendicitis, and reported all the signs and symptoms that supported the diagnosis of appendicitis (eg, right-sided abdominal pain, vomiting, and a family history of appendicitis). When the APN examined the patient, she asked about last menstrual period, did an exam, ordered studies, and found life threatening ectopic pregnancy.

voices

All Problems Aren't Created Equal—Determine the Cause
To treat health problems, be sure that you understand the underlying causes. For example, studies support that chronic wounds are biologically different from acute wounds like surgical incisions, so they require different treatment. Acute wounds usually follow the body's "healing cascade" in a predictable and orderly way. However, chronic wounds such as pressure ulcers are usually "stalled" in the inflammatory healing phase, requiring an intensive evidence-based treatment plan. Local wound care without the correct supportive care, based on etiology or cause, won't work!

—Elizabeth A. Ayello, PhD, RN, CS, CWOCN
(personal communication, 2008)

The Difference Between Expert and Novice Diagnosticians
There is an accumulation of evidence that expert problem-solving . . . depends on (1) a wealth of prior specific experiences which can be used in routine solution of problems by pattern recognition . . . and (2) elaborate conceptual knowledge applicable to the occasional problematic situation . . . The main difference between expert clinicians and students is that experts generate better hypotheses (from the beginning, they have better hunches about what the problems may be).[11]

—Dr. Geoffrey Norman

☺ **Placebos. . . . Cure Alls?**
One of my favorite cartoons shows a TV screen with a bottle of pills on it. The caption reads: Placebo™—For relief of high cholesterol, allergies, acid reflux, insomnia, arthritis, and restless leg syndrome. Ask your doctor if Placebo™ is right for you.[11]

CRITICAL THINKING EXERCISE VIII

Recognizing, Mapping, and Stating Nursing Diagnoses

To complete this session, read pages 114–130. Example responses start on page 242.

I. Recognizing Nursing Diagnoses. This session is designed for you to practice recognizing nursing diagnoses by comparing data with the defining characteristics and related factors of specific diagnoses.

   The following are eight common nursing diagnoses (letters a to h). After the diagnoses are eight imaginary people who have been admitted to the hospital (numbers 1–8). For each number, write the letter of the diagnosis that best matches the available patient data. To make the diagnosis: (1) study the data; (2) choose a possible nursing diagnosis from the available choices; then (3) look up the diagnosis in the section on Quick Reference to Nursing Diagnoses starting on page 223 and compare the data with the defining characteristics and related factors for the chosen diagnosis. Each letter should be used only once.

a. Risk for Aspiration
b. Activity Intolerance
c. Anxiety
d. Risk for Impaired Skin Integrity
e. Fear
f. Ineffective Breathing Pattern
g. Ineffective Airway Clearance
h. Impaired Skin Integrity

1. _____ Assessment data for Mrs. Ballard:
Subjective data (SD): Says she feels tired all the time.
Objective data (OD): Lungs clear; becomes short of breath after walking 5 yards; heart rate increases to 130 beats per minute after walking 5 yards; anemic (hemoglobin 7 g/dL).

2. _____ Assessment data for Jim Riley:
SD: States his jaws were wired closed yesterday; complains of nausea.
OD: Jaws wired shut.

3. _____ Assessment data for Charles Lindsay:
SD: States he feels "sort of nervous" but can't pinpoint why.
OD: Restless, glances about, doesn't make good eye contact.

4. _____ Assessment data for Daryl Laird:
SD: States he's afraid of giving himself an injection; states he lives alone and is worried that something might go wrong when he's alone giving himself an injection.
OD: Doesn't maintain good eye contact; restless.

5. _____ Assessment data for Tim Dydo:
SD: States he's had a cold for 2 weeks and now has pain in lower right rib cage; states he feels like he needs to cough, but finds it too painful.

(critical thinking continues on page 132)

OD: Respiration 34 breaths per minute; pulse 128 beats per minute; able to cough if rib cage is splinted by me; coughs up thick white mucus.

6. _____ Assessment data for Beth Hendrix:
   SD: States she has problems with urinary incontinence.
   OD: Wears perineal pad; perineal area red and excoriated.

7. _____ Assessment data for Mary Eipert:
   SD: States she's had mild emphysema for 5 years, but now it seems to be getting worse; states she gets out of breath when going up one flight of stairs; says she never learned adaptive breathing techniques.
   OD: Expiratory wheezes heard in both lungs; unable to demonstrate pursed-lipped breathing; respiratory rate up to 48 breaths per minute after going up one flight of stairs.

8. _____ Assessment data for Margaret Wolartowski:
   SD: Says she's afraid of moving because of pain in her hip.
   OD: 92 years old; very thin; had a hip pinning yesterday; skin very dry, no obvious breakdown at present.

II. Mapping Nursing Diagnoses

1. In three to five sentences, explain why mapping and diagramming diagnoses promotes critical thinking.
2. Draw a map of the diagnostic process. (No example response available. Compare your map with a peer or explain your map to someone.)

III. Stating Nursing Diagnosis: Summary Statements

Part A

1. **Practice identifying problems, related factors, and signs and symptoms (PRS).** Study the following nursing diagnoses. Circle the problem, underline the cause (etiology, or related factors), and let the signs and symptoms stand as is.
   a. Urge Incontinence related to inability to hold large amounts of urine as evidenced by voiding immediately upon realization of need to void.
   b. Anticipatory Grieving related to impending death of mother as evidenced by statements of extreme sadness over impending death.
2. **In one to three sentences,** explain why you don't address signs, symptoms, or defining characteristics when you write risk diagnoses.

Part B. Practice Using the PES (or PRS) System for Stating Diagnoses

The data presented in each of the following clinical situations matches one of the following diagnoses: Powerlessness; Imbalanced Nutrition (Less than Body Requirements); Ineffective Airway Clearance. Study each case, choose the matching diagnosis, and write a three-part diagnostic statement using the PES (or PRS) format.

1. Stuart demonstrates the following cues (signs and symptoms):
   Subjective (SD): Asks for help clearing secretions; states he can clear airway with help from suction.

Objective (OD): Copious secretions from tracheostomy tube.
Nursing Diagnosis:

2. Bob demonstrates the following cues (signs and symptoms):
   SD: Reports that he's had no appetite for 2 weeks because of depression.
   OD: Ten-pound weight loss since last visit; 15 lb under recommended weight.
   Nursing Diagnosis:

3. Lilly demonstrates the following cues (signs and symptoms):
   SD: Reports she's depressed and has no control over daily activities.
   OD: Quadriplegic—has a rigorous schedule of daily physical therapy.
   Nursing Diagnosis:

Part C

The data presented in each clinical situation below match one of the following diagnoses: *Risk for Ineffective Airway Clearance; Possible Ineffective Individual Coping; Risk for Fluid Volume Deficit; Possible Ineffective Sexual Pattern.* Study each situation, choose the matching diagnosis, and write a two-part statement, stating the problem and its cause.

1. Mr. Reardon has been confined to bed with casts on both his legs. He seems angry and has stated that he does not want to talk to anyone. You're aware that he's had a fight with his girlfriend.
   Nursing Diagnosis:

2. Mrs. Cappelli has a temperature of 101°F. She sleeps a lot and has a poor appetite. She drinks about 2000 milliliters a day if you offer frequent fluids and encourage her to drink.
   Nursing Diagnosis:

3. Mr. Rogers has just had his gallbladder removed today under general anesthesia. His nursing assessment form shows that he has smoked a pack of cigarettes a day for the past 20 years. He has a productive cough.
   Nursing Diagnosis:

4. You see Mrs. Jackson in clinic 3 months after a hysterectomy. She states that she feels well physically, but that emotionally she just doesn't feel like herself yet. She states that she gets angry easily, cries a lot, and that she's concerned the hysterectomy is affecting her emotionally and physically.
   Nursing Diagnosis:

Try This on Your Own

1. **Problem-Based Learning**—a way of learning that helps you learn about specific clinical problems though hands-on experience—is a great way to improve your ability to make diagnoses and identify clinical problems. Ask your instructor, mentor, or manager for the ten most common diagnoses/problems you're likely to encounter in the clinical setting. Then assess every patient you have for those common problems. You'll find that you'll quickly have these problems "in your head." You'll be able to

(critical thinking continues on page 134)

readily recognize when your patient has one of these common problems and you'll remember them for NCLEX. For some great references on problem-based learning, go to http://www.pbli.org/bibliography/articles.htm#n

2. **With a partner or in a group,** discuss the *Think About It* and *Voices* on page 130.

Identifying Potential Complications

An important part of identifying actual and potential problems is predicting potential complications (PC). Remember the following definition from earlier in the chapter.

Potential Complications. Problems that may occur because of current diagnoses, treatment, invasive monitoring, or diagnostic studies (see examples on inside back cover and facing page).

> **R U L E**
>
> **Preventing potential complications (PCs) requires early recognition of signs and symptoms seen when the complication happens.** For example: If you have someone with fractured ribs, look up fractured ribs and find out what the commonly related complications are (pneumothorax and hemothorax). Then look up the signs and symptoms of pneumothorax and hemothorax (chest pain, increased respirations, feeling of inability to get enough air, decreased breath sounds), as these are signs and symptoms you need to be looking for.

Your ability to predict and detect PCs will grow as your nursing knowledge expands and you have repeated experiences assessing people with different types of problems. Some knowledge can be gained only by clinical experience. For example, you have to listen to many lungs before you can readily recognize *abnormal breath sounds*. The following guidelines can help you to act in your patients' best interest, making sure that PCs are prevented, detected, and managed in a timely way.

Guidelines: Identifying Potential Complications

❏ **Until you feel confident identifying potential complications, report all abnormal data.** What may seem like an isolated cue to you may prompt a more experienced person to be concerned.

❏ **Remember that the onset of complications often is subtle.** Signs and symptoms gradually worsen over a period of time. Always compare your data with data charted by others over the past 24 to 48 hours (sometimes longer). For example if you get a temperature reading of 99.6°F, compare the reading with temperatures over the past 24 to 48 hours.

❑ **Look up all medications taken.** Often medications contribute to complications. Use the memory-jog **TACIT** as described at the top of page 73.

❑ **Consider the possibility of allergic responses** (to new medications, dyes used in diagnostic studies, or other environmental factors). If you identify an allergy, follow facility policies for recording the allergy in ways that flag this problem for other caregivers (you will probably need to put a special wrist band on the patient, as well as record the allergy in a specific place).

❑ **Review critical paths, policies, procedures, protocols, and standards that address your patient's situations** (eg, management of chest tubes). These often guide you to assess for specific signs and symptoms you must report to monitor for potential complications.

❑ **Look up the common complications of the patient's current medical problems.**

❑ **Be aware of recent diagnostic or treatment modalities**—determine whether there are commonly associated potential complications (eg, thrombi, emboli, and bleeding are potential complications of cardiac catheterization).

❑ **Read patient records** (medical history and physical report, nursing history and physical report, progress reports, consultations, diagnostic studies). Be sure you're aware of past medical problems as they often point to future ones.

❑ **In complex situations, check with the primary care physician or APN.** For example, say something like, "There's a lot going on with this patient. Are there any specific signs and symptoms you want us to report?"

R U L E

To record potential complications, use "PC" followed by a colon, then name the potential complication.[9] Example: PC: pneumothorax.

Need a Mentor or an Online Reference for Drugs and Diseases?

Check out the U.S. Public Health Mentoring Program at http://phs-nurse.org/MentoringProgram.htm. For up-to-date clinical information on drugs and diseases—and for patient handouts—go to http://www.medscape.com/druginfo

---

Identifying Problems Requiring Multidisciplinary Approaches

The final thing we'll talk about in this chapter is identifying problems that require multidisciplinary approaches. Recognizing early that problems are so complex that you need to include other disciplines like occupational and physical therapy is the key to achieving cost-effective outcomes. The main question to ask to determine whether you have problems that require multidisciplinary approaches is this:

Looking at the big picture of this person's situation, is it likely that he or she will be able to reach the desired outcomes in the expected time frame using only nursing expertise or care management? If the answer is "no," initiate appropriate referrals.

For example, if the outcome for a healthy woman having a hysterectomy is "will ambulate the first day after surgery," you could expect to achieve this outcome using nursing resources alone. However, if the woman has other coexisting problems, for example, difficulty walking due to neuromuscular problems, you should consider requesting a physical therapist's involvement with planning and managing ambulation.

CRITICAL THINKING EXERCISE IX

Predicting Potential Complications/Identifying Problems Requiring a Multidisciplinary Approach, Pulling It All Together

To complete this session, read pages 134–136. Example responses to each question can be found on page 243.

Part I

Practice identifying potential complications. Imagine you're looking after someone with each of the problems below. After the letters "PC," put the complications that you need to consider (use the inside back cover and facing page as a guide).

1. Intravenous Therapy
   PC:
2. Concussion
   PC:
3. Myocardial Infarction
   PC:
4. Nasogastric Suction
   PC:

Part II

How would you decide if your patient's problems are such that they may require a multidisciplinary approach (one to three sentences)?

Part III

Get a piece of paper and list the nursing diagnoses, potential complications, and strengths you identify in the following admission data.

Admission Data for Mrs. Goode, who has been admitted with a cerebral concussion:

Subjective Data

❏ States she has a headache and feels dizzy when she lifts her head off the pillow.
❏ Expresses concern about having her husband look after her two children because "he is not good with them."

❏ States she is afraid of hospitals and needles.
❏ States she has never worked outside the home because her children need her.
❏ States, "I can't stay in bed and use the bedpan as the doctor said."

Objective Data

❏ Age: 31 Ht: 5′0″ Wt: 160 lb
❏ Temperature: 98.4°F
❏ Pulse: 78 and regular
❏ Respirations: 22 and nonlabored
❏ Blood Pressure: 128/72
❏ Moves all extremities with equal strength
❏ Pupils are equally reactive to light
❏ Large bruise over right forehead
❏ Abdomen soft, nontender, obese
❏ Peripheral pulses strong
❏ IV in right arm running at 30 mL/h

THIS CHAPTER AND NCLEX*

❏ When prioritizing diagnoses, physiologic needs rise above all others. Airway issues and abnormal lab values are top priority. Risks for suicide, safety, and infection are a priority too.
❏ Be sure to note and connect all the data in the question. Missing a key piece of information may point you to the wrong answer. *Analysis* and *application* are the highest-level questions.

❏ Expect questions on all major nursing specialties, as well as advance directives; infection, injury, and error prevention; family systems, cultural diversity, legal rights and responsibilities; bioterrorism, disaster response, human sexuality, and mental health.
❏ See also "This Chapter and NCLEX" on pages 42, 87, 177, 202, and 221.

SUMMARY / KEY POINTS

▪ Page 93 gives a visual summary of Diagnosis—the pivotal second step of the nursing process—in context of the Predict, Prevent, Manage, and Promote model.
▪ Nurses' diagnostic responsibilities continue to grow, with nurses at all levels taking on more accountability for preventing, diagnosing, and treating health problems.

▪ The term diagnosis has legal implications. It implies that there's a problem that requires qualified treatment. Unless you're an APN, state laws prohibit you from making medical diagnoses independently. You are, however, *accountable* for giving high priority to assessing for—and reporting—signs and symptoms that may indicate the need for attention from a

*The author acknowledges the help of Deanne Blach (www.deanneblach.com) and Judith Miller (www.judymillernclexreview.com) in developing NCLEX tips.

professional more qualified than you. This is called "activating the chain of command."

- Today's nurses' diagnostic roles are affected by use of critical pathways, computer-assisted diagnosis, multidisciplinary practice, society's changing needs, and nursing's expanding knowledge base.
- As the field of informatics grows, standard vocabularies continue to evolve; use the terms required by the facility where you work.
- Including patients as partners in diagnosis is a key to preventing errors and identifying the priority problems.
- To be a competent diagnostician—and know how to respond to NCLEX questions and elec-

tronic decision support programs—make the principles and rules of diagnosis, as addressed in this chapter, habits of thinking.

- Mapping diagnoses and considering all factors that contribute to the diagnoses is the key to identifying a comprehensive treatment plan.
- If you're required to write a summary statement to describe the diagnoses you make, use the PES or PRS system as described on page 128.
- Scan this chapter for important rules, maps, and diagrams highlighted throughout, then compare where you stand in relation to the expected learning outcomes on page 91.

References

1. American Nurses Association. (2004). *Nursing scope and standards of performance and standards of clinical practice.* Washington, DC: American Nurses Publishing.
2. American Nurses Association. (2004). *Nursing scope and standards of performance and standards of clinical practice.* Washington, DC: American Nurses Publishing.
3. Buppert, C. (2008). The legal distinction between the practice of medicine and the practice of nursing. *The Journal for Nurse Practitioners, 4*(1), 22–24.
4. American Nurses Association. (2003). *Nursing: A social policy statement* (2nd ed.). Washington, DC: American Nurses Publishing.
5. American Nurses Association. (2004). *Nursing scope and standards of performance and standards of clinical practice.* Washington, DC: American Nurses Publishing.
6. North American Nursing Diagnosis Association International (NANDA-I). (2008). *Nursing diagnoses: Definitions and classification 2007–2006.* Philadelphia: Author.
7. Herdman, H. (2007). President's message. *NANDA E-news.* Retrieved March 22, 2007, from http://www.fernley.com/nanda-enews/winter07/content.html#1
8. North American Nursing Diagnosis Association International (NANDA-I). (2008). *Nursing diagnoses: Definitions and classification 2007–2006.* Philadelphia: Author
9. Carpenito-Moyet, L. (2008). *Nursing Diagnosis: Application to clinical practice* (12th ed.). Philadelphia: Lippincott Williams & Wilkins.
10. Norman, G. (1988). Problem-solving skills, solving problems, and problem-based learning. *Medical Education, 22,* 279.
11. Margulies, J. (2008). Cartoon in *The (Hackensack, NJ) Record.* Retrieved May 8, 2008, from www.northjersey.com/margulies

chapter 4

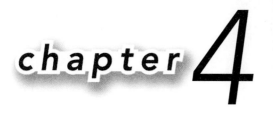

Planning

what's in this chapter?

Having a recorded plan that's clear, focused, and up-to-date makes the difference between safe, effective care and care that's haphazard (even dangerous). This chapter helps you gain the skills you need to be able to record a plan that meets key standards and promotes safe, efficient care. Here, you learn the four main purposes of the plan of care and explore how to set priorities and decide which problems *must* be documented. You learn principles and rules of developing patient-centered outcomes and individualized nursing interventions. You also clarify your responsibilities related to recording a comprehensive plan, including how to use standard and electronic plans.

ANA standards related to this chapter[1]

Standard 3 Outcome Identification. The registered nurse identifies expected outcomes for a plan individualized to the patient or the situation.

Standard 4 Planning. The registered nurse develops a plan that prescribes strategies and alternatives to attain expected outcomes.

critical thinking exercises

■ **Critical Thinking Exercise X** Applying Standards, Setting Priorities, and Clarifying Expected Outcomes

■ **Critical Thinking Exercise XI** Determining Interventions and Making Sure the Plan Is Adequately Recorded

expected learning outcomes

After studying this chapter, you should be able to:

- Describe the four main purposes of the plan of care.
- Explain how the memory-jog EASE helps you remember the four main care plan components.
- Explain the difference between initial and ongoing *Planning*.
- Name five things that influence priority ratings.
- Decide how to set priorities the next time you're in the clinical setting.
- Give four reasons why specific, measurable outcomes are the key to effective planning.
- Address the relationship of outcomes to accountability.
- Make decisions about taking accountability
- Explain the importance of considering clinical, functional, and quality-of-life outcomes.
- Discuss how to use standard plans (eg, critical paths, guidelines, electronic plans).
- Explain the role of case management in planning efficient, cost-effective care.
- Discuss how to weigh risks and benefits when determining nursing interventions.
- Develop and record a comprehensive plan of care.
- Evaluate patient records to determine if the plan of care is adequately documented.

(continued on next page)

Thinking Critically During *Planning*

We examined what it takes to think critically during *Assessment* and *Diagnosis*. Let's go on to explore the thinking you need to do during *Planning*—the step where you develop and record the plan of care. Keep in mind that having a recorded plan that's focused, clear, and up-to-date makes the difference between care that's safe and effective and care that's haphazard—even dangerous. Whether you're developing your own plans or using standard plans, this chapter helps you learn how to ensure that your patients' plans meet today's standards and keep them safe.

Four Main Purposes of the Plan of Care

The recorded plan of care serves the following purposes:

1. Directs care and documentation
2. Promotes communication among caregivers, thereby facilitating continuity of care.
3. Creates a record that can later be used for evaluation, research, and legal reasons.
4. Provides documentation of health care needs for Medicare, Medicaid, and other insurance reimbursement purposes.

To meet the above purposes, the plan of care must have the components listed in the following box.

> ### Major Care Plan Components
>
> The word **EASE** helps you remember the four main care plan components.
>
> **E** **E**xpected outcomes
> **A** **A**ctual and potential problems
> **S** **S**pecific interventions
> **E** **E**valuation/progress notes

Initial Versus Ongoing Planning

Remember the diagram from Chapter 1 that shows how *Planning* is a key part of *Implementation* (putting the plan into action):

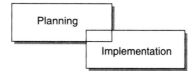

This chapter focuses on *initial planning*, helping you learn how to develop and record a plan of care that meets practice standards and communicates care management to all those involved in your patient's care. The next chapter addresses the *ongoing*, day-to-day planning you do during *Implementation*. As you read through this chapter, keep the following in mind.

> ### R U L E
> **The plan you record during this phase guides interventions performed during *Implementation*.** It's YOUR responsibility to make sure that the plan is:
>
> 1. Individualized to the patient, considering each patient's unique circumstances (eg, their age, health state, culture, values, capabilities, desires, and resources); and
> 2. Recorded according to facility policies and procedures (remember from Chapter 2 that promoting critical thinking requires recording information in a standard way).

> ### R U L E
> **Your ability to establish relationships and communicate well verbally and in writing makes the difference between competent, efficient care—and care that's sloppy, unprofessional, and prone to errors.**

The following shows the phases of *Planning* in context of developing an initial plan of care.

PLANNING

> ❑ Attending to Urgent Priorities
> ❑ Clarifying Expected Outcomes (Results)
> ❑ Deciding Which Problems Must Be Recorded
> ❑ Determining Individualized Nursing Interventions
> ❑ Making Sure the Plan is Adequately Recorded

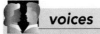 **voices**

Patients' Well-Being Depends on Communicating and Relating
Nursing is incredibly relational. . . . We're invited into the most intimate moments of the lives of people who minutes before were strangers . . . We cannot truly care for people without knowing them, without knowing their values, fears, beliefs, relationships, and plans for their lives. So each day we are thrust deep into relational work that touches our own humanity in ways we often cannot anticipate. . . . We need each other not just for support and understanding, but because the care requirements of patients are not limited to our shift or our day of assigned work. For us to do good work, to make a difference in the lives of our patients and their families, our work must be continuous, coordinated and well communicated—shift-to-shift and nurse-to-nurse.
—*Gladys Campbell, RN, MSN*[3]

Applying Standards

Before going on to address how to develop an initial plan, let's look at *applying standards*—something that applies to all the phases of *Planning*.

The standards you must apply are determined by:

❑ The law: Your state's nurse practice act outlines the scope of nursing practice. Your state board of nursing also outlines what you are and are not allowed to do.

❑ National practice standards, such as those of ANA or the Canadian Nurses Association.

❑ Specialty professional organizations, such as the Emergency Nurses Association and the Critical Care Nurses Association, which develop standards for specialty practice.

❑ The Joint Commission: This powerful accrediting body has developed detailed standards that must be followed to keep accreditation.

❑ The Agency for Healthcare Research and Quality (AHRQ): This organization develops, reviews, and updates clinical guidelines to aid health care providers to prevent, diagnose, and manage common clinical conditions.

❑ Your employer. Each place usually develops its own unique set of standards (standards of care, guidelines, policies, procedures, critical pathways, standard care plans, and so forth) that reflect how nursing care should be given in specific situations.

Clinical Decision Making

As you read through this chapter, remember that the ultimate goal of *Planning* is to make clinical decisions that are in your patients' best interest. Study the following map that helps you decide when you should make an independent plan and when you need to get help.

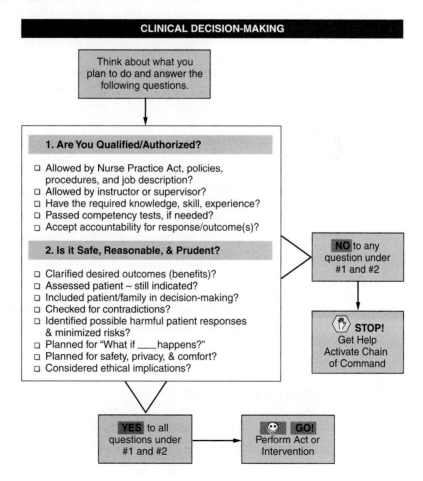

CLINICAL DECISION-MAKING

Think about what you plan to do and answer the following questions.

1. Are You Qualified/Authorized?

❑ Allowed by Nurse Practice Act, policies, procedures, and job description?
❑ Allowed by instructor or supervisor?
❑ Have the required knowledge, skill, experience?
❑ Passed competency tests, if needed?
❑ Accept accountability for response/outcome(s)?

2. Is it Safe, Reasonable, & Prudent?

❑ Clarified desired outcomes (benefits)?
❑ Assessed patient – still indicated?
❑ Included patient/family in decision-making?
❑ Checked for contradictions?
❑ Identified possible harmful patient responses & minimized risks?
❑ Planned for "What if ___ happens?"
❑ Planned for safety, privacy, & comfort?
❑ Considered ethical implications?

NO to any question under #1 and #2

STOP! Get Help Activate Chain of Command

YES to all questions under #1 and #2

GO! Perform Act or Intervention

Pain Management, Restraint Management, and Patient Safety Standards

As we continue to focus on evidence-based care, national standards for common patient problems such as pain management, restraint management, infection control, and patient safety are constantly refined and updated. These standards give focused, comprehensive approaches to preventing unnecessary patient suffering. They also help reduce costs. When you go to a new clinical setting, ask for policies and procedures related to things like pain management; use of restraints; and prevention of infection, falls, and errors. Be sure you incorporate these into the plan of care.

think about it

Be Sure Your Plan Shows Patient Involvement in Pain Management
Pain management significantly improves your patient's ability to do what he needs to do to heal. The American Pain Society's quality improvement initiatives and Joint Commission Standards stress that you must: (1) promise patients that pain management will be a key part of the plan; (2) determine a way to monitor pain, treat it promptly, and evaluate the response; and (3) make information about analgesics and nondrug interventions readily available for patients, families, and staff. For more information, go to www.thejointcommission.com, or www.ampainsoc.org—the Web site of the American Pain Society, which is a multidisciplinary educational and scientific organization dedicated to serving people in pain.

Standard and Electronic Plans

In many cases today, you'll have standard and computer plans to guide your care. These tools are helpful because they spot trends and jog your mind to think about key things you need to include in the plan. For example, if you enter the diagnosis of diabetes, the computer asks you to consider whether you need to send a consultation to the dietary department to have someone come and discuss nutritional needs with the patient. However, keep in mind the following rule.

RULE
Standard and electronic plans are guides that generally—but not always completely—apply to individual patient situations. YOU are responsible for discriminating about what does and doesn't apply, and for individualizing care accordingly.

Attending to Urgent Priorities

Some nurses will tell you *Planning* starts with *setting priorities*. Others will tell you it starts with *clarifying outcomes*. In a way, they're both right. To start, you do two things:

1. Determine urgent problems (eg, those requiring immediate attention) before taking the time to clarify outcomes.

2. After you handle urgent priorities, determine *overall* expected results—usually called discharge outcomes—so you know how to prioritize in context of the big picture of patient care.

For example, think about how your priorities might differ if you were planning care for patients with the two following discharge outcomes.

❑ Three days after surgery, the patient will be discharged home, able to demonstrate wound care.

❑ Three days after surgery, the patient will be discharged to a skilled nursing facility for wound care and medical management.

If your patient will manage his own wound care at home, you give teaching about wound care a high priority. But if your patient is being discharged to a skilled nursing facility, teaching about wound care is a lower priority—it may even be inappropriate, depending on patient capabilities.

You can see that identifying desired outcomes early in the planning phase is crucial to setting priorities. Before going on to the section on clarifying expected outcomes, study Box 4.1 (next page), which gives basic principles on setting priorities, Box 4.2 (page 149) which outlines critical thinking during *Planning,* and Box 4.3 (page 150), which lists critical thinking indicators (CTIs) related to *Planning.* Also take a few moments to think about where you stand in relation to each of the CTIs.

Clarifying Expected Outcomes (Results)

ANA standards stress the importance of identifying outcomes early in the nursing process.[1] In fact, some nurses consider *outcome identification* to be a "sixth step" in the nursing process. As with NCLEX, in this book, we address it as an integral part of *Planning.*

> **R U L E**
>
> **Early clarification of expected outcomes (the benefits expected to be seen in *each particular patient* after interventions are done) is the key to safety and efficiency.** If you don't know the expected outcome of interventions—and the evidence that supports that you're likely to achieve those outcomes—then you shouldn't be intervening at all, because you haven't *thought it through.*

Expected (desired) outcomes are descriptions of what the patient will be able to do by when. Outcome descriptions serve three main purposes:

1. Outcomes are the "measuring sticks" for the plan of care. You determine the success of the plan by finding out if the patient achieved the expected outcomes. For example, suppose you have the expected outcome of "*the patient will be discharged*

---

box 4.1 Attending to Urgent Priorities: Basic Principles

1. **Choose a method of assigning priorities and use it consistently.** For example, for identifying initial urgent priorities, some nurses use the **ABC** method (make sure the patient has no threats to his **A**irway, **B**reathing, or **C**irculation).
2. *Maslow's Hierarchy of Needs* is also a good model for setting priorities:
   - ❏ **Priority 1.** Physiologic needs—Life-threatening problems (or risk factors) posing a threat to physiologic needs (eg, problems with breathing, circulation, nutrition, hydration, elimination, temperature regulation, physical comfort)
   - ❏ **Priority 2.** Safety and security—Problems (or risk factors) posing a threat to safety and security (eg, environmental hazards, fear)
   - ❏ **Priority 3.** Love and belonging—Problems (or risk factors) posing a threat to feeling loved and a part of something (eg, isolation or loss of a loved one)
   - ❏ **Priority 4.** Self-esteem—Problems (or risk factors) posing a threat to self-esteem (eg, inability to perform normal activities)
   - ❏ **Priority 5.** Personal goals—Problems (or risk factors) posing a threat to the ability to achieve personal goals
3. **Problems usually present in a cluster—study the *relationships* among the problems to determine major priorities.** Assign high priority to problems that contribute to other problems. For example, if someone has chest pain and difficulty breathing, pain management is a high priority because pain causes increased stress and oxygen demand.

The following tips offer additional strategies for setting priorities:

- ❏ **Ask, "What problems need immediate attention and what could happen if I wait until later to attend to them?"** Take immediate appropriate action to initiate treatment as indicated (eg, notify the charge nurse and initiate actions to reduce the problem).
- ❏ **Identify problems with simple solutions and initiate actions to solve them** (eg, correcting someone's position to improve breathing, calling a friend or family member to come in). Sometimes, simple actions have a big impact on physiologic and psychological status.
- ❏ **Develop an initial problem list, identifying actual and potential problems, and their causes, if known.** This method gives you a visual record you can reflect on to check whether you're missing anything and also to think about whether one problem might be contributing to another.

---

able to change his own dressing by the third day after surgery." On the third day after surgery, is he able to do this?

2. **Outcomes direct interventions.** For example, in the above case, you need to make sure that the patient gets the teaching and practice needed to do dressing changes.
3. **Outcomes are motivating factors.** Having a deadline for getting things done gets everyone working toward the same deadline.

Outcomes Versus Indicators

Although the terms *outcomes* and *indicators* are sometimes used interchangeably, these two terms are slightly different: Indicators are the *specific, measurable data that indicate that an outcome has been achieved.* To better understand this definition, study the examples in the box at the bottom of page 150.

box 4.2 Critical Thinking During *Planning:* Ten Key Questions

1. **What major outcomes (observable beneficial results) do we expect to see in this particular person, family, or group when the plan of care is terminated?** Example: Three days after surgery, the person will be discharged, free from signs of infection, able to care for him- or herself.

2. **What problems, risks, or issues must be addressed to achieve the major outcomes?** Answering this question will help you set priorities. Study your problem list and narrow down to those that *must* be addressed.

3. **What are the circumstances (what is the context)?** Consider things like who's involved (eg, child, adult, group), whether the problems are acute or chronic, what factors are influencing the problems (eg, when, where, and how the problems developed), and the patient's values, beliefs, and culture.

4. **What knowledge is required?** All the Knowledge CTIs listed in Chapter 1 (page 34) are required. You must also be clearly aware of the circumstances, as addressed in number 3 above.

5. **How much room is there for error?** For example: In which of the following cases do you think you have more room for error?
   ❏ You're trying to decide whether to give a healthy child a one-time dose of acetaminophen for heat rash without checking with the doctor.
   ❏ You have a child who's been sick for 3 days with a fever and the mother wants to know if she should continue giving acetaminophen without checking with the doctor.
   If you thought the first one above, you're right. In the second case, the symptoms have continued for 3 days without a diagnosis. If you make the mistake of continuing to give acetaminophen without checking with a physician, you might be masking symptoms of a problem requiring medical management.

6. **How much time do I/we have?** Be realistic about the amount of time you have with the patient. Accomplish what you can and consider referrals for follow-up care.

7. **What resources can help?** Human resources include clinical nurse educators, nursing faculty, preceptors, more experienced nurses, advance practice nurses, peers, librarians, and other health care professionals (pharmacists, nutritionists, physical therapists, physicians). The patient and family are also valuable resources (they know themselves best). Information resources include texts, articles, computer data bases and decision-support software; national practice guidelines; facility documents (eg, guidelines, policies, procedures, assessment forms). Also consider financial resources, such as free community programs and services.

8. **What perspectives must be considered?** The most significant perspective to consider is that of the patient. Other important perspectives include those of key stakeholders (eg, significant others, caregivers), relevant third parties (eg, insurers), plus standards that apply to the patient's problems.

9. **What's influencing thinking?** Recognize personal values and beliefs, as well as biases and motivations of key stakeholders (eg, families, insurance companies).

10. **What must we do to prevent, manage, or eliminate the problems, issues, and risks identified in #2 above?** Identify specific interventions aimed at achieving the outcomes; managing the problems, issues, and risks; and promoting function, independence, and well-being.

box 4.3 Major Critical Thinking Indicators (CTIs) Related to Intellectual Skills Required for *Planning*

Nursing Process and Decision-Making Skills:

- ❏ Applies standards and principles when planning, giving, and adapting care
- ❏ Considers multiple explanations and solutions
- ❏ Determines individualized outcomes; focuses on results
- ❏ Manages risks, predicts complications, promotes health, function, and well-being; anticipates consequences and implications—plans ahead accordingly
- ❏ Sets priorities and makes decisions in a timely way; includes key stakeholders in making decisions
- ❏ Weighs risks and benefits; individualizes interventions
- ❏ Communicates effectively orally and in writing
- ❏ Identifies ethical issues and takes appropriate action
- ❏ Identifies and uses technologic, information, and human resources

Other Related Skills:

- ❏ Facilitates teamwork (focuses on common goals; helps and encourages others to contribute in their own way)
- ❏ Delegates appropriately; leads, inspires, and motivates others
- ❏ Demonstrates systems thinking (shows awareness of the interrelationships existing within and across health care systems)
- ❏ Establishes empowered partnerships with patients, families, peers, and coworkers
- ❏ Teaches patients, self, and others
- ❏ Organizes and manages time and environment
- ❏ Addresses conflicts fairly; fosters positive interpersonal relationships
- ❏ Facilitates and navigates change

Note: The knowledge CTIs listed on page 34 also apply.

Source: *Critical Thinking Indicators (2008 Evidence-Based Version).* © 2008 R. Alfaro-LeFevre. All rights reserved. Do not copy without written permission. Available: www.AlfaroTeachSmart.com

Example Outcomes	*Corresponding Indicators*
After 2 days, with the help of printed drug information, the person will demonstrate knowledge of medication regimen.	■ Gives all drug names, actions, doses, administration route, and side effects ■ Explains how and when drugs are to be taken, including whether to take them on an empty or full stomach, and what to do if dose is missed ■ Demonstrates special administration techniques (eg, injection technique, if applicable) ■ Lists reportable signs and symptoms
Maintains intact skin	■ Skin shows no signs of discoloration or irritation ■ Control of risk factors recorded on chart per protocol (eg, patient has adequate nutrition and hydration, repositioned hourly, skin care every 8 hours)

> **R U L E**
>
> **The terms goals, objectives, outcomes, and indicators often are used inter-changeably—but they are different.** *Goals* and *objectives* refer to *intent* (eg, "Our goal is to teach this person about diabetes."). *Outcomes* and *indicators* refer to specific *results* (eg, "How will we know if this person actually *learned* what he needs to know about diabetes?").

Principles of Patient-Centered Outcomes

To pass NCLEX and succeed in the clinical setting, be sure that you're familiar with the following principles of patient-centered outcomes.

1. **Outcomes describe the *specific benefits* you expect to see in the patient after care has been given.** In some cases, for example, with a newborn, outcomes may describe what you expect to see in a caregiver (eg, "Father will safely bathe the newborn.").
   - **Short-term outcomes** describe *early expected benefits* of nursing interventions (eg, "Will be able to walk to the bathroom unassisted by tomorrow.").
   - **Long-term outcomes** describe the benefits expected to be seen *at a certain point in time after the plan has been implemented* (eg, "Will be able to walk independently to the end of the hall three times a day within 10 days after surgery.").
2. **Outcomes may relate to *problems* or *interventions*.**
   - **Outcomes for problems** state what you expect to observe in the patient when the problems are resolved or controlled (eg, "The patient will have no signs or symptoms of infection.").
   - **Outcomes for interventions** state the benefit you expect to observe in the patient after an intervention is performed (eg, if you suction someone's tracheostomy, you expect that breath sounds will be clearer after suctioning). If you can't clearly identify the benefits you expect to see in the patient after nursing care, then you shouldn't be intervening.

   The next page gives a diagram for how to determine outcomes.
3. **To create very specific outcomes, include the following components.**

Five Components of Outcome Statements

Subject: Who is the person expected to achieve the outcome (eg, patient or parent)?
Verb: What actions must the person take to achieve the outcome?
Condition: Under what circumstances is the person to perform the actions?
Performance criteria: How well is the person to perform the actions?
Target time: By when is the person expected to be able to perform the actions?
Example: "Parents will bathe newborn in room independently by 5/8."

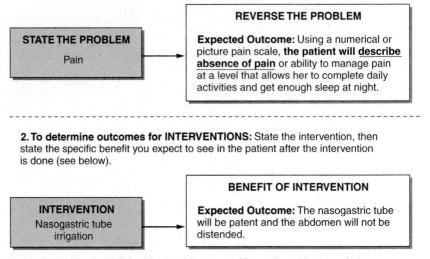

HOW TO DETERMINE OUTCOMES FOR PROBLEMS AND INTERVENTIONS

1. To determine expected outcomes for PROBLEMS: State the problem, then reverse the problem to show the specific desired improvement (see blelow).

STATE THE PROBLEM

Pain

REVERSE THE PROBLEM

Expected Outcome: Using a numerical or picture pain scale, **the patient will describe absence of pain** or ability to manage pain at a level that allows her to complete daily activities and get enough sleep at night.

2. To determine outcomes for INTERVENTIONS: State the intervention, then state the specific benefit you expect to see in the patient after the intervention is done (see below).

INTERVENTION
Nasogastric tube irrigation

BENEFIT OF INTERVENTION

Expected Outcome: The nasogastric tube will be patent and the abdomen will not be distended.

Source: Clinical Cards © 2008. AlfaroTeachSmart.com. No copying without permission.

4. **Use measurable verbs** (verbs that describe things you can see, feel, smell, or hear). For example, suppose you write an outcome for a woman that says, "Will understand how to use sterile technique." The word *understand* is vague and therefore not measurable. Ask yourself, How can we really know if she understands? The only way you can really know how well she understands is if she actually verbalizes or demonstrates sterile technique. The following are examples.

- **Measurable verbs (Use verbs like these to be specific.)**

identify	list	walk
describe	hold	cough
state	exercise	share
verbalize	perform	will lose
demonstrate	express	will gain
communicate	relate	has an absence of

- **Non-measurable verbs (Do not use.)**

know	understand	accept
think	appreciate	feel

5. **Consider affective, cognitive, and psychomotor outcomes, as described in the following bullets.**
   - **Affective domain:** Outcomes associated with changes in attitudes, feelings, or values (eg, deciding eating habits need to be changed).

- **Cognitive domain:** Outcomes dealing with acquired knowledge or intellectual skills (eg, learning the signs and symptoms of diabetic shock).
- **Psychomotor domain:** Outcomes dealing with developing motor skills (eg, mastering how to walk with crutches).

table **4.1** Examples of Verbs Representing the Three Domains

Cognitive	Affective	Psychomotor
Teach	Express	Demonstrate
Discuss	Share	Practice
Identify	Listen	Perform
Describe	Communicate	Walk
List	Relate	Administer
Explore		Give

Table 4.1 gives examples of verbs commonly used in affective, cognitive, and psychomotor outcomes. The following guidelines help you clarify expected outcomes.

Guidelines: Determining Patient-Centered Outcomes

❑ **Be realistic and consider:**

  ❑ Patient's health state, overall prognosis
  ❑ Expected length of stay
  ❑ Growth and development
  ❑ Patient values and cultural considerations
  ❑ Other planned therapies for the patient
  ❑ Available human, material, and financial resources
  ❑ Risks, benefits, and current scientific evidence
  ❑ Changes in status that indicate you need to modify usual expected outcomes

❑ **Partner with patients and families, determining outcomes together and involving other key members of the health care team.** If the outcomes are predetermined by standard plans, inform those involved what the outcomes are and seek agreement that the outcomes are attainable.

❑ **In complex cases, develop both short- and long-term outcomes.** Use short-term outcomes as stepping stones to the long-term outcomes.

❑ **Be sure the outcomes and indicators are measurable: that they describe something you can hear, see, feel, or smell in the person to demonstrate that the outcomes are achieved.** Use measurable, observable verbs (page 152).

❏ **Apply the principles of patient-centered outcomes as outlined on page 151.**

❏ **Identify only one behavior per indicator.** If you need to write two behaviors, write two indicators, so that you can evaluate each one separately.

E x a m p l e

Wrong: By 12/15, explains the role of insulin in carbohydrate metabolism and gives himself insulin.

Right: By 12/15, explains the role of insulin in carbohydrate metabolism.
By 12/15, administers own insulin.

❏ **Sometimes outcomes and indicators already will be developed for your patient's problems in standard plans.** Carefully compare your patient's actual situation with the standard plans and decide whether the indicators are appropriate to your patient's particular situation.

Relationship of Outcomes to Accountability

Determining outcomes helps you decide accountability for resolving problems. Study the following diagram, which shows the decision-making process after you identify expected outcomes.

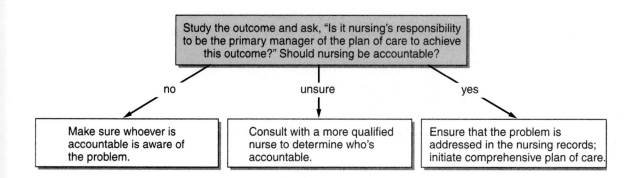

Study the outcome and ask, "Is it nursing's responsibility to be the primary manager of the plan of care to achieve this outcome?" Should nursing be accountable?

no → Make sure whoever is accountable is aware of the problem.

unsure → Consult with a more qualified nurse to determine who's accountable.

yes → Ensure that the problem is addressed in the nursing records; initiate comprehensive plan of care.

Clinical, Functional, and Quality-of-Life Outcomes

Because nurses focus holistically on the patient, it's your role to consider clinical, functional, and quality-of-life outcomes, as explained here.

Clinical outcomes describe the expected status of medical, nursing, or multidisciplinary problems at certain points in time, after treatment has been given. They address whether the problems are resolved or to what degree they are improved.

Examples:

❑ Chest tube out 3rd postoperative day
❑ Lungs clear, absence of signs of infection 2 days after admission
❑ Able to demonstrate wound care 3 days after surgery

Functional outcomes describe the person's ability to function in relation to desired usual activities.

Examples:

❑ Four days after total knee replacement, Mr. Palmer will be discharged to a rehabilitation facility able to perform straight-leg raises and range-of-motion exercises twice daily.
❑ Six months after total knee replacement, Mr. Palmer will return to his job as a police officer, able to perform usual job description as a policeman (able to walk two to three flights of stairs, participate in a chase on foot, and so forth).

Quality-of-life outcomes focus on key factors that affect someone's ability to enjoy life and achieve personal goals. Some examples are:

❑ Relates that pain is tolerable during key activities and sleep.
❑ Absence of depression
❑ States that usual sleep patterns are back to normal
❑ Able to perform work and leisure activities

With some health problems, we have very specific indicators that have been developed for problems that measure whether the patient's life is being positively impacted by care. For example, pediatric asthma indicators include decreased emergency-room visits and improved attendance at school.

Discharge Outcomes and Discharge Planning

Identifying discharge outcomes and starting discharge planning early are the hallmarks of efficiency. Today, the best discharge planning begins with outpatient education before admission and follows the patient throughout the continuum of care, including after discharge.[2]

Discharge outcomes are written in broad terms, describing the level of assistance the person is likely to need at home (eg, "Will be discharged home with care managed by wife and biweekly visits by home care nurse"). These statements may be followed by the indicators that describe the expected status of patient problems upon discharge (eg, "Abdominal drains out," "Demonstrates wound care," and so forth). Box 4.4 (next page) shows an discharge planning questionnaire that helps you begin discharge planning early. The next page also shows a pathway for home care that's discussed with patients before they're admitted for heart surgery. You can see how this pathway helps patients to know what to expect when they leave the hospital.

box 4.4 Discharge Planning Questionnaire

1. Is there a problem at home with any of the following?
   - ❏ Heat   Yes   No   Possibly
   - ❏ Hot/cold water   Yes   No   Possibly
   - ❏ Electricity   Yes   No   Possibly
   - ❏ Refrigeration   Yes   No   Possibly
   - ❏ Cooking   Yes   No   Possibly
   - ❏ Bathroom facilities   Yes   No   Possibly
   - ❏ Stairs   Yes   No   Possibly
   - ❏ Wheelchair accessibility   Yes   No   Possibly
2. Is necessary transportation available?   Yes   No   Possibly
3. How can the patient be reached by phone?
4. Will the person require:
   - ❏ Assistance with activities of daily living   Yes   No   Possibly
   - ❏ Assistance with medications   Yes   No   Possibly
   - ❏ Assistance with treatments   Yes   No   Possibly
   - ❏ Additional teaching   Yes   No   Possibly
   - ❏ Ongoing nursing assessment   Yes   No   Possibly
   - ❏ Community resources or referrals   Yes   No   Possibly
5. List available support systems (eg, family, neighbors willing to help).

'AT HOME' PATH TO RECOVERY FROM CARDIAC SURGERY: THINGS TO DO EACH DAY

Activity	*Health*	*Medications*	*Self-Care*	*Reasons to Call for More Information*
❏ Walk four times/day	Do each of the following items around the same time each day:	❏ Take your medications as prescribed	❏ Keep your feet up while at rest	The nursing station phone number is (910) 716-6658.
	❏ Check your incisions			
	❏ Take your temperature by mouth (call if over 100°F)		❏ Shower/bathe as instructed	*Call your doctor if:* ❏ your heart rate (pulse) is less than 60 beats/minute or greater than 120 at rest, or
❏ Do exercises as prescribed			❏ Practice reading food labels for fat intake, cholesterol, and sodium levels	❏ you have severe chills, or
❏ Rest				❏ unusual shortness of breath, or
❏ Limit visitors the first week or so (three to four people for 30 minutes/day)	❏ Check your pulse for one minute (normal: 60 to 120 beats/minute)	❏ Drink several glasses of water each day	❏ Eat healthy! Try new recipes	❏ fever greater than 100°F (by mouth), or ❏ weight gain over 2 lb. in one day or 5 lb. in one week, or
❏ Resume sexual activities when ready				❏ red or draining incisions, or
				❏ chest pain, or
❏ After two weeks, help with light housework	❏ Weigh yourself (call if you gain over 2 lb. in one day)		❏ Wear stockings if ordered	❏ if you have *any* questions or concerns

Source: Adapted from path developed by *The North Carolina Baptist Hospitals*, Winston-Salem, NC.

Case Management

Case management—a method of care delivery that aims to improve outcomes and reduce costs through optimum use of resources—is an essential piece of *Planning.* Today, nurses in hospitals and communities are expected to recognize early when patients demonstrate problems that might require additional resources to achieve outcomes in a timely way. For example, suppose your patient is paraplegic who is having a routine cholecystectomy. This person is likely to have additional needs that an able-bodied person would not have. Early in the planning phase, ask, "Does this person have unusual or multiple health problems or disabilities?" If so, consider whether you should be asking your manager about getting additional resources, such as a case manager involved in the plan of care.

Deciding Which Problems Must Be Recorded

Deciding which problems must be recorded is influenced by your understanding of:

❑ The person's overall health status and expected discharge outcomes.
❑ The expected length of contact with the patient (you have to be realistic about what problems can (and must) be tackled within the allotted time).
❑ The patient's perception of priorities. If the patient doesn't agree with your priorities, it's unlikely the plan will succeed.
❑ Whether there are standard plans that apply. For example, are there critical pathways, guidelines, protocols, procedures, or standard plans that address daily priorities for this particular patient's situation?

RULE

Always follow policies and procedures for recording the plan of care—these are designed to keep patients safe and to protect you from legal liability. Patient records must communicate nurses' awareness of, and response to, all major care priorities. Some problems may not need to be recorded on the care plan because they are addressed in other parts of the record (eg, Foley catheter care usually is addressed in policy and procedure manuals).

There are three main steps to determining which problems must be recorded.

1. Make a list of your patient's problems.
2. Decide which problems must be managed in order to achieve the *overall outcomes* of care.
3. Determine what documentation will guide how each problem will be managed (eg, Doctor or APN orders? Following protocols? Critical pathway? Nurse-developed individualized plan? Patient self-manages?)

box 4.5 Example Multidisciplinary Problem List		
Problem	**Onset**	**Status**
Diabetes	2/05	See insulin and BS flow sheet. Gives own insulin.
Anxiety/Coping	2/05	Sees APN for counseling once a week
Right knee replacement	4/05	Ambulatory, PT twice a week
Arthritis	1995	Managed well (no meds)
Hypertension	1992	Stable—see med sheet
Asthma	1995	Stable—see current inhalers
Laminectomy	1996	Symptom free

To communicate all major problems to the entire health care team, make sure that an up-to-date problem list with a summary of past and current problems is in a prominent place on the patient record. For example, notice how the problem list in Box 4.5 above gives you a picture of the status of all the patient's problems.

RULE

Be sure that any problems, diagnoses, or risk factors that may impede progress toward outcome achievement are addressed somewhere on the patient record. Doing this may require you to add a standard plan, modify a standard plan, or develop an individualized plan of your own.

think about it

Asking Negative Questions Helps Set Priorities
When making decisions about what to record on the plan, ask yourself negative questions. Negative questions begin with, *What could happen if I **don't** . . . * For example, *What could happen to this person if I **don't** address this problem on the plan of care?* or *What could happen if I **don't** report this problem?* Asking yourself these types of questions helps you focus on what's most important. If the answer is *Not much can happen,* you know the problem has a low priority. If the answer causes you concern, then you know the problem has a high priority.

CRITICAL THINKING EXERCISE X

Applying Standards, Setting Priorities, and Clarifying Expected Outcomes

To complete this session, read pages 144–158. Example responses can be found on pages 243–244.

Part I. Applying Standards and Setting Priorities

1. Give at least three types of standards that apply to your nursing practice.
2. What are the four main purposes of the plan of care?

3. Using the memory-jog EASE, name the four components of a plan of care, giving an example of each.
4. List five factors that may influence how you set priorities.
5. If you had someone with the following problems, which problem would you need to treat immediately and why?
   a. Diarrhea
   b. Severe dyspnea
   c. Risk for Fluid Volume Deficit
6. What is the relationship between *identifying expected discharge* outcomes and *setting priorities?*

Part II. Clarifying Expected Outcomes

1. What are the three main purposes of outcomes?
2. What four words are sometimes used interchangeably and usually mean the desired result of interventions?
3. Of the four terms you listed in number 2, which two terms are considered to be most specific?
4. **a.** If you identify an outcome and decide it's *not* within nursing's responsibility to manage the problems to achieve the outcomes, what must you do?
   b. What must you do if it *is* within nursing's responsibility?
5. What are your responsibilities during planning in relation to case management? (Three sentences or less)

Part III. Developing Outcome Statements

1. Why is it important to use measurable verbs when identifying outcomes? Give three examples of measurable verbs.
2. What are the five components of outcome statements?
3. Determine which of the following outcomes are written *correctly*. Identify what's wrong with the statements that are written *incorrectly*.
   a. Knows the four basic food groups by 1/4.
   b. Demonstrates how to use the walker unassisted by Saturday.
   c. Improves appetite by 11/5.
   d. Lists the equipment needed to change sterile dressings by 9/5.
   e. Walks independently in the hall the day after surgery.
   f. Understands the importance of maintaining a salt-free diet.
   g. Ambulates to the bathroom using her cane by 3/4.
   h. Loses 5 lb by 1/9.
   i. Feels less pain by Thursday.
4. For each diagnosis/problem, write an appropriate outcome:
   a. Impaired Oral Mucous Membrane related to poor oral hygiene
   b. Risk for Impaired Skin Integrity related to constant diarrhea
   c. Impaired Verbal Communication related to inability to speak English

(critical thinking continues on page 160)

Part IV. Practice Recognizing Affective, Cognitive, and Psychomotor Outcomes

Determine whether each of the following outcomes is in the affective, cognitive, or psychomotor domain. Use "a" for affective, "c" for cognitive, and "p" for psychomotor. (There may be more than one domain for each outcome.)

a. Demonstrates how to sterilize her baby's formula
b. Relates feelings concerning going home
c. Discusses the relationship between blood sugar levels and eating
d. Administers own insulin according to the results of morning blood sugar readings

Determining Nursing Interventions

Nursing interventions are actions performed by the nurse to:

1. Monitor health status and response to treatments
2. Reduce risks
3. Resolve, prevent, or manage problems
4. Help with activities of daily living (bathing and so forth)
5. Promote optimum sense of physical, psychological, and spiritual well-being
6. Give patients the information they need to make informed decisions and be independent.

Nursing interventions are classified into two categories:

❏ **Direct care interventions:** Actions performed through direct interaction with patients. Examples include helping someone out of bed and teaching someone about diabetes.
❏ **Indirect care interventions:** Actions performed away from the patient but on behalf of the patient. These actions are aimed at managing the health care environment and promoting interdisciplinary collaboration. Some examples include monitoring results of laboratory studies and contacting a social worker.

Considering both direct and indirect interventions helps account for nurses' time. If you focus only on what the nurse does directly with the patient, you miss a lot of nursing time that's spent on other crucial nursing activities.

Assessment—Monitoring Health Status and Responses to Care

When planning care, it's important to consider what assessments need to be done to monitor status. *Assessment* may be planned specifically to detect or evaluate problems or to monitor responses to interventions. In fact, *Assessment* is a part of every intervention. Your plan should reflect awareness of the need to assess the person at three key points:

1. **Before you act,** to be sure the action is safe and appropriate
2. **As you act,** to monitor for adverse reactions
3. **After you act,** to monitor the response

Teaching—Empowering Patients and Families

Teaching patients about their health and treatment plan, and motivating them to become involved in their own care, is the key to empowering them to become their own best advocate and caregiver. Teaching may be planned to enhance someone's knowledge about a specific problem (eg, teaching about diabetes) or as part of an intervention to explain why it's being done (eg, reinforcing the rationale for coughing and deep breathing as you're assisting the person to cough and breathe deeply). At every patient encounter, seize teaching opportunities. In complex situations, carefully plan what you're going to teach, and how you're going to teach it. Because teaching is a complex skill that includes paying attention to many different factors, the following guidelines are suggested to help you plan teaching.

Guidelines: Planning Teaching

❏ Assess readiness to learn and previous knowledge before developing a teaching plan.
❏ Ask about preferred learning styles (for example, a person who is a "reader" might want to read a pamphlet first, whereas someone who is a "doer" might want to handle equipment first). Adapt to the patient's preferred style rather than your own.
❏ Determine expected learning outcomes mutually with the patient, so that you both know what must be learned and mastered (eg, "How would you feel about learning how to give an injection by Thursday?").
❏ Plan an environment that's conducive to learning, without interruptions.
❏ Identify active learning experiences. Use examples, simulations, games, and audiovisuals.
❏ Use simple terms, and teach *basic concepts* before moving on to more complex material.
❏ Plan learning experiences to build on successes.
❏ Encourage asking questions and verbalizing understanding of what is being taught (eg, "I want you to feel free to ask questions no matter how insignificant you think they are. It's not easy learning something new. It is very important that you understand this.").
❏ Plan to pace learning. Don't give too much information at one time; progress at the person's learning pace.

❑ Allow time to discuss progress (eg, to ask the person how he feels he's progressing) and to summarize what has been taught.

❑ Find ways to include significant others in the teaching session. For people with English as a second language, get a translator and look for handouts in their language.

Download Patient Teaching Handouts (In English and Spanish) on Various Common Health Problems From
http://nursing.advanceweb.com/SpecialPages/NW/PatientHandouts.aspx (English) and http://nursing.advanceweb.com/Editorial/Content/editorial.aspx?CTIID=1497 (Spanish)

Counseling and Coaching: Helping People Make Informed Choices

Counseling and coaching people to help them make needed changes in their lives—or to help them make choices about their health care—is another important nursing intervention that may be part of the plan. Counseling and coaching often include teaching and reinforcing key points in the plan of care (eg, checking how diabetics are doing with following their diet and medication plan). Counseling and coaching also include exploring motivations and offering support during periods of adjustment to new circumstances. By using teaching and therapeutic communication techniques, you can offer valuable psychological and intellectual support, thereby reducing the stress associated with making choices about health care management. As you counsel people, apply ethics principles (pages 26–27) and promote autonomy. Point out to people that being informed is the key to being able to make good decisions, based on their own values and beliefs.

Consulting and Referring: Key to Multidisciplinary Care

Making appropriate consultations and referrals is the cornerstone for care delivery in multidisciplinary practice. For example, suppose you have someone who has trouble swallowing pills. You should be thinking, I wonder if the pharmacist might know a better way to give medications (eg, a liquid form). If someone isn't eating because she dislikes hospital food, think about referring this problem to the dietitian so different meals can be served. Be sure that you recognize when your patient's care would benefit by your consulting with other nurses and health care professionals.

Even when there is no need for formal consultations or referrals, with today's complex situations, you're likely to find yourself consulting with other experts on a regular basis.

Individualizing Interventions

The interventions you identify should aim to:

❏ Detect, prevent, and manage health problems and risks.
❏ Promote optimum function, independence, and sense of well-being.
❏ Achieve the desired outcomes safely and efficiently.

Determining individualized interventions requires you to answer following questions, in context of each particular patient situation:

1. What can be done to prevent or minimize the risks or causes of this problem?
2. What can be done to manage the problem?
3. How can I tailor interventions to include patient preferences and meet the expected outcomes?
4. How likely are we to get desired versus adverse responses to the interventions (and what can we do to reduce the risks and increase the likelihood of beneficial responses)?
5. What needs to be recorded about this intervention and how often should it be recorded?

Figure 4.1 maps the process of determining interventions for a patient with a nursing diagnosis and a potential complication. Page 164 gives a worksheet to guide you when identifying specific interventions.

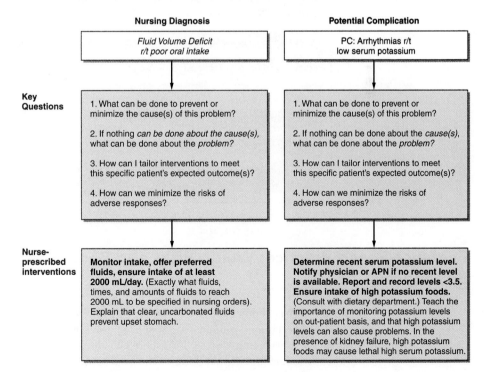

FIGURE 4.1 Example of how to determine nursing interventions.

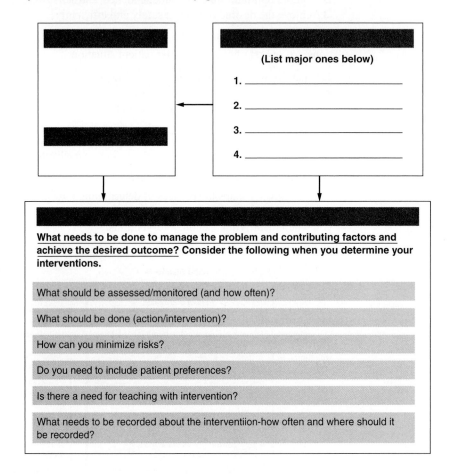

HOW TO DETERMINE SPECIFIC INTERVENTIONS

INSTRUCTIONS: Make sure interventions are *specific* to each situation by remembering <u>PCO</u> (<u>P</u>roblem, <u>C</u>ontributing factors, and <u>O</u>utcome). What needs to be done about the problem and contributing factors? How can you best achieve the outcome? Complete the boxes below. Use back of page as needed.

(List major ones below)

1. _____
2. _____
3. _____
4. _____

<u>What needs to be done to manage the problem and contributing factors and achieve the desired outcome?</u> Consider the following when you determine your interventions.

What should be assessed/monitored (and how often)?

What should be done (action/intervention)?

How can you minimize risks?

Do you need to include patient preferences?

Is there a need for teaching with intervention?

What needs to be recorded about the interventiion-how often and where should it be recorded?

Evidence-Based Practice: Weigh Risks and Benefits— Be Proactive

Evidence-based practice requires you to be aware of research that supports the use of the interventions you identify: If you're asked the question, "How do you know that this intervention works?" you should be able to answer by saying something like, "The textbook says it does," "This is according to our protocols and procedures here in the hospital," or "This is recommended by national clinical practice guidelines." The point is that you should know the strength of the evidence that supports your interventions.

Before you choose an intervention, weigh the risks of causing *harm* against the probability of getting the *desired results.* To do this, ask the following questions:

1. How reliable is the evidence that supports that the intervention(s) I plan to use is likely to work?
2. How likely are we to see the desired response in this particular patient and situation?
3. What is the worst thing that can happen if this intervention is performed, and how likely is it to happen?
4. What measures can we take to minimize the chances of causing harm?
5. What could happen if we do nothing about this problem or these risk factors?

Looking for Evidence-Based Care for the Elderly?

Visit ConsultGeriRN.org, the web site of The Hartford Institute for Geriatric Nursing, where you can find online resource for nurses in clinical and educational settings.

Guidelines: Individualizing Nursing Orders

The following guidelines help you individualize your nursing orders.

❏ **Assess the person to determine a baseline** of current signs, symptoms, and risk factors of the problem.
❏ **Check for medical orders** (eg, medications, diet, activity, diagnostic studies, and so forth).
❏ **If you use standard plans (eg, critical path, protocol, preprinted or electronic plan), remember that you're responsible for:**
  • Detecting changes in patient status that may contraindicate using the plan.
  • Using good judgment about which parts of the plans apply and which do not.
  • Recognizing when problems aren't covered by the plan and finding other ways to address them (for example, some facilities have an additional page that can be placed on the record to address "out-of-the-box" situations).
  • Adding unique patient requirements (eg, walker) in appropriate places.

R U L E

To protect patients from errors and yourself from legal problems, use standard and electronic plans with a critical mind. Compare your patient's circumstances with the standard or electronic plan. Decide what applies, what doesn't, and what's missing. Then modify (add, delete, or modify) interventions as indicated.

❏ **Decide monitoring regimens for potential complications:** What focus assessments need to be done to monitor the status of signs and symptoms? How often do assessments need to be recorded to spot trends?

❏ **Identify interventions that prevent or minimize the underlying causes or risk factors of the problem and help achieve the expected outcome.** For example, if you have "risk for injury related to chronic muscle weakness" with an outcome of "demonstrates safe ambulation with the use of a walker," tailor interventions to reflect that the person will be using a walker (eg, have the person practice using the walker for ambulation in various circumstances, like going up and down stairs and going to the bathroom).

❏ **If you can't do anything about the causes or risk factors, decide what can be done about the problem.** For example, if someone is terminally ill and has anxiety, you can't do anything about the fact that the person is going to die, but you can do something about the anxiety through counseling and therapeutic communication.

❏ **Be sure the interventions are congruent with other therapies (eg, allowing rest after physical therapy).**

❏ **Consider the person's preferences.** Get input from the patient about how and when the interventions are performed. Individualize as much as possible.

❏ **Determine the scientific rationale** (evidence) for planned actions.

❏ **Create opportunities for teaching** (eg, explain rationale for all actions).

❏ **Consult with other professionals when indicated** (physician, APN, physical therapist).

❏ **Before prescribing any actions:**

1. Weigh the risks and benefits of performing the actions.
2. Decide whether you're willing to be accountable for the responses to the interventions you delegate (see Boxes 5.1 and 5.2 on page 189).
3. Make your orders specific: Keep in mind "see, do, teach, record" (ie, what to assess [see], what to do, what to teach, and what to record). For example, suppose you're caring for someone who's had abdominal surgery and you identify Risk for Ineffective Airway Clearance related to chronic smoking and incision pain. Your orders might look like this:
   • Assess breath sounds every 4 hours.
   • Help the person to perform coughing and breathing exercises with pillow and hand over incision every 4 hours.
   • Reinforce the importance of coughing and deep breathing.
   • Record breath sounds and sputum production once a shift and as needed.
   • Encourage the person to use current illness as a way to begin quitting smoking.

The following box summarizes what to include in your nursing orders.

What to Include in Your Nursing Orders

Date: The date you write the order.
Verb: Action to be performed.
Subject: Who is to do it.
Descriptive phrase: How, when, where, how often, how long, or how much?
Signature: Be consistent in how you sign.
Example: (Today's date) Assist patient to stand by the side of the bed for 10 minutes twice a day wearing her back brace. R. Alfaro-LeFevre, RN.

Making Sure the Plan Is Adequately Recorded

The final phase of *Planning* is making sure that the plan is adequately recorded: You must be sure that all problems and risks that must be managed in order to achieve the overall outcomes of care are recorded somewhere in the patient record.

Forms for—and methods of—recording the plan of care are tailor-made to meet the needs of the nurses and patients in each unique setting. As you go from working in one place to another, remember the following rule.

R U L E

You are accountable for making sure your patient's plan meets each facility's specific standards. Be certain that somewhere on the patient record, people can find evidence of the four required components of the plan of care as addressed by the memory-jog **EASE** (page 143).

Box 4.6 gives key points to evaluate the plan of care to decide how it "measures up" compared with current standards.

---

box 4.6 Checklist to Evaluate the Plan of Care

1. Was the plan developed with the patient (and, if appropriate, significant others and other involved health care providers)?
2. Have you addressed:
   ❏ Actual and potential problems that must be managed to achieve the overall outcomes in a safe and timely way?
   ❏ Problems that require individualized, not routine, nursing interventions?
3. If you identified problems that aren't on the plan of care, have you made sure that they are addressed somewhere in the patient's record (eg, chest tube management might be addressed by physician's orders)?
4. Are the outcomes:
   ❏ Derived from the diagnoses or problems?
   ❏ Measurable?
   ❏ Mutually formulated with the patient and other key players?
   ❏ Realistic and attainable?
   ❏ Written according to the rules (patient-centered; measurable verbs; clear about who, what, when, how, and where)?
5. Do the nursing orders:
   ❏ Include interventions that focus on controlling the *underlying cause* or risk factors of the problem (or, if that's not possible, treating the *problem*)?
   ❏ Clearly direct interventions (addressing who, what, when, how, and how much)?
   ❏ Incorporate use of resources and strengths?
   ❏ Show the signature of the prescriber?
6. Does the plan:
   ❏ Reflect current policies and practice standards?
   ❏ Apply research and scientific principles?
   ❏ Address developmental, psychosocial, spiritual, cultural, and biologic needs?
   ❏ Include interventions for health promotion and teaching?
   ❏ Provide for continuity (eg, is it easily accessible, clear, and concise)?
   ❏ Aim to reduce costs while promoting convenience and comfort?

Multidisciplinary Plans

With multidisciplinary plans, all disciplines (nursing, medicine, dietary, and so forth) work from the same plan. Multidisciplinary approaches bring "the best of all worlds" together. Keep in mind, however, that as the nurse, you're the one at bedside the most. It's your job to stay focused on human responses—how the person is likely to respond as a whole to the plan—and to see that your patients' individual needs and desires are considered in the plan.

Box 4.7 gives an example of a multidisciplinary plan showing a problem list and SOAP charting (a charting method that addresses subjective data, objective data, analysis, and plan of care). Pages 171–176 show examples of various plans of care (Figures 4.2 to 4.4). Remember that student plans are usually longer, more theoretical, and very comprehensive, because they're used to assess students' knowledge of various theories and all details of the nursing process.

---

box 4.7 Multidisciplinary Record and SOAP Charting

Description: Example of a multidisciplinary record, with all disciplines charting on the same record, creating an interdisciplinary problem list (see I below) and sample of SOAP charting (see II below).

I. Example problem list

Date of Diagnosis	Problem	Date Resolved
1/5	**1.** *Cerebrovascular accident* (identified by physician)	
	2. *Risk for Impaired Skin Integrity related to immobility* (identified by nursing)	
	3. *Unsteady gait* (identified by physical therapist)	
1/7	**4.** *Body Image Disturbance* (identified by nursing)	
1/8	**5.** *Urinary tract infection* (identified by physician)	1/13

II. Example SOAP charting*

S: Subjective Data	"I can't feel anything on the right side."
O: Objective Data	Absent reflexes on the right side. Slouched in bed, leaning toward right. Has reddened area about 5 cm on the right hip
A: Analysis	*Risk for Impaired Skin Integrity related to right-side loss of sensation and immobility*
P: Plan	Prevent skin breakdown. Monitor back and hips for signs of decreased circulation from pressure point every 2 hours. Reposition side, back, side every 2 hours. Place air mattress and sheepskin on bed.

*After initial planning, some facilities add I (implementation) and E (evaluation), making the acronym SOAPIE.

CRITICAL THINKING EXERCISE XI

Determining Interventions and Making Sure the Plan Is Adequately Recorded

To complete this session, read pages 160–168. Example responses can be found on pages 244–245.

Part I. Determining Interventions

1. What's the point of classifying interventions into direct and indirect interventions? (Three sentences or less.)
2. How do the words "see, do, teach, record" help you remember what you need to consider when determining interventions?
3. After you identify a problem, what two questions do you need to ask to determine interventions?
4. Explain how to weigh risks and benefits. (Five sentences or less.)

Part II. Practice Individualizing Interventions Based on Problems and Outcomes

For each problem and outcome listed here, list some appropriate nursing interventions that might achieve the outcome.

1. Risk for Impaired Skin Integrity related to prescribed bed rest and loss of sensation in lower extremities
   Outcome: Maintains intact skin
   Indicators: Absence of redness or irritation; management of risk factors recorded daily on skin protocol
   List appropriate nursing interventions:
2. Risk for Ineffective Airway Clearance related to thoracic, incision pain
   Outcome: Demonstrates effective airway clearance
   Indicators: Coughs effectively every 3 hours; lungs clear
   List appropriate nursing interventions:
3. Constipation related to insufficient exercise and inadequate fluid and roughage intake as evidenced by no bowel movement in 4 days
   Outcome: Reports or demonstrates no constipation
   Indicators: Daily soft bowel movements; exercises 20 minutes every day; drinks minimum of 2000 milliliters daily; demonstrates adequate roughage intake
   List appropriate nursing interventions:

Part III. Monitoring to Detect Potential Complications

For each of the following problems, identify potential complications and determine a plan to monitor for the problems. (You may need to use an additional resource, such as a medical–surgical textbook for this section.)

1. Intravenous infusion at 25 mL/h
   Potential complications:
   Plan for monitoring to detect potential complications:

(critical thinking continues on page 170)

CRITICAL THINKING EXERCISE XI *(continued)*

2. Insulin-dependent diabetes
   Potential complications:
   Plan for monitoring to detect potential complications:
3. Foley catheter
   Potential complications:
   Plan for monitoring to detect potential complications:

Part IV. Ensuring the Plan Is Adequately Recorded

Using the memory-jog EASE, what four things do you need to check on the plan to be sure that the plan has been adequately recorded?

Try This on Your Own

Practice weighing risks and benefits and making decisions about interventions. Consider the interventions in the following situations and decide whether you would prescribe them and whether there is anything you could do to minimize the risks involved.

1. Your neighbor calls at 10 pm and tells you her 9-year-old has chickenpox and generally is irritable and uncomfortable. She asks you if you think it would be okay to give her Children's Tylenol®. What would you tell her? What would you have told her if it were aspirin? Be sure to look up these drugs before answering.
2. Mr. Evans is weak from being on bed rest. He reports being depressed because he's become so dependent on others. He's now allowed to go to the bathroom on his own and requests that he be allowed to do his daily hygiene unsupervised in the bathroom. You are concerned that he might tire in the bathroom. Would you prescribe for him to be allowed to do his morning care alone in the bathroom? If so, what would you do to minimize the risks?
3. Your patient has a left chest tube and doesn't want to lie tilted to his left side because it's painful. Even though his right lung is compromised from previous disease process, he insists on being turned only to the right side. Would you allow him to turn only to his right side? If so, what would you do to minimize the risks?
4. With a peer or in a group, discuss the implications of the *Voices* and *Think About It*s in this chapter.

(text continues on page 177)

INTERDISCIPLINARY REHABILITATION CARE PLAN

Patient Name: Robert Kirk

Primary Diagnosis:

R-THA 7/1/05

Primary Physician: McGwire

Age: 75
Diet: ADA
Allergies: Sulfa

Ht. 5'7" **Wt.** 187
Religion: Cath.

Date Admitted: 7/7/05
Exp. Discharge: 7/21/05

CARE REVIEW

Week of: 7/14/05

Primary Problems	Care Management	Status	Comments
Pain Management	Rehab Team	Current	Controlled. See flowsheet.
Impaired Mobility	Rehab Team	Current	Participating in therapy. Ambulation with walker with assistance 3 X day.
ADL Dysfunction	Rehab Team	Current	Minimal assistance.
Delayed wound healing	Wound Care Team	Current	(r) hip incision open 2 cm. Small amount pink drainage.

Co-Morbidities

Parkinson's	Dr. Kostyo	Current	Stable with meds since 1995
Chronic A-fib with pacer (left side)	Dr. Foster	Current	On Coumadin since 2001. See anticoagulant flow sheet. Pacer rate set at 60. Rate controlled. Last checked pre-op 6/15
Glaucoma both eyes	Dr. Bell	Current	Stable with meds since 1999
Diabetes	Dr. Flynn	Current	Manages own BS and insulin

Discharge Planning

Expected Discharge: 7/21/05 **Discharge outcome:** To home; primary caregiver wife; independent with walker; skilled care visits twice a week.	**Consults:** Case Manager: Home Health:	J. Knox VNA	**Other:** Anticoagulant reports to Dr. Foster

FIGURE **4.2** Example first page of interdisciplinary care plan. (© 2004 Terri Patterson, RN, MSN, CRRN, FIALCP, www.nursingconsultation.com)

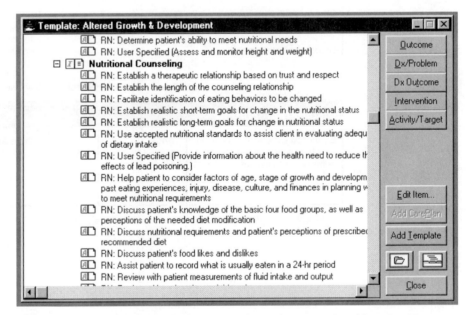

FIGURE 4.3 Two sample screens of a computerized care plan. (Reproduced from CareManager software by permission of Ergo Partners, LC, www.ergopartners.com)

PHYSICAL ASSESSMENT & TREATMENT

TKR Day of Surgery (date) _____	TKR Post-op Day 1 (date) _____	TKR Post-op Day 2 (date) _____
_____ Possessions labeled and secured	_____ AM care completed	_____ AM care completed
_____ VS Q15 min × 3 until stable, then Q1h × 4, then Q4h	_____ VS Q4h	_____ VS Q4h
_____ **VS normal, Temp <101°F**	_____ **VS normal, temp <101°F**	_____ **VS normal, temp <101°F**
_____ Lungs clear, non-productive cough, no dyspnea	_____ IS, cough & deep breathing Q1h W/A	_____ IS, cough & deep breathing Q4h W/A
_____ Oxygen as ordered	_____ Lungs clear, non-productive cough, no dyspnea	_____ Lungs clear, non-productive cough, no dyspnea
_____ IS, cough & deep breathing Q1h W/A	_____ Oxygen saturation >92%, oxygen discontinued	_____ I/O Q Shift
_____ I/O Q Shift	_____ I/O Q Shift	_____ Saline lock site w/o redness
_____ Nausea and vomiting tolerable w or w/o meds	_____ IV line converted to saline lock, site w/o redness	_____ Wearing TEDs
_____ Emesis without blood	_____ Nausea and vomiting tolerable w or w/o meds	_____ TEDs removed ½ hr, heels w/o redness
_____ Wearing TEDs	_____ Emesis without blood	_____ Skin without breakdown
_____ Skin without breakdown	_____ Wearing TEDs	_____ Pneumatic boots or stockings when in bed
_____ Pneumatic boots or stockings on when in bed	_____ TEDs removed ½ hr, heels w/o redness	_____ CPM settings
_____ Begin CPM setting	_____ Skin without breakdown	_____ Brace applied (if ordered)
_____ IV patent, site without redness	_____ Pneumatic boots or stockings on when in bed	_____ **Alert and Oriented × 3, speech clear**
_____ **Alert and Oriented × 3, speech clear**	_____ CPM Settings	_____ **Normal Neurovascular checks (Q shift)**
_____ **Normal Neurovascular checks (Q2h)**	_____ Measured for brace/applied (if ordered)	_____ Wound dsg change time: _____
_____ **Hemovac patent and vacuum intact**	_____ **Alert and Oriented × 3, speech clear**	_____ Staples/sutures intact
_____ **Hemovac drainage <500 cc in 8 hrs**	_____ **Normal Neurovascular checks (Q shift)**	_____ Wound drainage min amt, serous/serosanguinous
_____ **Wound bandage clean, dry and intact**	_____ Hemovac discontinued	
	_____ Wound dsg change time: _____	
	_____ Staples/suture intact	
	_____ Wound drainage min amt, serous/serosanguinous	

PSYCHOSOCIAL ASSESSMENT

_____ Oriented to room	_____ Coping effectively	_____ Coping effectively
_____ Coping effectively	_____ Sleeping well: ☐ with medication ☐ without medication	_____ Sleeping well: ☐ with medication ☐ without medication
_____ Sleeping well: ☐ with medication ☐ without medication		

TESTS/LABS

_____ Other tests WNL _____	_____ H&H ≥ 9/26	_____ H&H ≥ 9/26
	_____ Chem 7 WNL	_____ Other: _____
	_____ T/K Revision cultures no growth	_____ Final T/K Revision cultures without growth
	_____ Other: _____	

PAIN CONTROL/MEDICATION

_____ IV antibiotics given	_____ Transfusion given if ordered ☐ AB ☐ BB ☐ DD	_____ **Offer oral meds for pain 30 minutes before therapy prn**
_____ Ice pack to surgical site	_____ # of transfusions _____	_____ Patient reported pain level 3 (0–10)
_____ Pain control: ☐ Spinal ☐ Epidural ☐ PCA	_____ IV Antibiotics completed	
_____ Patient reported pain level 3 (0–10)	_____ ☐ Spinal ☐ Epidural ☐ PCA discontinued	
	_____ Patient reported pain level 3 (0–10)	

NUTRITION

_____ Offered liquids	_____ Diet advanced and tolerated	_____ No nausea or vomiting, usual diet

FIGURE 4.4 A portion of a clinical pathway for Total Knee Replacement (TKR). This section of the pathway indicates the type of clinical treatment or patient care activities to be carried out during the day of surgery and on the first 2 days after surgery for a patient undergoing total knee replacement. The accompanying pathway documentation form is used to document any variances from the pathway that occur. (Reproduced with permission from Inova Mount Vernon Hospital, Alexandria, VA.) Key: T/KI=total knee, EOB=edge of bed; SAQ=short arc quad; UE=upper extremity; LE=lower extremity; TJR=total joint replacement; RK=right knee; LK=left knee; 3:1 Commode= commode used at bedside, over toilet, and as a shower chair.

ELIMINATION

___ Foley catheter in place
___ Urine clear, output ≥30 cc/hr
___ Bowel sounds present, abdomen soft

ACTIVITY & THERAPY

___ General plan & comorbidities documented
___ Trapeze in place
___ Heels elevated while in bed
___ Dangled/stood at bedside 6–12 hrs after surgery
___ Ambulate Uni-knee

Instruction and practice:
___ Ankle pump.
___ Quad/glut sets

ELIMINATION

___ Foley catheter discontinued
___ Voiding QS
___ Bowel sounds present, abdomen soft

ACTIVITY & THERAPY

___ Trapeze in place
___ Heels elevated while in bed/knee extended
___ Ambulates to bathroom (BR) with walker or crutches uses 3:1 commode
___ PT/OT eval completed, Plan of Care established
___ Goals established (Outcomes/Rehab Rounds Form)
___ Evaluation same as pre-op
___ Chart reviewed

Instruction and practice:
___ Supine to sit
___ Transfers to EOB
___ Dangle/Stand
___ Sit to stand
___ OOB in chair
___ Gait on level surface
___ Device
___ Distance

Exercises in gym:
___ Ankle pump, quad/glut sets
___ Heelslide
___ Straight Leg Raise
___ SAQ (right)
___ SAQ (left)
___ Eval for UE group

	Extension	HS	Sitting flexion	Quad leg
___ RK				
___ LK				

___ Endurance
___ Instruction in set up of elevated toilet seat

ELIMINATION

___ Voiding QS
___ Normal bowel sounds, abdomen soft

ACTIVITY & THERAPY

___ Trapeze removed
___ Heels elevated while in bed/knee extended
___ Dressed in gym clothes
___ OOB for 2 of 3 meals
___ Ambulates to BR with walker or crutches/assist: uses 3:1 commode

Instruction and practice:
___ Supine to sit
___ Transfers to EOB
___ Sit to stand
___ Curbs and steps

Tech treatment
___ Gait on level surface
___ Device
___ Distance
___ Toilet transfer
___ Toilet hygiene
___ Grooming
___ Wash UE/trunk/LE
___ Dressing (LE)
___ Dressing (UE)
___ Shoes/socks
___ Brace on/off

Exercises in gym:
___ Ankle pumps, quad/glut sets
___ Heelslide
___ Straight Leg Raise
___ SAQ (right)
___ SAQ (left)
___ Abduction/adduction

	Extension	HS	Sitting flexion	Quad leg
___ RK				
___ LK				

___ Endurance
___ Instruction in set up of elevated toilet seat

FIGURE 4.4 Continued.

TKR Day of Surgery (date) _____

____ TJR packet given to patient
____ Post do's and don'ts, exercises at bedside

Patient instructed in/demonstrates understanding of
____ IS, cough & deep breathe
____ Weight bearing
____ Bed mobility, use of bedpan
____ Pain management, PCA/CADD

____ Family Participation reinforced
____ RN completes discharge outcomes form

Operative Note in Progress Notes

PATIENT IDENTIFICATION

	Initials	Time
RN D or A		
RN E		
RN N or P		
PT		
OT		
CM		
Physician		
Tech		
Other		

TKR Post-op Day 1 (date) _____

EDUCATION

Patient instructed in/demonstrates understanding of
____ IS, cough & deep breathe
____ Ankle pump and quad/glut exercises
____ Pain management
____ Weight bearing
____ **Family teaching scheduled for:**

DISCHARGE PLANNING

____ Plan reviewed with patient/family
____ D/C transportation identified _____
____ Discharge orders confirmed

OTHER

SURGEON NOTES

____ Examination as above, variances noted
____ Reviewed previous day's charting
____ Plan: continue pathway

	Initials	Time
TKR POST-OP DAY 1		
RN D or A		
RN E		
RN N or P		
PT		
OT		
CM		
Physician		
Tech		
Other		

TKR Post-op Day 2 (date) _____

Patient instructed in/demonstrates understanding of
____ IS, cough & deep breathe
____ Pain management
____ Do's and Don'ts
____ Weight bearing
____ Family present for teaching

____ Home equipment discussed and ordered
____ Patient adhering to pathway
____ Referrals completed: __ ICF __ HHC __ OP __ Sub acute Rehab

____ Examination as above, variances noted
____ Reviewed previous day's charting
____ Plan: continue pathway

	Initials	Time
TKR POST-OP DAY 2		
RN D or A		
RN E		
RN N or P		
PT		
OT		
CM		
Physician		
Tech		
Other		

FIGURE 4.4 Continued.

General Plan

Knee
- ☐ Right
- ☐ Primary
- ☐ Left
- ☐ Revision

Diagnosis: _____
- ☐ Bilateral
- ☐ Uni-compartmental

Major Releases:

Weight bearing status: (with walker or 2 crutches)
- ☐ Non-weight bearing
- ☐ 25%
- ☐ 50%
- ☐ Full Weight Bearing as tolerated

Brace: _____

CPM _____

Anticoagulation medication: ☐ YES   ☐ NO

Comorbidities: (Date ID/Initials)
- ___/___ Diabetes
- ___/___ Hypothyroidism
- ___/___ Obesity
- ___/___ Hypertension
- ___/___ Asthma
- ___/___ CABG
- ___/___ HF
- ___/___ BPH
- ___/___ CAD
- ___/___ COPD

Variance From General Plan:

☐ **Yes**

See Variance Documentation Pathway

Day _____

Date/Time	Pathway Day	Variance/Problem	Action Taken/Outcome	Initials

FIGURE **4.4** Continued.

THIS CHAPTER AND NCLEX*

❏ Essential = Safety. When you see the word *essential* in the question (eg, *What essential actions must you plan?*), the answer usually addresses something you must do to keep the patient *safe*.

❏ Expect questions on the monitoring (assessment) role related to procedures and drug administration. For example, *What will you assess pre-procedure, intra-procedure, and post-procedure? What will you assess before, during, and after drug administration?*

❏ Pay attention to "time frame" words. For example, *upon admission, prior to discharge, immediately*

prior to surgery, or *just returned from* (these determine the correct answer)

❏ Visualize and identify the outcomes (results) of each answer (is this desired?).

❏ Be prepared for many questions on setting priorities (page 148) and delegating care (page 169 in the next chapter). Ask, if I can only do one thing for this patient what should it be? Remember, "Keep them breathing and keep them safe." When a question is unclear, think "safety."

❏ See also "This Chapter and NCLEX" on pages 42, 87, 137, 202, and 221.

SUMMARY / KEY POINTS

■ The recorded plan of care serves four main purposes: (1) Directs care and documentation; (2) Promotes communication and continuity of care; (3) Creates a record that can later be used for evaluation, research, and legal reasons; and (4) Provides documentation of health care needs for insurance purposes.

■ Whether you develop your own plan or use a standard plan, you are responsible for following policies and procedures to make sure the plan is individualized.

■ The memory-jog **EASE** helps you to remember the four main care plan components (**E** xpected outcomes; **A** ctual and potential problems; **S** pecific interventions; **E** valuation/progress notes).

■ Applying local and national standards is the key to developing a safe, effective plan; page 145 shows a map for making clinical decisions.

■ Initial planning involves attending to urgent priorities, and then determining expected out-

comes of care. Outcomes for *problems* state what you expect to observe in the patient when the problems are resolved or controlled. Outcomes for interventions state the benefit you expect to observe in the patient after an intervention is performed (eg, if you suction someone's tracheostomy, you expect that breath sounds will be clearer after suctioning). If you can't clearly identify the benefits you expect to see in the patient after nursing care, then you shouldn't be intervening.

■ You determine the success of the plan by finding out if the patient achieved the expected outcomes. When writing outcomes, use measurable verbs (see page 152). Outcomes may be written for affective, cognitive, or psychomotor domains (see number 5 on page 152).

■ Patient records must communicate nurses' awareness of, and response to, all major care priorities; some problems may not need to be recorded on the care plan because they are

---

*The author acknowledges the help of Deanne Blach (www.deanneblach.com) and Judith Miller (www.judymillernclexreview.com) in developing NCLEX tips.

SUMMARY / KEY POINTS

addressed in other parts of the record (eg, Foley catheter care usually is addressed in policy and procedure manuals).

■ The interventions you identify must be individualized to the patient and aim to: (1) Detect, prevent, and manage health problems and risks; (2) Promote optimum function, independence, and sense of well-being; and (3). Achieve the desired outcomes safely and efficiently.

■ Evidence-based practice requires you to know the strength of the evidence that supports the use of the interventions you choose.

■ Scan this chapter for important rules, maps, and diagrams highlighted throughout, then compare where you stand in relation to the expected learning outcomes on page 141.

References

1. American Nurses Association. (2004). *Nursing scope and standards of performance and standards of clinical practice.* Washington, DC: American Nurses Publishing.

2. Merriman, M. (2008). Pre-hospital discharge planning: Empowering elderly patients through choice. *Critical Care Nursing Quarterly, 31*(1), 52–58.

3. Campbell, G. (1997). President's note. *AACN News, 14*(8), 2.

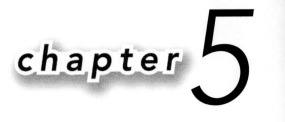

chapter 5

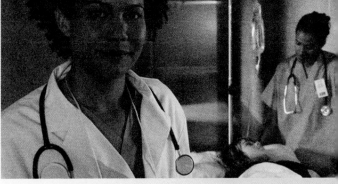

Implementation

what's in this chapter?

Whereas the last chapter addressed how to develop an *initial* plan of care, this chapter helps you understand your responsibilities related to *putting the plan into action*. Here, you learn principles of giving and taking shift reports (shift hand-offs), and how to get organized, set priorities, and make the most of your time. You explore two important topics you need to know for both NCLEX and clinical practice: (1) How do you prioritize care? and (2) When is it appropriate to delegate care to others, and how can you do this safely and effectively? You study your role as coordinator of care and gain insight into the importance of implementing the plan with an open, active mind that monitors patient responses and reflects on ways to improve care. Finally, you learn key principles that help you chart effectively, whether you're using handwritten or electronic charting systems.

ANA standards related to this chapter[1]

Standard 5	Implementation. The registered nurse implements the identified plan.
Standard 5a	The registered nurse coordinates care delivery.
Standard 5b	The registered nurse employs strategies to promote health and a safe environment.
Standard 6	Evaluation. The nurse evaluates progress toward attainment of outcomes.

critical thinking exercises

■ **Critical Thinking Exercise XII**   Delegating, Case Management, Critical Paths, and Care Variances
■ **Critical Thinking Exercise XIII**   Principles of Effective Charting

expected learning outcomes

After studying this chapter, you should be able to:

- Discuss how to prepare for getting change-of-shift (hand-off) report the next time you're in the clinical setting.
- Identify strategies for getting organized and setting priorities the next time you're in the clinical setting.
- Explain how the key words "assess, re-assess, revise, record" apply to performing interventions.
- Describe how to weigh risks and benefits to reduce the likelihood of harm from an intervention.
- Discuss how to build "safety nets" to keep patients safe during *Implementation*.
- Apply delegation principles when deciding how to delegate actions to an unlicensed helper.
- Address your role related to case management and variances in care.
- Describe the characteristics of effective charting systems.
- Chart effectively, following policies and procedures of each facility where you work.
- Discuss how to give a factual, organized change-of-shift (hand-off) report the next time you're in the clinical setting.

Implementation: Putting the Plan into Action

Critical Thinking Indicators (CTIs) Related to Implementation

Preparing for Report and Getting Report (Shift Hand-off)
Preparing for Report (Shift Hand-off)
Getting Report (Shift Hand-off)

Setting Daily Priorities
Strategies: Prioritizing Care for Several Patients

Delegating Care, Not Accountability

Coordinating Care

Monitoring Responses: Assessing and Reassessing

Performing Nursing Interventions
Be Proactive—Promote Safety, Comfort, and Efficiency

Implementation and Evidence-Based Practice

(continued on next page)

Implementation: Putting the Plan into Action

The following diagram shows how *Implementation*—putting the plan into action—is like "a bridge" between *Planning* and *Evaluation* (you plan, you implement, you evaluate).

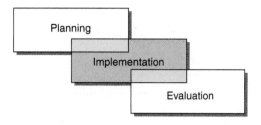

Planning is part of *Implementation* for two main reasons:

1. The plan developed during *Planning* guides what you *do* during *Implementation*.
2. Putting the plan into action means making sure the plan is still appropriate, setting priorities, and fine-tuning the plan as indicated. You don't just put the plan into action—you monitor patients closely to determine responses to interventions.

   Evaluation is a part of *Implementation* because monitoring responses means *evaluating* how your patient is responding to treatment. On a daily basis, you need to be asking, How well is my patient progressing toward overall expected outcomes?

   In this chapter, you learn how to put the plan into action in a safe, effective, organized way—a way that increases the likelihood of getting the results you need, while preventing errors and other undesirable results. It focuses on the following key activities.

IMPLEMENTATION

❑ Preparing for report and getting report (shift hand-off)
❑ Setting daily priorities
❑ Assessing appropriateness of (and readiness for) interventions
❑ Performing interventions and reassessing to determine responses
❑ Making immediate changes (revising approaches) as needed
❑ Charting to monitor progress and communicate care
❑ Giving report (shift hand-off)

R U L E

Your ability to communicate (listen, speak, and write effectively) with patients, families, peers, and other professionals makes the difference between competent, efficient care—and care that's sloppy, unprofessional, and prone to errors.

Critical Thinking Indicators (CTIs) Related to Implementation

Implementation is challenging because it often requires you to put all five steps of the nursing process together while "thinking on your feet" to make quick decisions. On a routine basis, you have to:

1. Assess patients to be sure their status hasn't changed and interventions are still appropriate.
2. Recognize when diagnoses or problems have changed.
3. Plan before you act.
4. Perform nursing actions (interventions).
5. Evaluate responses carefully, and revise your approach as indicated.

> **R U L E**
>
> **Remember "assess, re-assess, revise, record":** *Assess* patients before you perform nursing actions. *Re-assess* them to determine their responses after you perform nursing actions. *Revise* your approach as indicated. Record patient responses and any changes you made in the plan.

Because of the complexity of *Implementation,* all of the CTIs listed in the boxes on pages 33–35 relate to this phase.

Preparing for Report and Getting Report (Shift Hand-off)

Getting change-of-shift (hand-off) reports is the first thing you do in *Implementation.* Change-of-shift reports are called "shift hand-offs" because you pass care from one nurse's hands to another.[2] Being prepared and staying focused is essential to getting a factual, relevant report—a report that helps you get organized and set priorities early in the day.

Preparing for Report (Shift Hand-off)

Preparing for shift hand-off—learning about patient problems, looking up common treatments, reading charts, and getting to the unit early—is the key to efficiency. Too often, there's little time for reading charts and looking up management of common problems during the course of the day. When you make time to prepare yourself for the day, you feel more confident, are more competent, and can begin giving care in a timely way.

Getting Report (Shift Hand-off)

Getting a factual, relevant shift hand-off is challenge for several reasons:

1. There often are interruptions and distractions as one shift ends and the other begins.
2. There's so much information to get that it's hard to write quickly enough.

3. Nurses giving report often are fatigued or they know the patients so well that they forget to tell you the unique aspects of care that you really need to know.

Completing a standard tool that ensures that the most important information is communicated from one caregiver to another prevents omission errors. Even if you're interrupted or tired, the tool helps you stay focused and "on task."

R U L E

To promote effective communication between caregivers, in most cases, you'll be required to follow specific hand-off procedures for giving and taking report.[3] The SBAR communication tool (page 61) is an example hand-off tool. The following box gives resources for learning more about hand-off tools.

Learn More About Hand-off Tools

1. Download the following hand-off tool kit components free of charge from http://www.aorn.org/PracticeResources/ToolKits/PatientHandOffToolKit/
- Hand-off Tool Kit Executive Summary
- Research in the Health Care Industry
- Hand-off Communication Tools Overview
- Sample Patient Hand-off Tools
- Recommendations for Perioperative Patient Hand-off
- Policy Guidance for Hand-offs
- Presentation on Standardizing Hand-offs for Patient Safety
- Perioperative Hand-off Talking Points
- Additional Hand-off Resources

2. Learn about evidence-based strategies and tools to enhance performance and patient safety at http://www.ahrq.gov/qual/teamstepps/

If you don't have a standard tool you're required to complete for hand-off reports, develop one yourself, rather than work from a blank page. Figure 5.1 shows a personal worksheet that I developed for myself when I was working in an intensive care unit.

Setting Daily Priorities

Setting priorities during *Implementation* requires applying the same principles of priority-setting addressed on the box on page 148. Take a few moments to review that box now.

The following section gives additional strategies to help you set daily priorities when you're caring for more than one patient.

Strategies: Prioritizing Care for Several Patients

1. **Make initial quick rounds** of your patients, briefly checking the "big picture" of how they're doing (preferably, do this before you go to report or sit down to study

Name _Wm. French_	Room: _145_
Age _62_	Med Dx: _Angina_
Dr. _O'Hara_	Nsg Dx: _Activity Intolerance_

Mental Status: _ok_	Diet: _Reg. No Caf_
Airway: _ok_	IV: _Hep lock @ hand_
Lungs: _clear_	Pain? _None since yesterday_
Oxygen: _at 2 l per cannula_	Relevant History
Heart rhythm: _reg - no PVC's_	_Hypertension_
GI:	
GU:	Special Concerns
Skin: _ok_	_- For stress test tomorrow_
Activity Restrictions: _OOB to chair only_	_- Wants to see priest for communion_

EKG: _ok_   Na _ok_   Cl _ok_   K _3.5_ CO_2 _ok_

VITAL SIGNS: _98⁴-72-22_ $\frac{140}{90}$ BLD SUGAR: _ok_

BLOOD GASES: _ok_   O₂ SATURATION: _ok_

FIGURE 5.1 Personal Worksheet developed by the author when she was working in an intensive care unit. The worksheet was key to getting organized and identifying data that was missed during report. For example, the two blanks next to "GI" and "GU" above point to missing information in those categories.

voices

Including Nursing Assistants and Patients in Hand-offs Improves Outcomes
I REALLY want to stress the importance of RNs and nursing assistants (NA) doing shift hand-offs *together*. I've worked with about 160 hospitals and have seen some near-disasters. Shift report is the perfect time for giving effective initial direction and for collaborative RN and NA planning (the off-going NAs can be answering call bells). On one NA-to-NA report, I observed NA talking about the patient having what sounded to me like symptoms of a stroke. The off-going NA reported to the oncoming NA that there simply was a need for additional help with ambulation! This all of course begs the question about what care delivery model you are using . . . the assignments have to reflect good delegation and supervision principles. Some places are now doing bedside reports to ensure that patients and families are included in planning from the start.[3]

—*Ruth Hansten, RN, MBA, PhD, FACHE*[4]
(www.HanstenRROHC.com)

the plan of care). **Rationale:** This helps you to identify problems requiring immediate attention and helps you to connect the actual patients with what you hear during report or read in patient records.

R U L E

In accordance with national patient safety goals, when you do an assessment or give nursing care, use at least two unique identifiers to be sure you have the right name and patient.[5] For example, ask the person his name and birth date and also check the ID bracelet to make sure it matches.

2. **Immediately after shift report,** verify critical information such as IV infusions, operation of equipment, and so forth. **Rationale:** Verifying information you received during report prevents misunderstandings and helps you and the nurse who's leaving to settle problems while both of you are available for clarification.
3. **Do quick priority assessments and identify urgent problems** (those posing an immediate threat to the patient, eg, chest pain or a disconnected IV line) and take appropriate action (eg, get help if needed). **Rationale:** Setting the wheels in motion to correct severe problems takes priority over taking time to analyze all the patient's problems.
4. **List your patients' major problems** in relation to the expected outcomes for the day, and answer the following questions:
   • Which problems must be resolved today, and what happens if I wait until later?
   • Which problems must I monitor today, and what could happen if I don't monitor them?

• To achieve the overall outcomes of care, which are the key problems or ones that I must resolve or manage today?
• Which of the patient's problems can I realistically work on today?

Rationale: You can only do so much in a day. Answering these questions helps you decide what must be done *today.*

R U L E

Partner with patients to set priorities. Begin care by asking patients and families to identify their *own* priorities for the day (eg, stating, "Tell me three main things you want to accomplish today," or "What are the most important things you want me to help you with?"). This sets the tone for mutual goal-setting. It helps you to avoid making assumptions about what's important to your patients, and also helps you to identify assumptions your patients may have made (eg, they may have unrealistic expectations).

---

5. **Determine the interventions that must be done to prevent, resolve, or manage the problems on your problem list.** List these interventions along with routine tasks such as baths and meals. **Rationale:** This helps you to get a big picture of the tasks of the day, which helps you to answer questions such as, What must be done first? and How can I make the best use of my time? For example, you may give a routine bath to promote hygiene and, at the same time, discuss problems with coping.

6. **Decide what things the patient or significant others can do on their own, what things to delegate to others, and what things you must do yourself** (see Boxes 5.1 and 5.2). **Rationale:** Encouraging patients and families to be as independent as possible helps them take charge of their own care. Often, patients and families don't know what they are or aren't expected to do for themselves. Using less qualified help appropriately allows you to spend more time accomplishing tasks that require the expertise of a registered nurse.

7. **Make a personal worksheet for getting things done for the day and refer to it frequently.** Be sure to consider the daily routine of the unit (eg, when meals are served). **Rationale:** You're likely to experience many distractions during the course of the day. Don't rely on memory. Although the daily routine of the unit shouldn't dictate your activities, it's vital to consider it when setting the schedule. For example, it's frustrating to both nurses and patients when meals arrive during baths or patients are called to physical therapy at inconvenient times.

Delegating Care, Not Accountability

Because today's nurses are often placed in leadership roles, an important nursing competency is being able to delegate care appropriately. To pass state board exams (NCLEX®) and to be a safe, effective clinician, be sure that you're very familiar with the principles of delegation listed in Boxes 5.1 and 5.2.

box 5.1 Key Points of Delegation*

Delegation defined: Transferring to a competent individual the authority to perform a selected task in a selected situation while retaining accountability for results.

❑ **Remember the "five rights of delegation":**
1. **The right task**—One that doesn't fall only under the scope of nursing's practice.
2. **To the right person**—Someone qualified and competent to do the job.
3. **In the right situation**—See Box 5.2 (*When Is It Safe to Delegate?*).
4. **With the right communication**—Be clear and concise when describing the task, the goal, and what you want reported.
5. **Performing the right evaluation**—As indicated, timely evaluation of the patient's response and worker's performance as the task is being done and after the task is completed.

❑ **Delegate with full knowledge of:**
1. Your state practice act and applicable standards, policies, and procedures (eg, what you're allowed to delegate and to whom may vary from state to state and facility to facility).
2. The worker's specific job description and competencies.
3. (When delegating to patients or family caregivers) whether they have the required knowledge and skills.

*Recommended: Hansten R., Jackson M. (2009). *Clinical Delegation Skills: A Handbook for Professional Practice.* 4th Ed. Sudbury, MA: Jones and Bartlett Publishers.

R U L E

YOU are accountable for the outcomes of care you delegate.[6] For example, suppose you delegate care of a child to Jane, a nursing aid. Then Jane tells the mother to watch the child while she's at lunch. If the mother goes to the bathroom, and something happens to the child, YOU are accountable.

box 5.2 When Is It Safe to Delegate?

Delegate When:	**Don't Delegate When:**
❑ The patient is stable.	❑ Complex assessment, thinking, and judgment are required.
❑ The task is within the worker's job description and capabilities.	❑ The outcome of the task is unpredictable.
❑ The amount of RN time with the patient isn't significantly reduced.	❑ There's increased risk of harm (eg, taking blood from an artery can cause more severe complications than venipuncture).
	❑ Problem solving and creativity are required.

Source: R. Alfaro-LeFevre workshop handouts © 2008

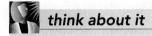 *think about it*

When You Delegate Care, Check the Results Yourself
Checking the results of care you delegated keeps patients safe, protects you from legal liability, and encourages good care (people you delegate care to are more likely to do a good job when they know you will be checking the *results*).

Coordinating Care

National practice standards stress that nurses are responsible for coordinating care during *Implementation,* and for documenting coordination of care.[1] As the nurse, you are with patients the most, so pay attention to the overall care patients receive. Reflect on their treatment schedule and how it's affecting them. Encourage patients to let you know if there are things that they would like to be organized differently (for example, patients who are "morning people" should have physical therapy treatments in the morning). Be sure to record how overall care can best be coordinated on the plan of care.

> **R U L E**
>
> **Remember the importance of thinking ahead, thinking in action, and thinking back (reflecting).[7,8] Think ahead** (be proactive—anticipate what might happen and how you can be prepared). **Think in action** (pay attention to what's going on in your head as you "think on your feet," gathering and putting information together). **Think back** (reflect on your thinking to decide what you can learn from what happened, what influenced your thinking, and what you can do better next time—this usually requires dialogue with others or journaling to make your thoughts explicit).

Monitoring Responses: Assessing and Reassessing

Monitoring patient status and responses to care—assessing patients before and after interventions are performed and revising your approach as needed—is a critical part of *Implementation.* To ensure patient safety, you must closely monitor responses to interventions: How is the patient responding? Are you getting the expected results? If not, why not? A recipe for disaster is blindly putting a plan into action without monitoring patient responses. Don't make assumptions. Recognize the importance of assessing with an open mind, as noted in the following example.

E x a m p l e
The Importance of Assessing With an Open Mind. During report, Jodi, the evening nurse, was told, "Mrs. Ross is a difficult patient—she won't ambulate." Later, when Jodi went to give Mrs. Ross her medications, she asked if there was something that was causing her to be so tired. Mrs. Ross responded that she hadn't slept well in

weeks because she had just found out her daughter had breast cancer and was afraid she might lose her. This was important information that hadn't been offered before. Jodi then was able to talk with Mrs. Ross about her fears and offer a positive outlook by explaining that breast cancer, when detected early, has a good prognosis. By later that evening, Mrs. Ross was ambulating and talking about how eager she was to go home.

> **R U L E**
>
> **Use every patient encounter as an opportunity to observe mental and physical status and to empower patients to care for themselves (through teaching, coaching, and so forth).** For example, if you're helping someone bathe, assess skin status (by observing the entire body) and mental status (by using therapeutic communication techniques). This is also an opportunity to teach good skin care.

Performing Nursing Interventions

Performing interventions entails getting prepared, performing interventions, determining responses, and making necessary changes.

Pages 163–165, in Chapter 4, give strategies for *individualizing* interventions. This section addresses how to *implement* interventions.

Be Proactive—Promote Safety, Comfort, and Efficiency

Adequate preparation before performing an intervention makes the difference between risky, haphazard care that taxes both you and the patient, and efficient, safe care that promotes comfort and gets results. Before you perform an intervention, ask the following questions:

❑ Am I qualified and is it prudent (see decision-making map on page 145)?
❑ What might I need?
❑ What could go wrong, what can I do to prevent it from happening, and am I prepared to deal with it, if it does happen?
❑ Is my patient ready?
❑ What can I do to make this easier?
❑ Are there any policies and procedures I need to check?

Implementation and Evidence-Based Practice

National practice standards stress the need to implement the plan of care using evidence-based interventions. As a thought-oriented, rather than task-oriented, nurse, be sure you can answer the question, "What evidence supports that these interventions are likely to work?" In some cases, you'll have several research studies cited in policies and procedures to support planned interventions. In others, you may only know that the interventions are recommended in a reliable text. Either way, don't settle for the answer, "This is how we always do it." Be sure you understand the strength of the evidence behind the interventions.

Guidelines: Preparing to Act

❏ **Review the plan and be sure you know the rationale and principles** behind the interventions. If you don't know the principles and rationale, you won't be able to adapt the procedure if you need to, and you may not even recognize if the intervention is no longer indicated.

❏ **Decide whether you're competent and qualified** to perform the interventions (if not, seek help).

❏ **Find out whether there are relevant facility procedures, protocols, guidelines, or standards** that address how you should perform the interventions.

❏ **Assess the patient's current status** and decide whether the interventions still are appropriate.

❏ **Predict possible outcomes.** Get a picture of what you're going to do, and think about what might come up, what could go wrong, and what you'll do about it.
   • Weigh risks and benefits (pages 164–165).
   • Identify ways to reduce risks of harm to the patient and yourself.
   • Determine how to promote comfort and reduce patient stress (eg, if someone is expected to sit for a long time, get a comfortable chair and offer distractions).

❏ **Obtain the required resources** (eg, equipment, personnel) and make sure you planned enough time and an environment conducive to performing the interventions.

❏ **Involve patients and significant others.** Explain what's to be done, why it's going to be done, and how long it will take. Encourage them to voice questions, suggestions, or concerns.

> **R U L E**
> **Before performing any intervention, ask yourself,** Am I clear about what I'm going to do, how I'm going to do it, and *why* it's indicated for this *specific* person?

Thinking Critically: What to Do If Things Go Wrong

Even when you're fully prepared, you may not get the desired response to your interventions. Let's look at what to do if you don't get the desired response, if the problem shows no improvement, or if the situation is aggravated by what you did.

If you don't get the desired response, a red flag that says "something's wrong" should go up in your mind. Stop and ask some key questions:

1. **Did I perform the interventions correctly?** For example, if you suctioned someone who sounded congested and there was no mucus, did you have enough suction and did you direct your tubing the way you needed to?

2. **Is the diagnosis correct, or has the problem or its cause changed?** For example, suppose you were caring for a woman with tachycardia, and her heart rate didn't come down as you expected after giving a medication to slow the heart rate. Your next questions should be something like, Could there be something else causing or contributing to the tachycardia? Could anxiety, fever, or a respiratory problem be causing this fast heart rate?
3. **Are there other interventions that may complement this intervention, increasing its effectiveness?** For example, a backrub and talking with someone who's anxious is likely to enhance the effect of an anti-anxiety agent.
4. **What could I be missing?** Should I get a second opinion?
5. **If you make a mistake,** take immediate steps to minimize patient harm; then follow policies and procedures for reporting errors.

R U L E

Monitor patient responses carefully as you carry out nursing actions. If you don't get the desired response, find out *why* and make corrections before continuing to act.

R U L E

Institute of Medicine competencies stresses the need to collaborate to keep patients safe. Work to create "safety nets" that prevent and minimize mistakes. Just as baseball players position themselves to back each other up if the ball is missed, pay attention to the possibility of human error. Collaborate to find ways to prevent mistakes, catch mistakes, and keep patients safe.

Case Management: Critical Paths and Care Variances

If you use a critical path like the one on pages 173–176 to guide your patient's care, it sets priorities for you on a day-by-day basis—that is, it does unless you identify a care variance. A care variance is said to have occurred when a patient hasn't achieved outcomes by the time frame noted on a critical path. For example, if the critical path states "By the second day after surgery, the patient will be out of bed in a chair three times a day," but your patient isn't well enough to be out of bed three times a day, this is a care variance.

What do you do if you identify a care variance? Care variances should trigger you to do additional assessments to determine whether the delay is justified or whether actions need to be taken to improve the likelihood of achieving the outcome.

R U L E

When using critical paths or other standard plans, never assume your patient is ready to progress as planned: look for care variances. If you identify a care variance, consider whether you need to contact additional professional resources for in-depth assessment and treatment.

***table* 5.1** Critical Paths Don't Replace Thinking

Examples of Thinking Critically When Using a Critical Path	Examples of Not Thinking Critically When Using a Critical Path
"I'm familiar with this path. . . . I wonder how this particular patient is doing in relation to the predicted care for this problem."	"I have a path for this patient, so this should be easy and straightforward because I already know what the problems are going to be."
"It's going to take time to think through what's really going on with this patient, but I'd better make time."	"There's no way I have time to go through everything I need to really understand this patient. I'd better just follow the path."

Table 5.1 gives examples of thinking critically and *not* thinking critically when using critical paths.

Ethical/Legal Concerns

We already addressed the fact that legally and ethically, you're responsible for protecting patients' privacy. Ethically (and in some cases, legally), you're responsible for emotional outcomes of your interventions, as well as physical outcomes. For example, in some states, it's against the law to tell people they have AIDS over the phone. You must tell them in person and provide counseling and support. Here's another example: Suppose your patient is having a facial tumor removed, and the standard plan is to give a pamphlet with graphic pictures of reconstructive surgery. As a prudent nurse, you must anticipate this response, stay with the person, and provide support.

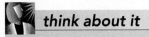 *think about it*

Evidence-Based Practice Challenges Assumptions About Restraints
Many people assume that restraining agitated patients protects them from harm. On the contrary, evidence shows that physical and chemical (drug induced) restraints may actually cause serious injuries and emotional and physical problems.[9]

Nine Rights of Medication Administration
To promote critical thinking for all involved in patient care, follow the "nine rights of drug administration": right patient; right drug; right dose; right route; right reason; right frequency; right documentation; patient's right to refuse and be educated about medications.

Caring Means More Than Being Nice. Caring means more than being friendly and nice. Patients do value this type of caring. But, what they want even more are knowledgeable, competent nurses who closely monitor their care. They want nurses who carefully double-check care management and advocate when something is wrong or could be improved.

CRITICAL THINKING EXERCISE XII

Delegating, Case Management, Critical Paths, and Care Variances

To complete this session, read pages 183–194. Example responses can be found on page 245.

1. Suppose one of the many tasks that had to be accomplished today was getting a 30-year-old woman who has had a routine cholecystectomy out of bed for the first time.
   a. Would you delegate this task?
   b. Why or why not?
2. Read the Rule on page 189.
   a. Why is the nurse accountable for the child slipping away? (One to two sentences.)
   b. What could the nurse have done to decrease the likelihood of the child slipping away? (One to two sentences.)
3. Answer each letter below, using three to five sentences.
   a. How do you assess a patient for a care variance?
   b. What would you do if you identified a care variance and why?
   c. What can happen to the patient if you miss the fact that your patient is demonstrating a care variance?
   d. What can happen to you if you miss the fact that your patient is demonstrating a care variance?

Try This On Your Own

In a personal journal, with a peer, or in a group, discuss the implications of the *Voices* and *Think About It*s in this chapter.

Charting

After you give nursing care, your next priority should be charting assessments, interventions, and patient responses to care. Two reasons for this are:

1. **Writing down what you've observed and done often jogs your memory about something else you need to assess or do.** For example, you may be charting an abdominal assessment and realize that you forgot to check whether the nasogastric tube equipment is functioning properly.
2. **You're likely to be more accurate and thorough when your memory is fresh.**

Six Purposes of Charting

The main purposes of your charting are to:

1. **Communicate care** to other health care professionals who need to be able to find out what you did and how the person is doing.
2. **Help you and others to identify patterns** of responses and changes in status (you identify patterns by reviewing charting over time).
3. **Ensure evidence-based care.** Most charting systems prompt you to record information and interventions that evidence has shown must be done within specific time frames (eg, giving an antibiotic within a certain amount of time of doing blood cultures).

4. **Provide a basis for evaluation,** research, and improvement of care quality.

5. **Create a legal document** that later may be used in court to evaluate the type of care rendered. Your records can be your best friend or worst enemy. The best defense that you actually observed or did something is the fact that you made a note of it.

6. **Supply validation** for re-imbursement from Medicare, Medicaid, and other insurance companies for the cost of care. The saying goes, "if it's not recorded, they won't pay."

R U L E

In many cases today, standards dictate what information is recorded and by when it must be recorded. Be sure to review each facility's policies and procedures for record, as well as the rules and content addressed in the section on Reporting and Recording Data beginning on page 82–86.

---

 voices

We Don't Make Charting Rules, But We MUST Follow Them
All patients admitted with a diagnosis of pneumonia need to have an antibiotic in the first 4 hours, or Medicare won't pay us. Check once, check twice, check three times. If your patient has CHF (congestive heart failure), be sure you record that you gave him CHF discharge instructions, even if he only has a *history* of CHF or we won't get paid!!! YES!!! YES!!! Patient care is always the most important part of nursing! We just have to "play the game" as well. In the end, it means better patient care!
—*Posting on a Staff Development Listserv*

Various Ways of Charting

There are various ways of charting, as charting systems seem to be changing almost as quickly as you can say "computer." Depending on the type of setting you work in, you may use any or a combination of the following charting methods (these methods are often incorporated into electronic health records, addressed in the last bullet here).

❏ **Source-oriented charting:** Nurses use separate records from other disciplines. You record a narrative, chronological account of the patient's day (see Figure 5.2, page 203).

❏ **Focus charting:** You use key words to identify the problem or issue you're addressing in the record and apply the memory-jog DARA to guide you to chart *data, action, response, action* (see Figure 5.3, page 204).

❏ **Multidisciplinary charting:** All health care professionals—nurses, physicians, nutritionists, etc. —chart on the same record (see Figure 5.4, page 204).

❏ **Flowsheet charting:** You use specific sheets or computer fields to enter focus assessments to track the status of specific patient conditions (see Figure 5.5, page 205)

❏ **Charting by exception (CBE):** You refer to unit standards, policies, and protocols in the patient record, charting narrative notes only when the patient's data change or care deviates from the norm. For an example, see Figure 5.6 (page 206).

❏ **Addendum sheet charting:** You use supplemental records, adding separate sheets for each type of situation (eg, discharge summary sheets, teaching sheets). For an example, see Figure 5.7 (page 207).

❏ **Electronic Health Records (EHR), also called Electronic Medical Records (EMR).** You chart directly on the computer and usually have mandatory fields that you must complete. The goal of EHR is to increase productivity and make information easy to record and retrieve. The use of EHR is still developing, and most places are in various stages of development. You can expect that there will be "growing pains" as EHR continues to evolve into records that are developed based on standards.[10] These standards will ensure streamlined, evidence-based care.

Whatever charting method you use, the goal is the same—to have charting that is:

❏ Accurate, factual, and complete
❏ Organized and standardized
❏ Timely and easily accessible (it should be easy for you to chart in a timely way, and easy for others to find the information they need).

Principles of Effective Charting

Because you're likely to work with a broad range of charting methods—from handwritten to electronic charting—it's important for you to learn principles of effective charting that are universal. Applying the following principles will help you adapt from one charting method to another. It will also help you to answer questions related to documentation on NCLEX.

1. **When others read your charting, they should see evidence of the following:**
   • **Initial and ongoing assessments:** What did you observe when you first encountered the patient and at subsequent encounters (especially before and after interventions)?
   • **Status of patient problems:** What are the patient's current signs and symptoms?
   • **Interventions and nursing care performed:** What did you do to meet the person's needs?
   • **Patient response (outcomes of care):** What results did you observe?
   • **Any specific attention given to safety or undesirable outcomes:** What did you do to ensure patient safety? If you didn't get the desired response in the patient, what did you do?
   • **The person's ability to manage care needs after discharge:** What did you observe and do in relation to the likelihood that the patient is able to manage his own care?
2. **Effective charting systems should:**
   • **Be tailored to the types of problems frequently seen** in the patient population of the facility—they should direct nurses to chart key aspects of care.
   • **Reflect use of the nursing process and be legally sound**
   • **Discourage double documentation** (charting the same thing in two different places).
   • **Increase the quality of patient records** while reducing the amount of time spent charting.

- **Be designed so that key patient information (eg, assessments and interventions) is easily retrievable,** thereby facilitating communication, evaluation, research, and quality improvement.

Chapter 2 (pages 84–86) gives additional guidelines for charting.

Avoiding Dumping Syndrome With Electronic Charting

When using electronic charting systems, it's important to avoid the dumping syndrome. Dumping syndrome is the tendency to dump information into a computer and forget about it: data goes from your brain to the computer, and there it sits, lost to the brain.

Find ways to reflect on your charting, either through printouts or cues in the system. If you don't make time to look for patterns, consider the big picture, and think about what you might be missing—you're not thinking critically. You're simply dumping data into a computer.

Learning to Chart Effectively

Charting effectively requires knowledge, experience, and application of principles of effective charting. As you improve your ability to perform assessments and discriminate between normal and abnormal findings, your charting will improve.

It's also important to do two things:

1. Practice using whatever type of charting you'll be using before you go to the clinical setting.
2. Read charts to learn from actual situations. As you read the charts, ask yourself questions like, What are the diagnoses? Where's the evidence that the diagnoses exist? What are they doing to treat them? and How is this person responding?

Guidelines: Charting During Implementation

❏ **To identify omissions and changes is patient status,** chart as soon as possible, following policies and procedures carefully.
❏ **Reflect on what you chart,** asking questions like, Am I missing anything? and How does what I'm charting compare with what the people before me charted? This helps you recognize changes in status early.
❏ **Record important actions immediately** to be sure that others know the action has been completed.
❏ **Record all variations from the norm** (eg, abnormalities in respiration, circulation, mental status, or behavior) and any actions taken related to the abnormalities (eg, if you reported the abnormality or if you intervened in some way).
❏ **Be precise.** Your notes should give a description and timeline for sequence of events, answering the questions of what happened and when, how, and where it happened.

❏ **Focus on significant problems or events that communicate *what's different*** about this person today. For example, don't record "went to the bathroom unassisted" unless this is unusual.

❏ **Stick to the facts.** Avoid judgmental language.

E x a m p l e
Right: "Shouting, 'Everyone had better stay away from me, or I'm going to hit someone.' "
Wrong: "Angry and aggressive."

❏ **Be specific.** Don't use vague terms.

E x a m p l e
Right: "Abdominal dressing has an area of light pink drainage about 6 inches in diameter."
Wrong: "Noted moderate amount of drainage on abdominal dressing."

❏ **Be concise, yet descriptive.** You don't have to write complete sentences. Use adjectives and accepted abbreviations to give a good picture of activities and observations. For example, "OOB to chair for a half hour—c/o slight dizziness on standing up but moved well."

R U L E

Check "Do Not Use" Lists and use only accepted abbreviations.

❏ **Sign your name consistently** using your first initial, last name, and credentials after each entry that you complete (eg, "R. Alfaro-LeFevre, RN").

❏ **If you forget to chart something, record it as soon as you can,** following procedures for making late entries.

E x a m p l e
"5/17 3:00 pm, Late entry: Stool was positive for blood at 10 am this morning. Notified Dr. Eyler. R. Alfaro-LeFevre, RN."

❏ **If you make a mistake on a chart, correct it according to facility policies.** Do not hide mistakes. Rather draw a line through them, mark them as errors and put your initials to indicate it was a mistake.

E x a m p l e
5/17 3pm. ~~Went to xray.~~ Error RAL.

❏ **Record refusal to follow prescribed regimen,** as well as any actions you took. For example: "Refuses to go to physical therapy. Says it 'doesn't do any good.' Notified Dr. Frazier and Rochelle Hutton in physical therapy."

Memory-Jogs for Charting

The following memory-jogs can help you remember some common approaches to charting narrative notes.

AIR-A (Assessment, Intervention, Response, Action). Chart the assessment data you observe, the interventions performed, the patient's response to interventions, and any actions you took based on the response.

DARA (Data, Action, Response, Action). This has the same meaning as the above.

SOAP, SOAPIE (Subjective data, Objective data, Analysis, Plan; Subjective data, Objective data, Analysis, Plan, Intervention, Evaluation). Chart the subjective and objective data you collected, your analysis of what the data indicate (your conclusion), and the plan. With SOAPIE, you also add the intervention(s) you performed and the evaluation (patient response) after the intervention(s) were performed. See example on page 168.

CRITICAL THINKING EXERCISE XIII

Principles of Effective Charting

To complete this session, read pages 195–200. Example responses can be found on page 245.

1. List the six main purposes of charting.
2. Give two reasons why you should chart as soon as possible after giving nursing care.
3. Get a piece of paper and write a note that records the following events using the mnemonic AIR-A.

   A patient calls you into the room and tells you that she feels like she's choking on mucus but is afraid to cough because of incisional pain. You help her to get in a better position and then teach her to splint the incision with a pillow. She coughs up a gray mucus plug and thanks you for your help. You listen to her lungs, and they sound clear. You emphasize the importance of reporting pain so that it can be managed to promote her ability to cough to clear lungs.
4. What's wrong with the following two excerpts from nurses' notes?
   a. 5/8 Patient is difficult and uncooperative. R. Alfaro-LeFevre, RN.
   b. 5/8 Patient seems confused. R. Alfaro-LeFevre, RN.
5. Pretend you wrote the nurse's note below on the wrong chart. Correct it using an accepted method for correcting charting errors.

   5/8 N/G tube draining light green drainage.

Giving Report (Shift Hand-off)

Just as with getting change-of-shift (hand-off) reports, the reports you give should be accurate, factual, and organized. What you say and how you say it can make a big difference in the quality of care that your patient receives. The following guidelines are presented to help you establish good habits for giving report.

Guidelines: Giving Report (Shift Hand-off)

❏ **Follow policies and procedures and apply the same rules of *getting report to giving report*** (review *Preparing for Report and Giving Report* beginning on page 184).
❏ **Be specific.** Avoid vague terms.

E x a m p l e
Right: "Mrs. Wu has had an increase in her respiratory rate to 32/min. Her heart rate is up to 122, and her temperature is 101°F."
Wrong: "Mrs. Wu seems to be having respiratory difficulty."
Right: "I gave Mrs. Wu 8 mg of morphine IM at 5:10 pm for incisional pain."
Wrong: "I gave Mrs. Wu a pain med around 5 pm."

❏ **If you make an inference, back it up with evidence** (eg, "Seems upset with her husband—crying and saying that he doesn't support her.").
❏ **Describe the status of all invasive lines** (eg, IV lines, Foley catheters, nasogastric tubes).
❏ **Stress abnormal findings** (eg, rales in the lungs, abnormal vital signs) and variations from routines (eg, "This patient won't be medicated before surgery.").

Keeping the Plan Up-to-Date and Evaluating Your Day

Although the next chapter gives specific guidelines for evaluation, it's important to point out here that early on, during Implementation, you should be reflecting on how things are going, monitoring progress, and updating the plan as needed. Take time to reflect on how your day has gone, think about what you can do to reduce stress and improve your efficiency. Remember the following standards.

ANA Professional Performance Standards Related to Evaluating Care and Personal Performance[1]

Quality of care: The nurse systematically evaluates the quality and effectiveness of nursing practice.
Performance appraisal: The nurse evaluates [her or his] own nursing practice in relation to professional practice standards and relevant statutes and regulations.

Box 5.3 shows the type of questions you should be asking on a daily basis to make sure the plan of care is kept up-to-date. Box 5.4 (next page) lists questions to ask yourself to evaluate your workday.

---

box 5.3 Determining If the Plan of Care Is Up to Date

❏ Does your patient still exhibit the problems identified on the plan?
❏ Does your patient have problems that *aren't* addressed on the plan of care but that may impede progress to outcome achievement?
❏ Are the expected outcomes still realistic?
❏ Are the interventions still relevant?

---

box 5.4 Evaluating Your Workday

Ask yourself:

- ❏ How has the day gone in general?
- ❏ Have I completed everything I should have?
- ❏ Have I identified my learning needs (should I be looking up information or getting advice from a more experienced nurse)?
- ❏ Have I been organized and able to set priorities well?
- ❏ What factors are influencing how I set priorities and organize my day?
- ❏ How much time am I spending performing collaborative nursing interventions?
- ❏ How much time am I spending implementing independent nursing interventions?
- ❏ Could I be doing more? Am I trying to do too much?
- ❏ Am I acting in a collegial way? Have I been clear and specific when delegating actions and communicating with others?
- ❏ Am I including patients and families as partners in care?
- ❏ How would my patients evaluate me in relation to meeting their specific needs?
- ❏ What changes should I make tomorrow?

 voices

When I'm under stress, I take the advice of flight attendants: Put your own oxygen mask on first.

—*Randy Pausch,*
Author of The Last Lecture

Do Your Best and Leave the Rest
Too many of us burn ourselves out trying to do it all. I know I can't do all "little things" that I'd like to do. On the way home from work, I remind myself, "Do your best and leave the rest."

—*Jeanne Regn, RN,*
Staff Nurse (personal communication, 2008)

THIS CHAPTER AND NCLEX*

- ❏ Expect case scenario questions that ask you about delegation (what should you delegate, to whom, and when?) and prioritization (what should you do *first?*). For setting priorities, see pages 185–188. For delegation, see pages 188–191.
- ❏ When asked questions on performing interventions, remember "Assess, Re-assess, Revise, Record" as described in rule on page 184.
- ❏ Expect pharmacology questions that address patients rights related to drug administration (see *Think About It* on page 194).

- ❏ Remember patient safety standards—review the rules on pages 187 and 193.
- ❏ To answer questions about what to chart on the patient record, see the memory-jogs on page 200 and apply the principles of effective charting on page 197.
- ❏ See also "This Chapter and NCLEX" on pages 42, 87, 137, 177, and 221.

*The author acknowledges the help of Deanne Blach (www.deanneblach.com) and Judith Miller (www.judymillernclexreview.com) in developing NCLEX tips.

SUMMARY / KEY POINTS

- Whereas the last chapter focused mostly on developing and recording an initial plan of care, this chapter talks about how to *put the plan into action.* Page 183 shows a diagram of how *Implementation* is a like "a bridge" between *Planning* and *Evaluation.*

- *Implementation* requires you to put the plan into action with an active, open mind—a mind that's constantly assessing and reassessing both patient responses and your own performance.

- Human responses are unpredictable. Monitor them carefully—be flexible and change approaches as needed in a timely way. Record changes you make in the chart and on the plan of care.

- Be sure you know how to delegate effectively (pages 188–190).

- Knowing how to set daily priorities and develop positive relationships with patients, families, and peers is key to *Implementation.*

- Learning to chart effectively comes with practice and experience. *Always* follow policies and procedures for communicating care (charting and giving Hand-off reports).

- Avoid the dumping syndrome (dumping data into a computer and forgetting about it). Unless you reflect on what you chart—to identify patterns, consider the big picture, and identify things you may have missed—you're not thinking critically.

- An important part of *Implementation* is evaluating how your own day went and determining ways you can be more organized and less stressed.

- Scan this chapter for important rules, maps, and diagrams highlighted throughout, then compare where you stand in relation to the expected learning outcomes on page 181.

Date and Time	Problems and Diagnoses	Nursing Assessments and Comments
5/8/09 0800	#1 *Risk for Ineffective Airway Clearance related to thick secretions* #2 *Risk for Fluid Volume Deficit related to poor fluid intake*	Coughing up thick white mucus. He does this well, but needs to be reminded to work at it. Lungs have a few scattered rhonchi at both bases. Fluids encouraged, he does drink juices well. Apple juice on ice kept at bedside. _____ H. Laird, RN
1000		OOB to chair for 1/2 hour. States he feels very fatigued, but he is steady on his feet. Voided lge amount clear yellow urine. Allowed to rest before pulmonary function test. _____ H. Laird, RN
1100		To special studies via wheelchair for pulmonary function. _____ H. Laird, RN
1230		Returned via wheelchair. Assisted back to bed. Ate all of his lunch; said it was the first time he's been hungry. _____ H. Laird, RN

FIGURE 5.2 Examples of source-oriented narrative nurse's notes.

Date	Focus	Progress Notes
5/8		
07:00	Wound care	D—States he's changed his mind about having wife do wound care at home. Says he wants to be self-sufficient and do own wound care.
		A—Encouraged him to view wound care video today.
		R—Requested to view video after AM care.
		A—Given video for afternoon viewing.
		T. Patterson, RN

FIGURE **5.3** Examples of focus charting, using DARA to stand for data, action, response, action.

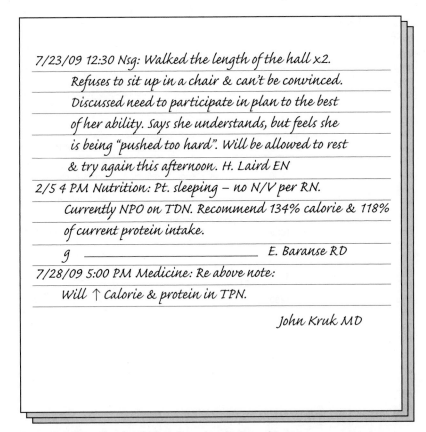

7/23/09 12:30 Nsg: Walked the length of the hall x2. Refuses to sit up in a chair & can't be convinced. Discussed need to participate in plan to the best of her ability. Says she understands, but feels she is being "pushed too hard". Will be allowed to rest & try again this afternoon. H. Laird EN

2/5 4 PM Nutrition: Pt. sleeping – no N/V per RN. Currently NPO on TDN. Recommend 134% calorie & 118% of current protein intake.

g E. Baranse RD

7/28/09 5:00 PM Medicine: Re above note: Will ↑ Calorie & protein in TPN.

John Kruk MD

FIGURE **5.4** Example of multidisciplinary handwritten charting.

FLOWSHEET: ABDOMINAL ASSESSMENT*						
Date/Time	8/8 7am	8/8 7pm	8/9 7am	8/9 7pm	8/10 7am	8/10 7pm
Abdominal girth Signs/symptoms	48" Pain at +3 feels bloated	52" NC	48" Pain at +2 Bloated	46" Pain at +2 Bloated	44" Pain free Bloated but less so	
Bowel sounds	Absent	NC	Distant	Distant	↑ activity	
N/G drainage	Small amt green	NC	NC	NC	NC	
Bowel movement	None	NC	NC	Passed gas	↑ passing gas	
RN Initials	RAL	DL	RAL	DL	RAL	

* If there is no change in finding chart "nc."

FIGURE 5.5 Example of flowsheet charting.

NORMAL INFANT ASSESSMENT PARAMETERS

NOTE: Normal findings for head-to-toe assessment are listed below. If your assessment of the infant yields data that match listed normal assessment parameters, place a check mark(√) and your initials to the right of the box. If assessment findings *vary* from listed normals, place an asterisk (*) in the box, mark your initials to the right of the box, and explain variance in the nurse's notes. Do NOT initial unless you have carefully assessed each area and compared it with the normal parameters.

HEAD: Soft, level, fontanelles; sutures approximated; normal hair; no infections, lice, lesions, cuts or bruises. ☐

EENT: PERLA. Focuses appropriately. Responds appropriately to voices. No ear pulling or drainage; TM's pearly and external canals clear. Nares patent without discharge. Mouth and throat without lesions. Moist, pink mucous membranes. Trachea midline and neck supple. Gag reflex present; normal swallowing & sucking. No lymphadenopathy. ☐

RESP: Rate normal for age. Breath sounds vesicular throughout lungs and bronchial over major airways without adventitious sounds. No nasal flaring or retractions. No cough. ☐

CARDIOVASCULAR: Regular heart rate within normal range for age. No extra heart sounds. Bilateral peripheral pulses satisfactory. No cyanosis (lips and nail beds). No edema, rapid capillary refill. ☐

SKIN: Skin warm, dry, & intact. Normal turgor. No red areas, rashes, bruises, lesions, lumps, or lacerations. Moist, pink mucous membranes. ☐

GI: Abdomen soft and non-tender with bowel sounds in all 4 quadrants. No hernias. tolerates diet. No nausea or vomiting. BM's normal (pattern, consistency, color). ☐

(See page two for neurological, orthopedic, and urologic parameters)

Nurse Signature: _____ Date: _____ Time: _____

FIGURE **5.6** Example nursing database showing normal infant assessment parameters, with directions for charting by exception (CBE).

ANTICOAGULANT TEACHING RECORD

Name: John Roch   **Age:** 75   **Diagnosis:** Chronic Atrial Fib

Primary care manager at home: Self   **Drug name:** Coumadin

	Teaching Done				Outcome Met
Note: Encourage patient to refer to patient information handouts, rather than trying to memorize. Give patient a blank copy of this page on first day of teaching and a copy of completed form at discharge.					
Expected outcomes:					
By _7/11_ , **you should be able to:**					
1. Produce a folder of teaching handouts to keep for reference, and identify where this folder will be kept at home.	7/7 RA	7/9 DL	—		7/9 DL
2. Explain why anticoagulant medication and close monitoring of anticoagulant blood level is essential.	7/7 RA	7/9 DL	—		7/9 DL
3. Relate when and where to go for first appointment for blood work (PT, INR)	7/7 RA	7/9 DL	—		7/9 DL
4. Describe: ❏ drug, action, and how dose will be determined ❏ drugs that may affect dosage (eg, ASA, NSAIDS, Vit K) ❏ foods that may affect dosage and must be avoided ❏ how to assess for unusual bleeding ❏ how to avoid injury or bruising (eg, using electric razor) ❏ how to treat cuts and bruise to minimize bleeding and injury ❏ the importance of reporting persistent headache	7/7 RA	7/9 DL	—		7/9 DL
5. Explain the need to report: ❏ unusual bleeding or bruising. ❏ to all doctors and dentists that anticoagulant is being taken.	7/7 RA	7/7 DL	—		7/9 DL
6. Carry a medic alert card or jewelry stating anticoagulant name.	7/7 RA	7/9 DL			

Comments/Progress Notes:

7/7 Teaching initiated pre-op. Uses handouts well RA
7/9 Waiting for medic alert ID. DL

Patient Signature _____ Discharge Nurse's Signature _____

FIGURE 5.7 Example addendum sheet charting showing patient teaching.

References

1. American Nurses Association. (2004). *Nursing scope and standards of performance and standards of clinical practice.* Washington, DC: American Nurses Publishing.
2. Haig, K., Sutton, S., & Whittington, J. (2006). SBAR: A shared mental model for improving communication between clinicians. *Journal of Quality and Patient Safety, 32*(3), 167–175. Retrieved April 22, 2008, from http://www.jcipatientsafety.org/fpdf/psp/SBAR.pdf
3. Caruso, E. (2007). The evolution of nurse-to-nurse bedside report on a medical-surgical cardiology unit. *MEDSURG Nursing, 16*(1), 18–22.
4. Hansten, R. (2008). Listserv posting.
5. The Joint Commission. (2008). *National safety goals.* Retrieved April 18, 2008, from http://www.jointcommission.org/PatientSafety/NationalPatientSafetyGoals/08_hap_npsgs.htm
6. Hansten, R.., & Jackson, M. (in press). *Clinical delegation skills: A handbook for professional practice* (4th ed.). Sudbury, MA: Jones and Bartlett Publishers.
7. Alfaro-LeFevre, R. (2008). *Critical thinking indicators: Evidence-based version.* Retrieved April 26, 2008, from http://www.alfaroteachsmart.com/cti.htm
8. Alfaro-LeFevre, R. (2009). *Critical thinking and clinical judgment: A practical approach to outcome-focused thinking* (4th ed.). Philadelphia: Saunders-Elsevier.
9. MSN Groups. (n.d.). *Side effects: Restraint and seclusion* [Web page]. Retrieved April 26, 2008, from http://groups.msn.com/SIDEEFFECTS/restraint.msnw
10. Yellowlees, P., Marks, S., Hogarth, M., & Turner, S. Standards-based, open-source electronic health record systems: A desirable future for the U.S. health industry. *Telemedicine and e-Health, 14*(3), 284–288.

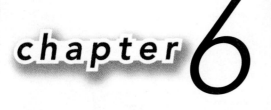

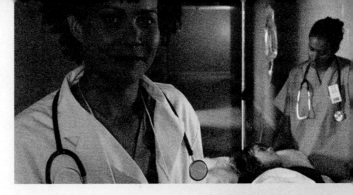

chapter 6

Evaluation

what's in this chapter?

Whereas Chapter 5 stressed the importance of doing *ongoing evaluation* during *Implementation* (assessing and re-assessing patients to monitor initial responses to care), here you learn how to do comprehensive evaluation that helps you decide whether the patient is ready for discharge. You also explore your responsibilities related to participating in quality improvement (QI) and Evidence-Based Practice (EBP) studies, as addressed by Institute of Medicine (IOM) core competencies. Finally, you gain insight into the importance of improving quality by studying outcomes (results), process (how you got the results), and structure (the setting, or environment) in which you got the results.

ANA standards related to this chapter[1]

Standard 7 Evaluation. The registered nurse evaluates progress toward attainment of outcomes.

critical thinking exercises

■ **Critical Thinking Exercise XIV** Determining Outcome Achievement, Identifying Variables Affecting Achievement, and Deciding Whether to Discharge the Patient

■ **Critical Thinking Exercise XV** Quality Improvement and Error Prevention

expected learning outcomes

After studying this chapter, you should be able to:

- Determine where your patients stand in relation to outcome achievement.
- Describe the steps involved in a comprehensive evaluation of an individual plan of care.
- Evaluate your patients to decide whether they're ready for discharge or whether you need to continue or revise the plan.
- Discuss the relationship between patient outcomes and how health care systems interact with one another.
- Explain why it's important to do all three types of evaluation studies—outcome, process, and structure—to improve care quality.
- Describe your four main responsibilities related to quality improvement (QI).
- Identify ways you can prevent errors and promote consumer satisfaction.
- Participate in research and evidence-based practice studies to improve care quality.

Critical Evaluation: Key to Excellence in Nursing

Evaluation and the Other Steps in the Nursing Process

Evaluating an Individual Plan of Care

Guidelines: Determining Outcome Achievement

Identifying Variables (Factors) Affecting Outcome Achievement

Deciding Whether to Discharge the Patient

Quality Improvement (QI)
Evidence-Based Practice
Consumer Satisfaction: Maximizing Value
Health Care Systems Interact and Affect Outcomes
Three Types of Evaluation: Outcome, Process, and Structure
Staff Nurses' Responsibilities

Preventing Mistakes and Infection Transmission

Critical Evaluation: Key to Excellence in Nursing

Critical evaluation—careful, deliberate, appraisal of various aspects of patient care—is the key to excellence in nursing. It make the difference between care practices that are doomed to repeat errors and care practices that are safe, efficient, and constantly improving.

Most often, you'll be involved in evaluating an individual plan of care. However, you also may be asked to help in another type of evaluation—quality improvement (QI). Quality improvement studies aim to evaluate groups of patients or specific aspects of care to improve care quality for all.

This chapter first looks at how to evaluate an individual plan of care, then it discusses what you need to know from a QI perspective.

Evaluation and the Other Steps in the Nursing Process

The following rule stresses the major relationship between *Evaluation* and *Planning*.

R U L E

Assuming that your diagnoses are accurate and the outcomes you developed are appropriate, the ultimate question to be answered during *Evaluation* is, Has the patient achieved the outcomes determined during *Planning*?

Evaluation involves examining all of the other steps of the nursing process, as shown in the following map.

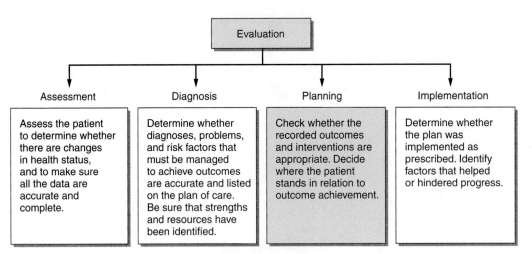

| Evaluation | | | |

Assessment	Diagnosis	Planning	Implementation
Assess the patient to determine whether there are changes in health status, and to make sure all the data are accurate and complete.	Determine whether diagnoses, problems, and risk factors that must be managed to achieve outcomes are accurate and listed on the plan of care. Be sure that strengths and resources have been identified.	Check whether the recorded outcomes and interventions are appropriate. Decide where the patient stands in relation to outcome achievement.	Determine whether the plan was implemented as prescribed. Identify factors that helped or hindered progress.

Evaluating an Individual Plan of Care

In context of evaluating an individual plan of care, *Evaluation* involves the following:

Evaluation

- Determining outcome achievement
- Identifying variables (factors) affecting outcome achievement
- Deciding whether to discharge the patient, to continue, or to change the plan

The following are suggested guidelines for evaluating outcome achievement.

Guidelines: Determining Outcome Achievement

❏ Assess the patient to determine current health status and readiness to test for outcome achievement.

❏ List the outcomes set forth in *Planning.*

E x a m p l e
Will walk unassisted with crutches the length of the hall by 7/3.

❏ Compare what the person is able to do in relation to the outcomes.

E x a m p l e
Can walk unassisted the length of the hall, but becomes unsteady toward the end of the hall.

❏ Decide the extent of outcome achievement by answering the following questions:
- Have the outcomes been completely met?
- Have the outcomes been partially met?
- Have the outcomes not at all been met?

❏ Record your findings on the patient or client record (progress notes, plan of care).

Identifying Variables (Factors) Affecting Outcome Achievement

Identifying the variables (factors) affecting outcome achievement means deciding what things influenced your patient's ability to get the desired results. This requires doing an in-depth patient assessment, analyzing the patient' chart, and involving the patient, family, and key caregivers to answer the following questions:

❏ To what level was the patient included in determining expected outcomes and fine-tuning interventions?

❏ Were the outcomes and interventions realistic and appropriate for this individual?

❏ Were the interventions consistently implemented as prescribed?

❏ Were problems and risks identified and managed *early?*

❏ What's the patient's opinion concerning outcome achievement and the plan of care?

❏ What factors impeded progress?

❏ What factors enhanced progress?

❏ Have we applied the most up-to-date evidence-based practice strategies?

Deciding Whether to Discharge the Patient

The final step is deciding whether to discharge the patient, to continue the plan as is, or to change it, incorporating new approaches that are more likely to succeed:

❑ **Continue the plan** if the person hasn't achieved outcomes, but you simply need more time.

❑ **Change the plan** when the person hasn't achieved outcomes and you've identified new problems or risks that need managing, or if you've identified more efficient interventions.

❑ **Terminate the plan and discharge the person** if he has achieved outcomes, has no new problems or risk factors that must be managed, and is able to manage his own care.

Box 6.1 gives steps for terminating the plan.

---

box 6.1 Steps for Terminating the Plan of Care

1. Ask the patient and family how health care will be managed at home (see Box 4.4, page 156, for the types of questions to ask for discharge).
2. Give verbal and written instructions for:
   ❑ Treatments, medications, activities, diet
   ❑ What signs and symptoms to report (when to call the doctor)
   ❑ How to reach relevant community resources
3. Ask the person to repeat (or show you) what has been learned (notes or instructions may be used to jog memory).
4. If the person (or caregiver) demonstrates knowledge of how to manage health care at home, terminate the plan and discharge the patient according to facility policy.

CRITICAL THINKING EXERCISE XIV

Determining Outcome Achievement, Identifying Variables Affecting Achievement, and Deciding Whether to Discharge the Patient

To complete this session, read pages 212–214. Example responses can be found on pages 245–246.

Part I

For each number below, compare the outcome criteria with the listed observable patient data. Put an "A" in the margin if the outcome has been achieved. Put a "P" if the outcome has only been partially met. Put an "N" if the outcome has not been met.

1. Outcome: Will demonstrate self-injection of insulin using aseptic technique.
   Observable data: Able to give actual injection well, but I had to first point out she had contaminated the needle without noticing it.

2. Outcome: Will demonstrate safe walking with crutches, including climbing and descending stairs.
   Observable data: Demonstrates ability to use crutches for walking, climbing, and descending without problems.
3. Outcome: Will relate the effect of increased exercise on insulin demand.
   Observable data: States that insulin demand is not affected by increased exercise.
4. Outcome: Will maintain skin free from signs of irritation.
   Observable data: Skin is intact with some reddened areas noted on both elbows.
5. Outcome: Will list the signs and symptoms of infection.
   Observable data: Lists pain, swelling, and drainage.

Part II

❑ How do you know whether to terminate, continue, or change the plan? (3 sentences)

Quality Improvement (QI)

The concept of QI is based on the philosophy that improving the quality of health care is a never-ending process—what's considered acceptable quality today may be substandard tomorrow, especially if you consider modern advances such as diagnostic and treatment modalities, electronic information management, and communication methods.

> **R U L E**
>
> At a basic level, QI studies aim to answer the question, "How can we apply the most up-to-date evidence to improve outcomes from a cost, quality-of-life, and consumer-satisfaction perspective?"

Evidence-Based Practice

Evidence-based practice (EBP)—moving from traditional approaches ("we do it this way because we've always done it this way") to evidence-based approaches ("we do it this way because the most up-to-date studies support that this is the best way to do it") is the cornerstone of quality improvement.[2] Think about the implications of the following example:

E x a m p l e
Traditionally, we have taught that mouth care must be done for hygiene and to prevent problems in the mouth. Research shows that poor mouth care can result in microbes colonizing the oropharynx. This colonization is a critical factor in the development of nosocomial (hospital-acquired) pneumonia. Evidence tells us that if we don't follow strict guidelines for giving oral hygiene, we put patients at risk for deadly *pneumonia*.[3]

Keep in mind that EBP means more than simply "applying research." It means integrating the *best research* with *expert opinions* and *patient values* to achieve the best outcomes.[4] Institute of Medicine (IOM) Core Competencies* stress that you must be able to participate in learning and research activities as much as feasible.[5] While you may not have the knowledge to do research projects, this chapter helps you to determine what contributions you can make toward research, QI, and EBP.

Learn More About Evidence-Based Practice. Visit the web sites below.

- **Agency for Healthcare Research and Quality (AHRQ),** the lead Federal agency charged with translating research findings to improve the quality, safety, efficiency, and effectiveness of clinical practices: www.ahrq.gov
- **The Academic Center for Evidence-Based Practice (ACE),** a university based center aiming to advance cutting-edge, state-of-the-art evidence-based practice, research, and education within an interdisciplinary context: http://www.acestar.uthscsa.edu/

voices

Rapid Response Teams Improve Care Quality and Patient Safety
"A review of the literature and our experience reveals that there are three main systemic issues that contribute to problems with safety and care quality: (1) Failures in planning (includes assessments, treatments, goals). (2) Failure to communicate (patient to staff, staff to staff, staff to physician, etc.). (3) Failure to recognize deteriorating patient condition

The Rapid Response Team—known by some as the Medical Emergency Team—is a team of clinicians who bring critical care expertise to the bedside (before the patient begins a downward spiral into a respirator or cardiac arrest). Simply put, the purpose of the Rapid Response Team is to bring critical care expertise to the patient's bedside (or wherever it's needed)."[6]
—*The Institute for Health Care Improvement*

Consumer Satisfaction: Maximizing Value

Evaluation gives us the feedback needed to assess consumer satisfaction and maximize the value of health care delivery. To improve and succeed as health care providers, we must consider both the needs and wants of consumers. Consider Box 6.2, which shows the types of outcomes to study to evaluate consumer satisfaction and demonstrate nurses' value.

Health Care Systems Interact and Affect Outcomes

To identify strategies to manage problems and achieve the best patient outcomes, you must look at how health care delivery systems are organized and how they all come together to affect patient care and outcomes. For example, if you work on a unit that

---

*For more information on the IOM go to http://www.iom.edu

> **box 6.2** Improving Care and Maximizing Value
>
> To improve care and maximize value, gathering, analyzing, and reporting data on the following health status outcomes is critical.
>
> ❑ **Quality of life:** Sense of well-being, whether depression is present, success of pain management.
>
> ❑ **Functional status:** Ability to work, be independent, and do favorite activities.
>
> ❑ **Patient satisfaction:** Convenience, efficiency, and cost of care; sense that staff is attentive and sees each person as an individual.
>
> ❑ **Compliance measures:** Things done to help patients comply with treatment plan.
>
> ❑ **Impact of educational interventions:** Ability to manage own care after teaching has been done.

has problems with delivery of linens, the worst situation these may create is not necessarily patients who are unhappy about their bedding. The worst problem may be wasted nursing time, as nurses spend their valuable time trying to find (or borrow) linens. Valuable nursing time is lost, and things that need to be done by nurses are omitted or done in a hurried way.

> **R U L E**
>
> **Patient outcomes—whether or not patients fare well—are greatly affected by how care delivery systems interact with one another.** For example, patients are directly affected by whether the dietary, pharmacy, and nursing departments come together to give essential nourishment and treatments in a timely way.

Three Types of Evaluation: Outcome, Process, and Structure

To ensure thorough monitoring of health care practices, QI studies consider three types of evaluation:

1. **Outcome Evaluation:** Studies the results, or outcomes of care (eg, Were outcomes achieved? Are people satisfied with care?).
2. **Process Evaluation:** Studies how the care was given (eg, Were assessments and interventions performed consistently and in a timely way?).
3. **Structure Evaluation:** Studies the setting in which the care takes place (eg, Were the physical environment, staffing patterns, and organization communication practices adequate for efficient care management?). Considering all three types of evaluation—outcome, process, and structure—provides a comprehensive examination of care management.

Box 6.3 (next page) shows example questions for all three types of studies.

Staff Nurses' Responsibilities

Staff nurses are accountable for participating in QI (most often for collecting data and tracking outcomes). Although QI studies may seem long and complicated, they're the

box 6.3 Examples of Questions to Ask for Three Types of QI Studies

❑ **Outcome Evaluation (focus on results):** How many of our patients undergoing emergency bowel surgery experience an infection severe enough to delay discharge?
❑ **Process Evaluation (focus on how care was given):** At what point was each of our patients undergoing emergency bowel surgery first given antibiotics?
❑ **Structure Evaluation (focus on setting):** In what setting were antibiotics given to each of our patients undergoing emergency bowel surgery (eg, emergency department, operating room, medical–surgical floor)?

voices

The significant problems we face today cannot be solved at the same level of thinking we were at when we created them.

—*Albert Einstein*

key to making your job more efficient and may make your next experience as a patient (or your family's next experience as a patient) better.

As a bedside nurse, you can make a valuable contribution to QI:

❑ **Get involved and think analytically about your practice.** As a nurse, you spend the most time with patients. If you see human problems or problems with hospital policies or procedures, report them to your supervisor.
❑ **Remember that how you document is important.** The records you create through ongoing documentation provide the basis for research that can benefit both health care consumers and nurses. If you're asked to do extra documentation for the purpose of these studies, realize that the information gained from the records is essential to improving quality.
❑ **Work on your own personal improvement.** Constantly reflect on how you can be more organized and prepared to meet your patients' needs. Be creative—think of ways you can overcome your limitations (eg, I developed the personal worksheet on page 186 to overcome my problem with getting organized during report; many nurses carry with them little notes and references that help them remember certain information).

Learn About How Nurses' Impact on Patient Outcomes. Explore the web page of National Database of Nursing Quality Indicators (NDNQI)®, a repository for nursing-sensitive indicators (http://nursingworld.org/MainMenuCategories/ThePracticeof ProfessionalNursing/PatientSafetyQuality/NDNQI/NDNQI_1.aspx). Here you find data that link nursing care and patient outcomes.

voices

Holistic and Complementary Therapies Improve Outcomes
Improving quality means considering all aspects of health care, including considering whether holistic and complementary therapies can improve results and reduce the need for treatments such as medications. For example, music therapy has been used to help children with cerebral palsy improve balance, to help stroke survivors learn how to walk again, and to help women in labor feel less pain. Music therapy can make the difference between withdrawal and awareness, between isolation and interaction, between chronic pain and comfort—between demoralization and dignity.[7]
—*American Music Therapy Association*

Preventing Mistakes and Infection Transmission

As we continue to make patient safety top priority, you can expect more QI studies to focus on how we can reduce risks of errors and infections. Be sure you follow policies for preventing infection transmission—especially hand-hygiene procedures. Realize that all cases of unanticipated death or major permanent loss of function associated with a hospital-acquired infection will be handled as major errors that qualify as sentinel events (Box 6.4).

---

box 6.4 Descriptions of Sentinel Event, Near Miss,
and Hazardous Condition

❑ **Sentinel event.** An unexpected incident that involves death or serious physical or psychological injury or the risk thereof. *Serious injury* specifically includes loss of limb or function. The phrase "or the risk thereof" means any variation from the usual process of care; that if it happens again, there is a significant chance of causing a serious adverse outcome. For example, a break in procedures that causes nurses to omit checking that the correct leg is marked for amputation and the wrong leg is removed. The term *sentinel* is used because of its relationship to a sentinel guard—a soldier who stands guard to keep his people safe. Sentinel events are so serious that they signal the need for immediate investigation to warrant care and ensure they don't happen again.
❑ **Near miss.** Anything that happens during the process of care that didn't affect the outcome, but for which a reoccurrence carries a significant chance of a serious adverse outcome. For example, if a physician almost operates on the wrong site, but this is caught just in time, it's a near miss. Near misses are considered sentinel events, but they may not be reviewed by the JCAHO under its Sentinel Event Policy.
❑ **Hazardous condition.** Any set of circumstances (exclusive of the disease or condition for which the patient is being treated) which significantly increases the likelihood of a serious adverse outcome.

Data from: http://www.jointcommission.org/SentinelEvents/

As a nurse, you—the one who spends the most time with patients—are in the best position to identify when there are system problems that increase the risk of errors (eg, when there are look-alike or sound-alike drugs). Stay alert for error-prone situations. Take responsibility and report them to your manager. Find ways to build "safety nets" into procedures so that you can catch mistakes early or make sure the big mistakes don't happen. Work collaboratively to prevent mistakes. In important situations, for example when calculating complicated math, ask a colleague to double-check you. Error prevention is *everyone's responsibility.* When mistakes happen, look for the root cause—the main underlying cause or contributing factors. For example, if someone gives a wrong medication, there could be many causes (eg, lack of knowledge, poorly marked bottles, stress from work overload, or fatigue from working overtime). Box 6.5 summarizes three ways to prevent mistakes.

R U L E

Evidence-based practice stresses the importance of keeping patients safe by looking for the root (main) cause of errors. Move from a "culture of blame" (where workers hide mistakes due to fear of punitive actions) to a "culture of safety" (where high priority is given to reporting mistakes, identifying systems that are error-prone, and working together to develop systems that keep patients safe).

---

think about it

Dietary and Housekeeping Are Your Job
Don't allow yourself to fall into the "it's not my job" mentality. If there's a problem that's delaying or compromising patient care—whether it's insufficient linens, meal trays that are consistently late, or transport people who come ill-equipped to take patients for studies—it is your job to be sure that these problems are addressed. Avoid "Band-Aid solutions," ones that are quick fixes only (eg, constantly borrowing linens or taking your time to call the dietary department about the same problem). Rather, report these types of problems to your supervisor so that department leaders can work together to address key issues.

---

box 6.5 Three Ways to Prevent Mistakes

Although studies show that most mistakes result from basic flaws in the way the health system is organized, we all share accountability for ensuring patient safety:

1. Pay attention to things that you're doing that may create risks for errors.
2. Report systems that fail to adequately protect patients (eg, let the risk management department know if you think of a potential change in a policy or procedure that could reduce chances for human error).
3. Empower your patients by teaching them what to expect and letting them know that the main thing they can do to prevent mistakes is to become actively involved in managing their own care.

CRITICAL THINKING EXERCISE XV

Quality Improvement and Error Prevention

To complete this session, read pages 215–220. Example responses are on page 246.

1. In five sentences (or phrases) or less, explain why QI studies are important.
2. Why is it important to consider outcome, process, and structure when performing QI studies?
3. Focusing on at least three different approaches to error prevention, write a personal plan for reducing risks of errors in your nursing practice.
4. What are the differences among a sentinel event, a near-miss, and a hazardous condition?
5. What are your three main responsibilities related to preventing mistakes?

Try This on Your Own

1. Visit http://www.ahrq.gov/, the home page of the Agency for Healthcare Research and Quality, where you can find a wealth of information for consumers (eg, how to quit smoking and assess health plans) and clinicians (eg, practice guidelines and information on outcomes and effectiveness of clinical practices). Pick a few topics that interest you and see what you can learn.
2. Check out the links to Patient Safety Indicators at http://www.qualityindicators.ahrq.gov/
3. With a peer or in a group, discuss: (1) The nursing process summary on the inside front cover; and (2) The implications of the *Voices* in this chapter.

THIS CHAPTER AND NCLEX*

❏ Questions that focus on evaluation are complex and require in-depth analysis and interpretation. Take your time and read keywords carefully to be sure you understand what's being asked. For example, evaluation questions tend to be written something like, "Which comment (behavior) indicates the client understands or does not understand the procedure (or diet or illness?)."

❏ For pharmacology questions, expect to be asked how to evaluate whether the medication has worked (eg, What data would tell you that the antibiotic has achieved the intended therapeutic effect?).

❏ When a question asks about evaluating care, look for an answer that addresses assessing the patient's RESPONSE.

❏ If a procedure is described, think about whether it's is it being done CORRECTLY or INCORRECTLY.

❏ When the stem of the question asks about what further teaching is necessary, this indicates the client has not met the goal.

❏ See also "This Chapter and NCLEX" on pages 42, 87, 137, 177, and 202.

*The author acknowledges the help of Deanne Blach (www.deanneblach.com) and Judith Miller (www.judymillernclexreview.com) in developing NCLEX tips.

SUMMARY / KEY POINTS

- Careful, deliberate, and detailed evaluation of various aspects of patient care is the key to excellence in nursing.
- Evaluation in the context of nursing process usually refers to determining the effectiveness of an individual plan of care (ie, Did the patient achieve the outcomes in a timely, efficient way?).
- Within the context of QI, Evaluation refers to ongoing studies of groups of patients to examine the effectiveness of care delivery practices.
- Comprehensive QI studies evaluate outcomes (results), process (how care was given), and structure (the setting in which care was given).
- Continuous improvement requires examining how health care delivery systems interact and impact on patient outcomes.

- As a nurse, you're in a great position to identify when there are system problems that increase the risk of errors. Stay alert for error-prone situations and report them to your manager.
- You're responsible for improving your own ability to serve patients and for recognizing and reporting problems related to other departments (eg, dietary and pharmacy). Collaborate with peers and others to identify and develop safety nets that prevent errors or catch them early.
- Scan this chapter for important rules, maps, and diagrams highlighted throughout, then compare where you stand in relation to the expected learning outcomes on page 211.

References

1. American Nurses Association. (2004). *Nursing scope and standards of performance and standards of clinical practice.* Washington, DC: American Nurses Publishing.
2. Alfaro-LeFevre, R. (2009). *Critical thinking and clinical judgment: A practical approach to outcome-focused thinking* (4th ed.). Philadelphia: Saunders-Elsevier.
3. American Association of Critical-Care Nurses. (2006). Practice alert: Oral care in the critically ill. *AACN News,* 23, 1–2. Retrieved April 29, 2008, from http://classic.aacn.org/AACN/aacnnews.nsf/GetArticle/ArticleThree 238.
4. Sackett, D., et al. (2000). *Evidence-based medicine: How to practice and teach EBM.* Edinburgh, Scotland: Churchill, Livingstone.
5. Institute of Medicine. (2003). *Health professions education: A bridge to quality.* Washington DC: Author.
6. Institute for Health Care Improvement. (n.d.) *Establish a Rapid Response Team.* Retrieved April 30, 2008, from http://www.ihi.org/IHI/Topics/CriticalCare/IntensiveCare/Changes/EstablishaRapidResponseTeam.htm
7. American Music Therapy Association. Retrieved April 30, 2008, from the AMTA Web site: http://www.music therapy.org/faqs.html#WHAT_IS_MUSIC_THERAPY.

Nursing Diagnoses

How This Section is Organized. Organized alphabetically, this section is designed to provide you with easy access to basic information about frequently seen diagnoses accepted for clinical testing by the North American Nursing Diagnosis Association International (NANDA-I). This section is divided into three parts:

Part 1. Frequently seen nursing diagnoses. This is an alphabetical list of the diagnoses listed in this section. For listing according to Gordon's Functional Health Patterns, see page 250. For in-depth information on *all* of the diagnoses, see the most up-to-date edition of *Nursing Diagnosis: Definitions and Classifications,* which is updated every 2 years by NANDA-I (www.nanda.org) and *Nursing Diagnosis: Clinical Application to Practice* by Lynda Carpenito-Moyet (LWW.com). Most diagnoses in this section are listed as *actual diagnoses* (eg, *Diarrhea,* rather than *Risk for Diarrhea*). Keep in mind that all the diagnoses in this section may be present as *actual or risk diagnoses.* Occasionally, the diagnosis is listed *only* as a *risk diagnosis* (this is because if the diagnosis were an *actual diagnosis,* it would be a *medical problem*—for example, *Risk for Aspiration* is a common diagnosis that nurses are accountable for managing independently. But if *Risk for Aspiration* becomes *Aspiration,* the diagnosis now needs immediate medical attention by a physician).

Part 2. Description of NANDA-I Taxonomy II domains

Part 3. Quick Reference Guide (starts on page 224). The definitions listed in this section are NANDA-I definitions, unless otherwise stated, with minor adaptation in some cases for clarity. The information listed under the headings Defining Characteristics, Related (Risk) Factors has been adapted from *Nursing Diagnosis: Definitions and* Classifications *2007–2008.**

PART 1. FREQUENTLY SEEN NURSING DIAGNOSES

Activity Intolerance
Airway Clearance, Ineffective
Anxiety
Aspiration, Risk for
Autonomic Dysreflexia
Body Temperature, Risk for Imbalanced
Breastfeeding, Ineffective
Breathing Pattern, Ineffective
Cardiac Output, Decreased
Caregiver Role Strain
Communication, Impaired*
Communication, Impaired Verbal
Confusion, Chronic
Constipation
Coping, Defensive
Coping, Ineffective
Diarrhea
Disuse Syndrome
Falls, Risk for
Family Processes, Altered
Fatigue
Fear
Fluid Volume Deficit

*Added by author; Not on NANDA-I list as of 2008.

Fluid Volume, Excess
Grieving
Growth and Development, Delayed
Health-Seeking Behaviors (Specify)
Health Maintenance, Ineffective
Home Maintenance, Impaired
Hopelessness
Infant Feeding Pattern, Ineffective
Infection, Risk for
Injury, Risk for
Knowledge, Deficit (Specify)
Memory, Impaired
Mobility, Impaired Physical
Nutrition, Imbalanced: Less than Body Requirements
Nutrition, Imbalanced: More than Body Requirements
Oral Mucous Membrane, Impaired
Pain, Acute
Pain, Chronic
Parent–Infant/Child Attachment, Risk for Impaired
Parenting, Impaired
Perioperative Positioning Injury, Risk for
Peripheral Neurovascular Dysfunction, Risk for
Post-Trauma Response
Rape Trauma Syndrome
Self-Care Deficit, Bathing/Hygiene
Self-Care Deficit, Dressing/Grooming
Self-Care Deficit, Feeding
Self-Care Deficit, Toileting
Self-Esteem Disturbance
Self-Mutilation, Risk for
Sexuality Patterns, Ineffective
Skin Integrity, Impaired
Sleep Pattern, Disturbed
Social Isolation
Spiritual Distress
Suicide, Risk for
Swallowing, Impaired
Therapeutic Regimen, Ineffective Management of
Thought Processes, Impaired
Unilateral Neglect
Urinary Incontinence, Stress
Urinary Incontinence, Total
Urinary Incontinence, Urge
Violence, Other-directed, Risk for
Violence, Self-directed, Risk for

PART 2. NANDA-I TAXONOMY II DOMAINS

Domain 1. Health promotion: the awareness of well-being or normality of function and the strategies used to maintain control of and enhancement of that well-being or normality of function

Domain 2. Nutrition: the activities of taking in, assimilating, and using nutrients for the purposes of tissue maintenance, tissue repair, and the production of energy

Domain 3. Elimination: secretion and excretion of waste products from the body

Domain 4. Activity/Rest: the productions, conservation, expenditures, or balance of energy resources

Domain 5. Perception/Cognition: the human information processing system including attention, orientation, sensation, perception, cognition, and comprehension

Domain 6. Self perception: awareness of the self

Domain 7. Role Relationships: the positive and negative connections or associations between persons or groups of persons and the means by which those connections are demonstrated

Domain 8. Sexuality: sexual identity, sexual function, and reproduction

Domain 9. Coping/Stress Tolerance: contending with life events/life processes

Domain 10. Life Principles: principles underlying conduct, thought, and behavior about acts, customs, or institutions viewed as having true or having intrinsic worth (eg, values and beliefs)

Domain 11. Safety/Protection: freedom from danger, physical injury, or immune system damage; preservation from loss; and protections of safety and security

Domain 12. Comfort: sense of mental, physical, or social well-being or ease

Domain 13. Growth/Development: age-appropriate increases in physical dimensions, organ systems, and attainment of developmental milestones

PART 3. QUICK REFERENCE GUIDE

Activity Intolerance

A state in which an individual has insufficient energy to endure or complete required or desired daily activities.

• Defining Characteristics

— *SUBJECTIVE DATA* reported —

Weakness or fatigue, exertional discomfort or dyspnea, reduced ability to perform desired activities

— *OBJECTIVE DATA* observed —

Abnormal heart rate and blood pressure response to activity, electrocardiograph changes reflecting arrhythmias or ischemia.

- **Related (Risk) Factors**

Deconditioned state (bed rest or immobility), generalized weakness, sedentary lifestyle, aging process, disease process (imbalance between oxygen supply and demand, acute or chronic illness), medication side effects

- **Clinical Alert**

Activity Intolerance often is related to compromised respiratory, cardiac, or circulatory function. Report sudden onset of Activity Intolerance immediately.

- **Compare With**

Disuse Syndrome, Fatigue

Airway Clearance, Ineffective

Inability to clear secretions or obstructions from the respiratory tract to maintain a clear airway

- **Defining Characteristics**

— *SUBJECTIVE DATA* reported —

Dyspnea

— *OBJECTIVE DATA* observed —

Diminished breath sounds; orthopnea; adventitious breath sounds (rales, crackles, wheezes); ineffective or absent cough; sputum; cyanosis; difficulty vocalizing; changes in rate, rhythm, or depth of respirations; restlessness

- **Related (Risk) Factors**

Environmental: Smoking, smoke inhalation, second-hand smoke; Obstructed airway: Airway spasm, retained secretions, excessive mucus, artificial airway, foreign body in airway, exudates in alveoli; Physiologic: Neuromuscular impairment, bronchial wall hyperplasia, chronic obstructive lung disease, asthma, allergies

- **Compare With**

Aspiration, Risk for; Breathing Pattern, Ineffective

Anxiety

Uneasiness (mild or intense), the source of which is often nonspecific or unknown to the individual

- **Defining Characteristics**

— *SUBJECTIVE DATA* reported —

Nervousness, tension; inability to relax, concentrate, or make decisions; lack of self-confidence; feelings of uncertainty, helplessness, or inadequacy; insomnia;

somatic discomfort (eg, diarrhea, headache, chest discomfort); changes in eating habits

— *OBJECTIVE DATA* observed —

Restlessness; increased perspiration, pulse rate, and blood pressure; pallor; tremors; extraneous movements; lack of initiative; self-deprecation; poor eye contact

- **Related (Risk) Factors**

Conflict about essential values or life goals; actual or perceived threat to self-concept, role function, security, or usual interaction patterns; situational or maturational crisis (eg, pregnancy, parenting); multiple stressors or demands; sleep deprivation; fear of pain, loneliness, physical or psychological harm; inability to cope with or control situations; loss(es)

- **Clinical Alert**

Sudden onset of anxiety, especially in the elderly, may be an early symptom of hypotension, hypoxemia, sepsis, or coronary disorders. Monitor vital signs carefully.

- **Compare With**

Fear

Aspiration, Risk for

The state in which a person is at risk for entry of gastrointestinal (GI) or oropharyngeal secretions, or solids or fluids into the tracheobronchial passages

- **Risk Factors**

Reduced level of consciousness; depressed cough and gag reflexes; impaired swallowing; presence of tracheostomy or endotracheal tube; incompetent lower esophageal sphincter; increased intragastric pressure; increased gastric residual; decreased GI motility; delayed gastric emptying; GI immaturity (infants); GI tubes; tube feedings; medication administration; situations hindering elevation of upper body; facial, oral, or neck surgery or trauma; wired jaws

- **Compare With**

Airway Clearance, Ineffective; Swallowing, Impaired

Autonomic Dysreflexia

The state in which a person with a spinal cord injury at T7 or above experiences a life-threatening, uninhibited, sympathetic response of the nervous system to a noxious stimulus

- Defining Characteristics

— *SUBJECTIVE DATA* reported —

Headache (a diffuse pain in different portions of the head and not confined to any nerve distribution area), chilling, paresthesia, blurred vision, chest pain, metallic taste, nasal congestion

— *OBJECTIVE DATA* observed —

Individual with spinal cord injury at T7 or above with: paroxysmal hypertension (sudden periodic elevated blood pressure, systolic pressure over 140 mm Hg and diastolic above 90 mm Hg); bradycardia or tachycardia (pulse rate of less than 60 or over 100 beats per minute); diaphoresis or red splotches on skin (above the injury); pallor (below the injury); conjunctival congestion; Horner syndrome (contraction of the pupil, partial ptosis of the eyelid, enophthalmos and sometimes loss of sweating over the affected side of the face); pilomotor reflex (gooseflesh formation when skin is cooled)

- Related (Risk) Factors

Bladder or bowel distention (nonpatent catheter, bladder infection, constipation, impaction); spastic sphincter; acute abdomen, abdominal or thigh skin stimulation; lack of knowledge of prevention

- Clinical Alert

This diagnosis requires immediate corrective measures (eg, raising the head of the bed, removing or correcting factors listed under Related (Risk) Factors). If the condition doesn't respond promptly to initial treatment, emergency treatment with pharmacologic intervention is likely to be required.

Body Temperature, Risk for Imbalanced

The state in which a person is at risk for failure to maintain body temperature within normal range

- Related (Risk) Factors

Extremes of age, extremes of weight, exposure to cold or hot environments, dehydration, inactivity or vigorous activity, medications causing vasoconstriction or vasodilation, impaired metabolic rate, sedation, inappropriate clothing for environmental temperature, illness or trauma affecting temperature regulation, infection

Breastfeeding, Ineffective

The state in which a mother and infant or child experience dissatisfaction or difficulty with the breastfeeding process

- Defining Characteristics

— *SUBJECTIVE DATA* reported —

Unsatisfactory breastfeeding process, inadequate milk supply, persistence of sore nipples beyond first week of breastfeeding

— *OBJECTIVE DATA* observed —

Mother: insufficient emptying of breast, no observable signs of oxytocin release (ie, let-down, or milk ejection, reflex), inadequate milk supply. **Infant:** inability to latch onto breast; arching and crying at the breast; non-sustained suckling; insufficient opportunity for suckling; fussing, crying, and unresponsiveness to comfort measures within the first hour after feeding; weight loss, or failure to gain

- Related (Risk) Factors

Mother: frequent supplemental feedings with artificial nipple, lack of basic breastfeeding knowledge, history of breastfeeding difficulty or failure, interrupted breastfeeding, previous breast surgery, inverted or painful nipples, engorged breasts, maternal diet inadequate in nutrients or fluids, nonsupportive partner or family, maternal anxiety or ambivalence. **Infant:** gestational age less than 34 weeks, structural anomaly, poor sucking reflex

Breathing Pattern, Ineffective

The state in which a person's inhalation or exhalation pattern does not promote adequate ventilation

- Defining Characteristics

— *SUBJECTIVE DATA* reported —

Dyspnea, shortness of breath

— *OBJECTIVE DATA* observed —

Changes in respiratory rate or depth of respirations; changes in pulse rate or rhythm; wheezing; fremitus; cough; nasal flaring; cyanosis; decreased diaphragmatic excursion; assumption of three-point position; use of accessory muscles; orthopnea; abnormal arterial blood gases; reduced vital capacity, forced-end expiratory volume, or oxygen saturation level; splinted or guarded respirations

- **Related (Risk) Factors**

Neuromuscular impairment, obstructive lung disease, restrictive lung disease, musculoskeletal impairment, decreased energy, Fatigue, Anxiety, Acute pain, medication side effects (respiratory depression)

- **Clinical Alert**

Report persistent Ineffective Breathing Pattern not responding to nurse-prescribed interventions immediately. This is especially important if confusion or severe anxiety is present, because both of these are signs of hypoxemia.

- **Compare With**

Activity Intolerance; Airway Clearance, Ineffective

Cardiac Output, Decreased

A state in which the heart is unable to pump blood with enough force to meet the body's metabolic demands

- **Defining Characteristics**

— *SUBJECTIVE DATA* reported —

Fatigue, vertigo, dyspnea, orthopnea

— *OBJECTIVE DATA* observed —

Low blood pressure; rapid heart rate; arrhythmias; angina; jugular vein distention; cyanosis of skin and mucous membranes; dependent edema; oliguria; decreased peripheral pulses; cold, clammy skin; rales; restlessness

- **Related (Risk) Factors**

Cardiac disease, myocardial infarction

- **Author's Note**

The defining characteristics of this problem represent a medical problem rather than a nursing diagnosis.

- **Compare With**

Activity Intolerance

Caregiver Role Strain

The state in which a caregiver perceives difficulty in performing the family caregiver role

- **Defining Characteristics**

— *SUBJECTIVE DATA* reported —

Inadequate resources; difficulty performing caregiving activities; concern regarding outcome for the care receiver; conflict with other role responsibilities; family conflict around issues of providing care; feelings of stress, nervousness, and depression

— *OBJECTIVE DATA* observed —

Reduction in quality of care, increased family discord, long hours of caregiving without time off

- **Related (Risk) Factors**

Care receiver: severity of or prolongation of illness, unpredictable illness course, early discharge from skilled nursing facility, complexity or amount of care needed. **Caregiver:** lack of preparation or experience, impaired physical or mental health, lack of respite or recreation, competing role commitments
Other Factors: inadequate physical environment, family dysfunction

Communication, Impaired

Decreased ability to send or receive messages (ie, has difficulty exchanging thoughts, ideas, or desires)

- **Defining Characteristics**

— *SUBJECTIVE DATA* reported —

Concern about being able to make self understood, or to understand directions, reluctance to speak, difficulty understanding or speaking dominant language

— *OBJECTIVE DATA* observed —

Repetition of questions without apparent understanding of answers; inappropriate (or absent) speech or response; incongruence between verbal and nonverbal messages; stuttering, slurring, word-finding problems; weak or absent voice; confusion; use of sign language

- **Related (Risk) Factors**

Effects of cerebral impairment (expressive or receptive aphasia), hearing or auditory comprehension deficits, decreased ability to speak words, language barriers, lack of privacy, Impaired Thought Processes

- **Compare With**

Communication, Impaired Verbal

Communication, Impaired Verbal

A decreased or absent ability to speak, but the person can understand others.

- Defining Characteristics

    — *OBJECTIVE DATA* observed —

Difficulty with dominant language, speech, or verbalization; does not or cannot speak

- Related (Risk) Factors

Physical barrier (tracheostomy, intubation), anatomic defect (cleft lip or palate), brain injury or disease causing expressive aphasia, psychological barriers (psychosis, fear), language barriers

- Compare With

Communication, Impaired

Confusion, Chronic

Irreversible, long-standing, or progressive deterioration of intellect and personality characterized by decreased ability to interpret environmental stimuli, decreased capacity for intellectual thought processes and manifested by disturbances of memory, orientation, and behavior

- Defining Characteristics

    — *OBJECTIVE DATA* observed —

Clinical evidence of organic impairment, impaired interpretation/response to stimuli, progressive/long-standing cognitive impairment, no change in level of consciousness, impaired socialization, impaired memory (short-term, long-term), impaired personality

- Related (Risk) Factors

Alzheimer disease, Korsakoff psychosis, multi-infarct dementia, cerebral vascular accident, head injury

Constipation

A state in which a person's bowel-elimination pattern is accompanied by difficult or incomplete passage of stool or passage of excessively hard stool

- Defining Characteristics

    — *SUBJECTIVE DATA* reported —

Feeling of rectal pressure or fullness, headache, abdominal pain, back pain, decreased appetite, nausea

    — *OBJECTIVE DATA* observed —

Decreased frequency of stools; hard, formed stools; straining at stool; palpable rectal mass

- Related (Risk) Factors

Bed rest, diet deficient in fluids or roughage, lack of exercise, lack of privacy, laxative dependence, painful defecation, pregnancy, medication side effects, neuromuscular impairment

- Clinical Alert

Chronic constipation may be a sign of bowel cancer. Untreated constipation can lead to fecal impaction and intestinal obstruction.

Coping, Defensive

The state in which a person repeatedly projects falsely positive self-evaluation based on a self-protective pattern that defends against underlying perceived threats to positive self-regard

- Defining Characteristics

    — *OBJECTIVE DATA* observed —

Denial of obvious problems or weaknesses, rationalization, hypersensitivity to criticism, grandiosity, projection of blame or responsibility, superior attitude toward others, difficulty establishing or maintaining relationships, hostile laughter or ridicule of others, difficulty in reality testing perceptions, lack of follow-through or participation in treatment or therapy

- Related (Risk) Factors

Loss of job or ability to work, financial problems, marital problems, failure in school, legal problems, institutionalization, fear, aging

- Compare With

Coping, Ineffective

Coping, Ineffective

Impaired adaptive behaviors and problem-solving abilities in meeting demands and roles of life

- Defining Characteristics

    — *SUBJECTIVE DATA* reported —

Inability to cope or inability to ask for help

— OBJECTIVE DATA observed —

Inability to meet role expectations or solve problems, impaired societal participation, destructive behavior toward self or others, inappropriate use of defense mechanism, change in usual communication patterns, manipulative behavior, high illness or accident rate

• Related (Risk) Factors

Situational or maturational crises, persistent stress, sensory overload, personal vulnerability, poor self-esteem, inadequate or unavailable support system, conflict with values or beliefs

Diarrhea

A state in which a person experiences a change in normal bowel habits characterized by the frequent passage of loose, fluid, unformed stools

• Defining Characteristics

— SUBJECTIVE DATA reported —

Abdominal pain, cramping, urgency

— OBJECTIVE DATA observed —

Loose liquid stools, increased frequency of stools, increased frequency of bowel sounds

• Related (Risk) Factors

Side effects of medications or radiation therapy, tube feedings, inflammatory or malabsorptive disorders, infectious processes, food intolerances, Anxiety

• Clinical Alert

Report excessive or persistent diarrhea, as this should be evaluated medically. This is especially important in young children.

Disuse Syndrome, Risk for

A state in which a person is at risk for deterioration of body systems as the result of musculoskeletal inactivity

• Related (Risk) Factors

Neuromuscular impairment (eg, paralysis, multiple sclerosis), musculoskeletal disorders, mechanical immobilization, prescribed immobilization, severe pain, altered level of consciousness, psychiatric disorders

• Author's Note

This diagnosis is appropriate when interventions are aimed at promoting physiologic and psychosocial integrity and preventing complications of immobility.

Falls, Risk for

Increased susceptibility to falling

• Related (Risk) Factors

Adults: History of falls, wheelchair use, aged 65 or older, lives alone, lower limb prosthesis, use of assistive devices such as canes or walkers, illness (acute or chronic), impaired mobility, diminished mental status, medications (causing dizziness, drowsiness, fatigue, or weakness), alcohol use, nighttime sedative use, restraint use, unfamiliar surroundings, dimly lit room, throw rugs, poorly fitted shoes, no anti-slip material in bathroom. **Children:** Age younger than 2 years old, boys younger than 1 year of age, lack of automobile restraints, lack of gate on stairs, lack of window guard, bed located near window, unattended infant on bed or changing table/sofa, lack of supervision

Family Processes, Altered

The state in which a family that normally functions effectively experiences dysfunction

• Defining Characteristics

— SUBJECTIVE DATA reported —

Family unable to express or accept wide range of feelings, unable to express or accept feelings of members

— OBJECTIVE DATA observed —

Family members: unable to meet physical, emotional, or spiritual needs; unable to relate to each other for mutual growth and maturation; unable to change or deal with traumatic experience constructively; unable to accept help; uninvolved in community activities; rigidity in functions and roles; absence of respect for individuality and autonomy of each other; failure to accomplish current or past developmental tasks; failure to send and receive clear messages; unhealthy decision-making processes; poor communication of family rules, rituals, symbols; perpetuation of family myths; inappropriate level and direction of energy; parents don't demonstrate respect for each other's views on child-rearing practices

- Related (Risk) Factors

Situation transition or crisis, developmental transition or crisis

Fatigue

An overwhelming, sustained sense of exhaustion and decreased capacity for physical and mental work

- Defining Characteristics

— *SUBJECTIVE DATA* reported —

Unremitting and overwhelming lack of energy; inability to maintain usual routines, need for additional energy to accomplish routine tasks; impaired ability to concentrate; decreased libido; disinterest in surroundings or introspection

— *OBJECTIVE DATA* observed —

Emotionally labile or irritable, decreased performance, lethargy or listlessness, increase in physical complaints, accident-prone

- Related (Risk) Factors (Etiology)

Decreased or increased metabolic energy production, overwhelming psychological or emotional demands, increased energy requirements to perform activities of daily living, excessive social or role demands, states of discomfort, altered body chemistry (eg, medications, drug withdrawal, chemotherapy), anemia

Fear

A feeling of dread the source or sources of which are identifiable

- Defining Characteristics

— *SUBJECTIVE DATA* reported —

Apprehension, terror, or panic in response to an identifiable source; insomnia; dry mouth; appetite loss

— *OBJECTIVE DATA* observed —

Aggression; irritability; vigilance; increased blood pressure, pulse, and respirations; increased perspiration, pallor, muscle tension; diarrhea, urinary frequency

- Related (Risk) Factors

Actual or perceived threat of pain, disability, disease, physical or psychological discomfort or harm, inability to control situations or cope effectively; loss (of objects, significant others, capabilities, role function, or independence); lack of knowledge

- Compare With

Anxiety

Fluid Volume Deficit

Decreased intravascular, extracellular, or intracellular fluid: This refers to dehydration—water loss alone without change in sodium.

- Defining Characteristics

— *SUBJECTIVE DATA* reported —

Dry mouth, thirst, weakness

— *OBJECTIVE DATA* observed —

Sudden weight loss except with third spacing; dry skin and mucous membranes; decreased skin turgor, oliguria, concentrated urine; increased body temperature, rapid pulse, decreased pulse volume/pressure; output greater than intake; elevated hematocrit; changes in mental state; decreased blood pressure

- Related (Risk) Factors

Active fluid volume loss, failure of regulatory mechanisms

- Clinical Alert

Report onset of confusion, hypotension, or arrhythmias (may indicate electrolyte imbalance or hypovolemia, which require immediate physician-prescribed interventions).

Author's Note: There is little, if any, difference between this term and the well-studied term *dehydration.*

Fluid Volume Excess

Increased fluid retention

- Defining Characteristics

— *SUBJECTIVE DATA* reported —

Anxiety, shortness of breath, orthopnea, ankle swelling, weight gain

— *OBJECTIVE DATA* observed —

Restlessness; edema; taut, shiny skin; effusion; anasarca; weight gain; intake greater than output; S3 heart sound; pulmonary congestion on chest radiograph; rales (crackles); change in respiratory pattern; change in mental status; decreased hemoglobin and hematocrit; blood pressure changes; central venous pressure changes; pulmonary artery pressure changes; jugular vein distention; positive hepatojugular reflex; oliguria; specific gravity changes; azotemia; imbalanced electrolytes

- Related (Risk) Factors

Compromised regulatory mechanism, excess fluid or sodium intake

- Clinical Alert

Report increasing edema, coughing, or shortness of breath immediately, as this may be a sign of congestive heart failure, which can progress to life-threatening pulmonary edema.

Grieving

The state in which a person or group experiences a normal pattern of extreme feelings of loss and sadness in response to an actual or perceived loss (of an object, relationship, loved one, pet, capability, body part, body function, or job status)

- Defining Characteristics

— *SUBJECTIVE DATA* reported —

During the first year after a loss: sadness in response to loss; guilt; unresolved issues; anger; mood swings; difficulty expressing loss; inability to stop crying, to concentrate, make decisions, or participate in meaningful activities or relationships

— *OBJECTIVE DATA* observed —

During the first year after a loss: idealization of lost object or person; changes in eating habits, activity level, libido, sleep or dream patterns; reliving of past experiences; interference with life functions; regression; labile affect; decreased ability to concentrate or pursue tasks

- Related (Risk) Factors

Actual or perceived loss

Growth and Development, Delayed

The state in which a child's growth or development is below the norm for his or her age group

- Defining Characteristics

— *OBJECTIVE DATA* observed —

Delay or difficulty in performing skills (motor, social, or expressive) typical of age group; altered physical growth; inability to perform self-care or self-control activities appropriate for age; regression in previously acquired skills; flat affect; listlessness; decreased responses

- Related (Risk) Factors

Inadequate caregiving (eg, indifference, neglect, abuse, inconsistent responsiveness, multiple caregivers); separation from significant others; environmental and stimulation deficiencies; physical illness or disability; prescribed dependence

Health Maintenance, Ineffective

Inability to maintain optimum health.

- Defining Characteristics

— *SUBJECTIVE DATA* reported —

History of lack of health-seeking behavior

— *OBJECTIVE DATA* observed —

Lack of knowledge regarding basic health practices; lack of adaptive behaviors to internal or external environmental changes; inability to take responsibility for meeting basic health practices in any or all functional patterns; failure to seek basic health information

- Related (Risk) Factors

Decreased communication skills (written, verbal, nonverbal); inability to make valid judgments; perceptual or cognitive impairment; complete or partial lack of gross or fine motor skills; developmental delay; ineffective coping skills; lack of resources; unavailable or inadequate support system; poor health habits

Home Maintenance, Impaired

The state in which a person or family is unable to maintain a safe, growth-promoting environment independently

- Defining Characteristics

— *SUBJECTIVE DATA* reported —

Difficulty in maintaining home in a comfortable fashion; seeking of assistance with home maintenance; outstanding debts or financial crises; history of accidents

— *OBJECTIVE DATA* observed —

Disorderly surroundings; unwashed or unavailable cooking equipment, clothes, or linen; accumulated dirt, food wastes, or unhygienic wastes; offensive odors; inappropriate household temperature; overtaxed family members (eg, exhausted, anxious); lack of necessary equipment or aids; presence of vermin or rodents; repeated hygienic disorders, infestations, or infections; hazards in the home

- Related (Risk) Factors

Individual or family member disease or injury; insufficient organization or planning; insufficient finances; unfamiliarity with available resources; impaired cognitive or emotional functioning; lack of knowledge, role models, or support systems; young children in home

Hopelessness

A state in which a person sees limited or no alternatives or acceptable choices and is unable to mobilize energy on his or her own behalf

- Defining Characteristics

— *SUBJECTIVE DATA* reported —

Inability to make choices, solve problems, or perform activity; apathy; indifference; decreased appetite

— *OBJECTIVE DATA* observed —

Passive anger, flat affect, sighing, decreased response to stimuli, decreased verbalization, turning away from speaker, closing eyes or shrugging in response to speaker, decreased or increased sleep, lack of initiative, lack of involvement in care or passively allowing care

- Related (Risk) Factors

Prolonged activity restriction creating isolation, failing or deteriorating physiologic condition, long-term stress, abandonment, lost belief in transcendent values or God.

- Compare With

Spiritual Distress

Infant Feeding Pattern, Ineffective

A state in which an infant demonstrates an impaired ability to suck or to coordinate the suck–swallow response

- Defining Characteristics

— *OBJECTIVE DATA* observed —

Inability to initiate or sustain an effective suck; inability to coordinate sucking, swallowing, and breathing; coughing or choking with feeding

- Related (Risk) Factors

Prematurity, neurologic impairment or delay, oral hypersensitivity, prolonged NPO status, anatomic abnormality

Infection, Risk for

The state in which a person is at increased risk for being invaded by pathogenic organisms

- Related (Risk) Factors

Inadequate primary defenses (broken skin, traumatized tissue, decreased ciliary action, stasis of body fluids, change in pH of secretions, altered peristalsis); inadequate secondary defenses (decreased hemoglobin, leukopenia, suppressed inflammatory response); immunosuppression; inadequate acquired immunity; chronic disease; malnutrition; environmental hazards (work, travel); treatment-related hazards (invasive lines or procedures, surgery, medications); extremes of age; Knowledge, Deficit (self-protection); high-risk behaviors (eg, unsafe sex, drug abuse)

Knowledge, Deficit (Specify)

The state in which a person lacks the skills or information to successfully manage his or her own health care

- Defining Characteristics

— *SUBJECTIVE DATA* reported —

Information seeking, dissatisfaction with ability to manage health care, incomplete or inaccurate information related to health care needs, difficulty performing skills

— *OBJECTIVE DATA* observed —

Inaccurate demonstration of skill, behavior inconsistent with instruction, inappropriate or exaggerated behaviors (eg, hysteria, hostility, agitation, apathy)

- Related (Risk) Factors

Cognitive limitation, lack of recall, lack of previous opportunity to learn, misinterpretation of information, lack of interest or motivation, unfamiliarity with information sources, inability to read or lack of access to written information, fear

Memory, Impaired

The state in which an individual experiences the inability to remember or recall bits of information or behavioral skills: Impaired memory may be attributed to pathophysiologic or situational causes that are either temporary or permanent.

- Defining Characteristics

— *SUBJECTIVE DATA* reported —

Reported experiences of forgetting, inability to recall recent or past events

— *OBJECTIVE DATA* observed —

Observed experiences of forgetting, inability to determine if a behavior was performed, inability to learn or retain new skills or information, inability to perform a previously learned skill, inability to recall factual information

- Related (Risk) Factors

Acute or chronic hypoxia, anemia, decreased cardiac output, fluid and electrolyte imbalance, neurologic disturbances, excessive environmental disturbances

Mobility, Impaired Physical

A state in which a person experiences a limitation of ability for independent movement

- Defining Characteristics

— SUBJECTIVE DATA reported —

Reluctance to attempt movement, pain with movement

— OBJECTIVE DATA observed —

Inability to move purposefully (confinement to bed; problems with transfer, ambulation; limited range of motion; decreased muscle strength, control, or mass)

- Related (Risk) Factors

Intolerance to activity or decreased strength and endurance, pain or discomfort, neuromuscular or musculoskeletal impairment, imposed restrictions of movement, medical protocol

- Compare With

Activity Intolerance; Disuse Syndrome, Risk for; Self-Care Deficit

Nutrition, Imbalanced: Less Than Body Requirements

The state in which a person is experiencing an intake of nutrients insufficient to meet metabolic needs

- Defining Characteristics

— SUBJECTIVE DATA reported —

Poor appetite; aversion to eating; lack of interest in food; impaired taste sensation; satiety immediately after ingesting small amount of food; abdominal pain with or without disease; abdominal cramping; frequent purging; perceived inability to ingest food; lack of information, misinformation; misconceptions regarding nutritional requirements

— OBJECTIVE DATA observed —

Food intake calculated to be less than metabolic requirements; body weight 20% below ideal; decreased serum albumin, muscle mass or tone, subcutaneous fat; pale

conjunctival and mucous membranes; excessive hair loss; weight inconsistent with perception of being fat.

- Related (Risk) Factors

Poor appetite, stomatitis, dysphagia, poorly fitting dentures, fad dieting, poor food choices, inability to obtain or prepare food (eg, physical or financial limitations), eating disorders (eg, anorexia nervosa, bulimia), increased metabolic requirements (eg, burns, infection, cancer), absorption disorders (eg, Crohn disease, cystic fibrosis), medication side effects

Nutrition, Imbalanced: More than Body Requirements

The state in which a person is experiencing an intake of nutrients that exceeds metabolic needs

- Defining Characteristics

— SUBJECTIVE DATA reported —

Eating in response to external cues such as time of day, social situation; eating in response to internal cues other than hunger (eg, Anxiety)

— OBJECTIVE DATA observed —

Excessive intake in relation to metabolic need; weight 20% over ideal for height and frame; triceps skin fold greater than 15 mm in men, 25 mm in women; percentage of body fat greater than that recommended based on age and sex; pairing food with other activities; concentrating food intake at end of day.

- Related (Risk) Factors

Obesity in one or both parents; rapid transition across growth percentiles during infancy and childhood; use of solid food as major food source before 5 months of age; use of food as reward or comfort measure; frequent, closely spaced pregnancies; higher baseline weight at beginning of each pregnancy; inadequate exercise or activity patterns; poor dietary habits (eg, snacking, unbalanced meals, high-fat foods); lack of knowledge of nutritional value of food; dysfunctional eating patterns; disease (thyroid problems, diabetes); medication side effects (eg, steroids, birth control pills)

Oral Mucous Membrane, Impaired

Disruptions in the tissue layers of the oral cavity

- Defining Characteristics

— SUBJECTIVE DATA reported —

Oral pain or discomfort

— OBJECTIVE DATA observed —

Coated tongue, stomatitis, lesions or ulcers, leukoplakia, edema, hyperemia, plaque, vesicles, hemorrhagic gingivitis, halitosis

• Related (Risk) Factors

Radiation to head or neck, oral surgery, periodontal disease, chemical irritants (eg, alcohol, tobacco, drugs), dehydration, ill-fitting dentures or braces, carious teeth, presence of endotracheal or nasogastric tube, NPO for more than 24 hours, ineffective oral hygiene, mouth breathing, malnutrition, infection, absent or decreased salivation, medication side effects (chemotherapy, immunosuppressants)

• Clinical Alert

Poor oral hygiene in hospitalized or debilitated people increases the risk of pneumonia.

Pain, Acute

A state in which a person experiences and reports the presence of severe discomfort or an uncomfortable sensation

• Defining Characteristics

— SUBJECTIVE DATA reported —

Description of pain or discomfort

— OBJECTIVE DATA observed —

Guarding or protective behavior; self-focusing; narrowed focus (altered time perception, withdrawal from social contact, impaired thought process); distraction behavior (moaning, crying, pacing, seeking out other people or activities, restlessness); facial mask of pain (eyes lack luster, beaten look, fixed or scattered movement, grimace); impaired muscle tone, autonomic responses (diaphoresis, blood pressure and pulse changes, pupillary dilation, changes in respiratory rate)

• Related (Risk) Factors

Injuring agents (biologic, chemical, physical, psychological), problems with structure or function of organ or systems, drug tolerance

• Clinical Alert

Report new onset of pain or unrelieved pain. Recognize that there are national guidelines for pain management available from the Department of Human Services.

• Compare With

Pain, Chronic

Pain, Chronic

A state in which a person experiences pain that continues for more than 6 months in duration

• Defining Characteristics

— SUBJECTIVE DATA reported —

Pain for more than 6 months; fear of re-injury; impaired ability to continue previous activities; poor appetite; changes in weight, behavior, or sleep patterns; depression; frustration; anger; Hopelessness.

— OBJECTIVE DATA observed —

Behavior changes, facial mask, guarded movement

• Related (Risk) Factors

Chronic physical or psychosocial disability, depression, problems with organ or system structure or function, drug tolerance

• Clinical Alert

People with Chronic Pain may not demonstrate usual autonomic response associated with pain (increased pulse and blood pressure). They may also appear to be pain-free (eg, smiling, laughing); however, this is usually a result of efforts to overcome pain through distraction and should not be considered a sign that the person really isn't in pain.

• Compare With

Acute Pain

Parent–Infant/Child Attachment, Risk for Impaired

A state in which there is a risk for disruption of the interactive process between parent/significant other and infant that fosters the development of a protective and nurturing reciprocal relationship

• Related (Risk) Factors

Inability of parents to meet the personal needs anxiety associated with the parent role, substance abuse, premature infant, ill infant/child who is unable to effectively initiate parental contact due to impaired behavioral organization, separation, physical barriers, lack of privacy

Parenting, Impaired

The state in which parent figure(s) experiences inability to create an environment that promotes the optimum growth and development of a child or children

- Defining Characteristics

— SUBJECTIVE DATA reported —

Inability to control child, disappointment in gender or physical characteristics of child, resentment toward child, disgust at body functions of child, feeling of inadequacy

— OBJECTIVE DATA observed —

Parental abandonment, child abuse or neglect, runaway child, absence of parental attachment, failure to make or keep appointments with health care providers, inattention to needs of child, inappropriate caregiving behaviors, inappropriate or inconsistent disciplinary measures, frequent accidents or illnesses, delay in growth and development of child (children)

- Related (Risk) Factors

Parent figure(s): lack of (or ineffective) role model, physical and psychosocial abuse, lack of support from significant other, unmet social or emotional needs, multiple pregnancies, lack of knowledge, Caregiver Role Strain.

Parent figure(s) or child(ren): actual or perceived threat to physical or emotional survival, unrealistic expectations, introduction of new family member(s) (eg, birth, adoption), mental or physical illness, stress. **Child(ren):** absent or inappropriate response

Parenting, Risk for Impaired

The state in which parent figure(s) is at risk for experiencing inability to create an environment that promotes optimum growth and development of a child or children

- Related (Risk) Factors

See Related (Risk) Factors for Impaired Parenting

Perioperative Positioning Injury, Risk for

A state in which the client is at risk for injury as a result of the environmental conditions found in the perioperative setting

- Related (Risk) Factors

Disorientation, immobilization, muscle weakness, anesthesia, obesity, emaciation, edema

Peripheral Neurovascular Dysfunction, Risk for

A state in which a person is at risk of experiencing a disruption in circulation, sensation, or motion of an extremity.

- Related (Risk) Factors

Fractures, trauma, burns, vascular obstruction, immobilization, orthopedic surgery, mechanical compression (eg, tourniquet, cast, brace, dressing, or restraint)

- Clinical Alert

Report changes from baseline neurovascular assessment findings that don't respond to nurse-prescribed interventions immediately, so that measures can be taken to prevent irreversible neuromuscular damage.

Post-Trauma Response

A sustained, painful emotional response to unexpected, extraordinary life event(s)

- Defining Characteristics

— SUBJECTIVE DATA reported —

Re-experience of the traumatic event that may be identified in cognitive, affective, or sensorimotor activities (eg, flashbacks, intrusive thoughts, repetitive dreams or nightmares, excessive verbalization of the traumatic event, survival guilt or guilt about behavior required for survival); psychic or emotional numbness (impaired interpretation of reality, confusion, dissociation, amnesia, vagueness about traumatic event)

— OBJECTIVE DATA observed —

Altered lifestyle: self-destructiveness, such as substance abuse, suicide attempt, or other acting-out behavior; difficulty with interpersonal relationships; phobia regarding trauma; poor impulse control; irritability and explosiveness; constricted affect

- Related (Risk) Factors

Disasters, wars, epidemics, rape, assault, torture, catastrophic illness, or accident

- Compare With

Rape Trauma Syndrome

Rape Trauma Syndrome

The person experiences an actual or attempted sexual penetration (vaginal, anal, oral) against his or her will or consent, resulting in an acute phase of disorganization of lifestyle and a long-term process of reorganization.

- Defining Characteristics

— *SUBJECTIVE DATA* reported —

Emotional reactions (anger, fear, embarrassment, humiliation, self-blame, desire for revenge); GI symptoms (nausea, vomiting, anorexia); genitourinary discomfort (pain, tenderness); muscle tension; insomnia; nightmares; changes in sexual behavior, relationship with opposite sex, or lifestyle; Anxiety; Fear

— *OBJECTIVE DATA* observed —

Changes in behavior, communication patterns, appearance, or lifestyle; reactivation of previous conditions (physical illness, psychiatric illness, alcohol or drug abuse). Additional data for Silent Reaction: lack of verbalization of the occurrence of rape.

- Related (Risk) Factors

Attempted or actual sexual assault

- Clinical Alert

Referral of this diagnosis to a qualified rape counselor improves outcomes.

Self-Care Deficit, Bathing/Hygiene

A state in which a person experiences an impaired ability to perform or complete bathing or hygiene activities for oneself

- Defining Characteristics

— *OBJECTIVE DATA* observed —

Inability to: wash body parts, obtain (or get to) water, regulate temperature or flow

- Related (Risk) Factors

Decreased mobility, strength, or endurance; pain, discomfort; perceptual, cognitive, neuromuscular, or musculoskeletal impairment; depression; Anxiety (severe); Activity Intolerance

Self-Care Deficit, Feeding*

A state in which a person experiences an impaired ability to perform or complete feeding activities for oneself.

- Defining Characteristics

— *OBJECTIVE DATA* observed —

Inability to bring food from a receptacle to the mouth

- Related (Risk) Factors

Decreased mobility, strength, or endurance; pain, discomfort; perceptual, cognitive; neuromuscular, or musculoskeletal impairment; depression; Anxiety (severe); Activity Intolerance

Self-Care Deficit, Dressing/Grooming*

A state in which a person experiences an impaired ability to perform or complete dressing and grooming activities for oneself

- Defining Characteristics

— *OBJECTIVE DATA* observed —

Impaired ability to: put on or take off necessary items of clothing, obtain or replace articles of clothing, fasten clothing, maintain satisfactory appearance

- Related (Risk) Factors

Decreased mobility, strength, or endurance; pain, discomfort; perceptual, cognitive, neuromuscular, or musculoskeletal impairment; depression; Anxiety (severe); Activity Intolerance

Self-Care Deficit, Toileting

Impaired ability to perform or complete toileting activities for oneself

- Defining Characteristics

— *OBJECTIVE DATA* observed —

Inability to: get to toilet, sit on or rise from toilet, manipulate clothing for toileting, carry out toilet hygiene, flush toilet or empty commode

- Related (Risk) Factors

Decreased mobility, strength, or endurance; pain, discomfort; perceptual, cognitive, neuromuscular, or musculoskeletal impairment; depression; Anxiety (severe); Activity Intolerance.

Self-Esteem Disturbance

Negative evaluation or feelings about self or about personal capabilities

- Defining Characteristics

— *SUBJECTIVE DATA* reported —

Shame or guilt; inability to deal with events; rejection of positive feedback or exaggeration of negative feedback;

hesitance to try new things or situations; lack of success in relationships, work, or other life events; difficulty making decisions

— *OBJECTIVE DATA* observed —

Dependence on others' opinions; poor eye contact; nonassertive, passive, or indecisive behaviors; excessive seeking of reassurance; being overly conforming; self-negating verbalization; difficulty making decisions

• Related (Risk) Factors

Relationships characterized by abuse (verbal, sexual, physical), parental neglect, helplessness

Self-Mutilation, Risk for

A state in which a person is at risk of performing an act upon the self to injure, not kill, which produces tissue damage and tension relief

• Risk Factors

Borderline personality disorder (especially females 16–25 years of age); psychotic state (frequently males in young adulthood); emotionally disturbed or battered children; mentally retarded and autistic children; history of self-injury; history of physical, emotional, or sexual abuse; inability to cope with increased psychological or physiologic tension; feelings of depression, rejection, self-hatred, separation anxiety, guilt, and depersonalization; fluctuating emotions; command hallucinations; need for sensory stimuli; parental or emotional deprivation; dysfunctional family

Sexuality Patterns, Ineffective

The state in which a person experiences, or is at risk for experiencing, a change in sexual patterns

• Defining Characteristics

— *SUBJECTIVE DATA* reported —

Difficulties, limitations, or changes in sexual behaviors or activities

— *OBJECTIVE DATA* observed —

Frequent sex-related questions

• Related (Risk) Factors

Knowledge or skill deficit about alternative responses to health-related transitions, altered body function or structure, illness or medical treatment, lack of privacy, lack of significant other, ineffective or absent role models, conflicts with sexual orientation or variant preferences, fear of pregnancy or of acquiring or transmitting a sexually transmitted disease, impaired relationship with a significant other

Skin Integrity, Impaired

A state in which a person's skin is damaged

• Defining Characteristics

— *SUBJECTIVE DATA* reported —

Itching, pain, numbness

— *OBJECTIVE DATA* observed —

Nonblanchable erythema, denuded skin, destruction of epidermal and dermal skin layers

• Related (Risk) Factors

Personal factors: extremes of age (infants, elderly). **External factors:** extremes of temperature, humidity, chemical substances, secretions or excretions, mechanical factors (shearing forces, pressure, restraints), trauma, radiation, immobilization, drainage, incontinence (stool, urine). **Internal factors:** imbalanced nutrition (obesity, malnutrition); metabolic problems; circulation problems, impaired sensation, skeletal prominence, developmental factors, immunologic deficits, medication side effects, edema, subcutaneous fat loss, decreased skin turgor; dehydration; edema

Sleep Pattern, Disturbed

Disruption of sleep time that causes discomfort or interferes with desired lifestyle

• Defining Characteristics

— *SUBJECTIVE DATA* reported —

Difficulty falling asleep, awakening earlier or later than desired, interrupted sleep, not feeling well-rested

— *OBJECTIVE DATA* observed —

Changes in behavior and performance (eg, increased irritability, restlessness, disorientation, lethargy, listlessness), nystagmus, hand tremor, eyelid ptosis, expressionless face, dark circles under eyes, frequent yawning, changes in posture, thick speech with mispronunciation and incorrect words

• Related (Risk) Factors

Internal sensory alterations: illness, psychological stress **External sensory alterations:** environmental changes, medication side effects, caregiving responsibilities

Social Isolation

The state in which a person experiences loneliness and perceives it as a negative or threatened state imposed by others

- Defining Characteristics

— SUBJECTIVE DATA reported —

Lack of satisfying personal relationships or significant purpose in life, feelings of rejection or being different from others, inability to meet others' expectations, insecurity in public

— OBJECTIVE DATA observed —

Absence of supportive significant other(s); sad, dull affect; communication deficits (eg, language barriers, withdrawal, poor eye contact); hostility in voice or behavior; preoccupation with own thoughts

- Related (Risk) Factors

Delay in accomplishing developmental tasks, immature interests, unusual physical appearance, chronic illness, impaired mental status, unacceptable social values or behavior, inadequate personal resources, absence of peers, inability to engage in satisfying personal relationships

Spiritual Distress

Distress of the human spirit, disruption in the life principle that pervades a person's entire being and integrates and transcends one's biologic and psychosocial nature

- Defining Characteristics

— SUBJECTIVE DATA reported —

Concern with meaning of life, death, or belief systems; anger toward God; seeking to understand meaning of suffering, own existence, or moral or ethical implications of therapeutic regimen; inability to participate in usual religious practices; desire to talk with a chaplain or priest; anger toward religious representatives; nightmares, sleep disturbances

— OBJECTIVE DATA observed —

Altered behavior or mood (eg, anger, crying, withdrawal, preoccupation, Anxiety, hostility, apathy, and so forth), use of gallows humor

- Related (Risk) Factors

Separation from religious or cultural ties, challenged belief and value system (eg, due to moral or ethical implications of therapy or intense suffering)

Suicide, Risk for

At risk for self-inflicted life-threatening injury

- Related (Risk)Factors

Behavioral: History of prior suicide attempt, impulsiveness, buying a gun, stockpiling medicines, making or changing a will, giving away possessions, sudden euphoric recovery from major depression, marked changes in behavior or attitude or school performance, threats of killing oneself, statements of desire to die or "end it all"

Situational: Living alone, retired, relocation, institutionalization, economic instability, loss of autonomy or independence, presence of gun in the home, adolescents living in nontraditional settings (eg, juvenile detention center, prison, halfway house)

Psychological: Family history of suicide, alcohol and substance use/abuse; psychiatric illness or disorder; history of childhood abuse; guilt; gay or lesbian youth

Demographic: Age (elderly, young adult males, adolescents); Race (Caucasian, Native American); Gender (male), widowed or divorced

Physical: chronic or terminal illness or pain

Social: Loss of important relationship, disrupted family life, grief, bereavement, poor support systems, loneliness, hopelessness, helplessness, social isolation, legal or disciplinary problem, cluster suicides

- Clinical Alert

Specifically ask those at risk for suicide whether there is a risk for suicide. Get them to make a promise or contract not to attempt suicide within a specific time frame (eg, "Can you promise me that you will call me if you feel like you might harm yourself before I see you in the morning?").

Swallowing, Impaired

The state in which a person has decreased ability to voluntarily pass fluids or solids from the mouth to the stomach

- Defining Characteristics

— SUBJECTIVE DATA reported —

Difficulty swallowing

— OBJECTIVE DATA observed —

Observed evidence of difficulty in swallowing, stasis or pocketing of food in oral cavity, coughing or choking with swallowing attempts, drooling, evidence of aspiration

- Related (Risk) Factors

Stroke, head injury, neuromuscular impairment (eg, decreased or absent gag reflex, decreased strength or excursion of muscles involved in mastication or swallowing, perceptual impairment, facial paralysis, postcerebrovascular accident); congenital anomalies (cleft palate, tracheoesophageal fistula); mechanical obstruction (eg, edema, tracheostomy tube, tumor); limited awareness; reddened, irritated oropharyngeal cavity; weakness, Fatigue

- Compare With

Aspiration, Risk for

Therapeutic Regimen, Ineffective Management of

A state in which a person has a pattern of regulating and integrating into daily living a program for treatment of illness (and sequelae) that is unsatisfactory for meeting specific health goals

- Defining Characteristics

— *SUBJECTIVE DATA* reported —

Desire to manage the illness and prevent sequelae; difficulty with regulation or integration of prescribed regimens for treatment of illness and its effects, or prevention of complications; report that no actions are being taken to include treatment regimens in daily routines or to reduce risk factors for progression of illness and sequelae

— *OBJECTIVE DATA* observed —

Acceleration or lack of improvement of symptoms, choices of daily living ineffective for meeting the goals of treatment or prevention program

- Related (Risk) Factors

Complexity of health care system or therapeutic regimen, mistrust of regimen or health care personnel, inadequate assistive resources (eg, written schedule to follow regimen, devices to make following regimen easier), economic difficulties, excessive demands on individual or family, family conflict or patterns of health care inconsistent with therapeutic regimen, social support deficits

Thought Processes, Impaired

Disruption in conscious thought, reality orientation, problem solving, judgment, and comprehension

- Defining Characteristics

— *SUBJECTIVE DATA* reported —

Inaccurate interpretation of internal or external stimuli, hallucinations, delusions, phobias, obsessions, Anxiety, Fear

— *OBJECTIVE DATA* observed —

Distractibility, cognitive dissonance, memory deficit, egocentricity, hyper- or hypovigilance, confusion, disorientation

- Related (Risk) Factors

Medication side effects, substance abuse, electrolyte imbalance, depression, dementia, bipolar disorders, borderline personality, multiple demands or stressors, sleep deprivation, sensory bombardment

Unilateral Neglect

The state in which a person is unaware of the hemiplegic side of his or her body, or unaware of objects, persons, or sounds on the hemiplegic side of the body

- Defining Characteristics

— *OBJECTIVE DATA* observed —

Failure to see, hear, or feel stimuli on affected side; failure to purposefully use extremities on affected side; lack of awareness of positioning of extremities on affected side

- Related (Risk) Factors

Effects of stroke, brain tumor, or brain injury (hemianopsia, one-sided blindness, perceptual disturbances)

Urinary Incontinence, Stress

A loss of urine of less than 50 mL occurring with increased abdominal pressure.

- Related (Risk) Factors

Weak pelvic muscles or structural supports associated with age, surgery, or childbirth; high intra-abdominal pressure (eg, obesity, gravid uterus, coughing); incompetent bladder outlet; overdistention between voiding

- Defining Characteristics

— *SUBJECTIVE DATA* reported —

Urinary urgency; urinary incontinence with coughing, sneezing

— OBJECTIVE DATA observed —

Dribbling with increased abdominal pressure, urinary frequency (more often than every 2 hours)

Urinary Incontinence, Total

A continuous and unpredictable loss of urine

• Defining Characteristics

— SUBJECTIVE DATA reported —

Unawareness of bladder filling or incontinence, decreased sensation of perineal area

— OBJECTIVE DATA observed —

Constant flow of urine at unpredictable times without urinary distention, incontinence not responding to treatment

• Related (Risk) Factors

Neuropathy preventing transmission of reflex indicating bladder fullness; neurologic dysfunction causing triggering of micturition at unpredictable times; independent contraction of detrusor reflex due to surgery, trauma, or disease affecting spinal cord nerves; anomaly (fistula)

• Compare With

Urinary Incontinence, Stress; Urinary Incontinence, Urge

Urinary Incontinence, Urge

Involuntary urine loss associated with a sudden, strong sensation of urgency

• Related (Risk) Factors

Decreased bladder capacity (eg, history of pelvic inflammatory disease, abdominal surgeries, indwelling urinary catheter), irritation of bladder stretch receptors causing spasm (eg, bladder infection), alcohol, caffeine, increased fluids, increased urine concentration, overdistention of bladder, enlarged prostate

• Defining Characteristics

— SUBJECTIVE DATA reported —

Urgency, inability to reach bedpan or commode in time, frequent voiding

— OBJECTIVE DATA observed —

Frequent urination, voiding immediately after urge to urinate

Violence, Self-Directed, Risk for

A state in which a person demonstrates behaviors that can be physically harmful either to the self or others

• Related (Risk) Factors

Antisocial character; history of aggressive acts; child or spouse abuse; organic brain syndrome; temporal lobe epilepsy; toxic reactions to medications, alcohol, illegal drugs; catatonic or manic excitement; panic states; hallucinations; rage reactions; suicidal behavior

References

1. North American Nursing Diagnosis Association-International. (2008). *Nursing diagnosis: Definitions and classifications 2007–2008.* Philadelphia: Author

Example Responses to
Critical Thinking Exercises

1. a. *Assessment* involves examining and interviewing the patient to determine health status. During *Diagnosis,* you analyze patient information and identify the problems requiring nursing or medical treatment. In *Planning,* the expected outcomes—expected results—are determined, and the treatment plan is developed and recorded. In *Implementation,* you put the plan into action. Finally, in *Evaluation,* you decide whether the patient achieved the expected outcomes, and modify or terminate the plan as indicated. **b.** Paraphrase any of the benefits listed in Box 1.1 on page 14. **2.** Use of the nursing process is a requirement set by national practice standards; it provides the basis for questions on state board exams; it promotes critical thinking in the clinical setting; it's required of nurses working in Magnet status hospitals. **3.** The problems identified in *Diagnosis* are based on the information collected during *Assessment.* The outcomes identified during Planning are based on the problems determined in *Diagnosis.* The interventions used in *Implementation* are based on the outcomes identified during *Planning.* **4.** *Diagnosis* depends on accurate assessment data. If she's good at *Diagnosis,* she must be good at *Assessment.* **5.** Make a poster addressing the top ten issues listed in the intext box on page 30 and post it at the nurses' station or lounge; have a conference on the importance of meeting patients' expectations; give patients short evaluation forms to evaluate satisfaction with their nursing care (nurses are more likely to pay attention to patient expectations if they are evaluated by them).

1. You can decide this by comparing yourself with the critical thinking indicators listed on page 33, 34, and 35.

Part I. 1. a. Tell me how you're feeling. **b.** How was your dinner? **c.** How do you feel about being here? **d.** Describe what you're feeling; tell me how you're feeling. **2. a.** So, you've been sick off and on for a month. What do you mean by sick off and on? **b.** You feel like nothing ever goes right for you. What's been happening? **c.** You have a pain in your side that comes and goes—can you explain more? d. You've had a funny feeling for a week. What do you mean by funny? **3. a)** C **b)** E **c)** S **d)** L **e)** O **f)** C **g)** S **h)** L **i)** O **j)** L **k)** E. **4. d.** How do you feel about feeding Susan? **h.** How would it be if your family visited? **j.** How do you feel about practicing more? **Part II. 1. a.** You have a lot of ground-in dirt here. What's it from? **b.** I feel a lump on the back of your head. How did it happen? Does it hurt when I touch it? **c.** Your breathing is a little fast. How do you feel? **d.** Your eye seems inflamed. How does it feel? **2. a.** Show me where (and examine that area). Is there anything you think causes it? **b.** Show me where (and examine that area). Tell me more about how it feels. **c.** That's a common symptom of infection. Let's get a urine sample (and examine it). **d.** Where do you feel this bloating? Your stomach? Ankles? Where? (and examine the area). **3. c**

C R I T I C A L   T H I N K I N G   E X E R C I S E   I V

Part I. 1. 51 years old, no pain, feels better, feels relieved, denies being weary. **2.** Lab study results, talking slowly, frequent sighing, vital signs. **Part II. a.** All the data listed under Part I, numbers 1 and 2. **b.** Physical condition seems to be improving. He is more comfortable. Seems weary/tired. **Part III. 1.** Certainly valid: Lab studies, talking slowly, frequent sighing. Probably valid: 51 years old, no pain, feels better, vital signs. Possibly valid: Weary/tired. **2.** Compare age with birth date. Ask probing questions to clarify comfort state (Are you sure you don't have any discomfort?). Look for nonverbal signs of discomfort (eg, rubbing hand on chest). Spend quality time with him discussing how he feels physically and psychologically. Recheck vital signs.

C R I T I C A L   T H I N K I N G   E X E R C I S E   V

1. You need to do both to facilitate recognition of both possible nursing problems and medical problems (see page 70). **2.** Body systems: **Resp:** 5, 6, 8, 10, 13, 14. **Card:** 6. **Circ:** 6, 15. GI: 9. **Neuro:** none listed. GU: none listed, although you might have chosen to put 11 (childbirth) here. **Skin:** None listed. Holistic nursing model: (this organizes data according to Functional Health Patterns, but you may have chosen another model) **Nutritional–Metabolic:** 5, 6, 9, 10, 11, 13, 14, 15. **Elimination:** None listed. **Activity-Exercise:** 3, 8. **Cognitive-perceptual:** None listed. **Sleep-rest:** 8. **Self-perception–self-concept:** 11 **Role-relationship:** 2, 3, 7. **Sexual–reproductive:** 1, 2. Coping-Stress: 10, 12. **Value–belief:** 4. **3.** You should think about how you can gain the missing information.

C R I T I C A L   T H I N K I N G   E X E R C I S E   V I

1. a) N **b)** A **c)** N **d)** A **e)** A **f)** N **g)** A **h)** A **i)** N **j)** A.

C R I T I C A L   T H I N K I N G   E X E R C I S E   V I I

1. a. You may perform an action if you're qualified to do so (if you've demonstrated competency and have been given the authority). **b.** See Table 3.3 on page 100. **2. 1)** q. **2)** f. **3)** b. **4)** a. **5)** g. **6)** c. **7)** k. **8)** m. **9)** l. **10)** o. **11)** d. **12)** j. **13)** e. **14)** p. **15)** n. **16)** h. **17)** i. **18)** r. **19)** t. **20)** s. **3. a.** 2,4,6 should have an "N." **b.** The following are nursing diagnoses: 2,3,5,6,9,11,12. **4.** Both models focus on treating health problems. The PPMP model has a stronger focus on early intervention to prevent or manage potential complications.

C R I T I C A L   T H I N K I N G   E X E R C I S E   V I I I

I. 1) b **2)** a **3)** c **4)** e **5)** g **6)** h **7)** f **8)** d. **II. 1)** Mapping and diagramming diagnoses promotes critical thinking because there are fewer rules, allowing you to focus on thinking rather than on rules of statements. Often, the brain handles maps better than words (this is especially so in right-brain dominant people). **III. Part A. 1. a.** Problem: Urge incontinence. Cause: inability to hold large amounts of urine. Signs and symptoms: voiding immediately upon realization of need to void. **b.** Problem: Anticipatory Grieving. Cause: related to impending death of mother. Signs and symptoms: statements of extreme sadness over impending death. **2.** Because if they had signs and symptoms, they'd be *actual* diagnoses. **Part B. 1.** Ineffective Airway Clearance related to copious secretions as evidenced by inability to clear tracheostomy without suction. **2.** Imbalanced Nutrition: Less than Body Requirements related to poor appetite as evidenced by 15 lb below recommended weight. **3.** Powerlessness related to quadriplegia and rigorous physical therapy schedule as evidenced by report of depression and feelings of having no choices. **Part C. 1.** Possible Ineffective Individual Coping. **2.** Risk for Fluid Volume Deficit related to fever. **3.** Risk for Ineffective Airway Clearance related to smoking history and recent general anesthesia. **4.** Possible Ineffective Sexual Pattern.

CRITICAL THINKING EXERCISE IX

Part I. 1. PC: thrombus formation, phlebitis, extravasation, fluid overload related to IV. **2.** PC: brain swelling, bleeding, increased intracranial pressure related to concussion. **3.** PC: arrhythmias, hypotension, shock, congestive heart failure, pulmonary edema, re-infarction, embolus, cerebrovascular accident, cardiac arrest related to MI. **4.** PC: electrolyte imbalance, abdominal distention, bleeding, misplacement of the tube related to nasogastric tube. **Part II.** You would ask a question like, Looking at the big picture of this patient's situation, is it likely that he/she will be able to reach the desired outcomes in the expected time frame using only nursing expertise for planning and management of care? **Part III.** Strengths: normal vital signs, moves all extremities with equal strength, strong peripheral pulses, abdomen soft, equal pupils. Nursing Diagnoses: Risk for Injury related to dizziness; Risk for Impaired Patterns of Urinary Elimination related to inability to use the bedpan; Fear related to hospitalization as evidenced by statements of fear of hospitals and needles. Potential Complications: increased intracranial pressure, bleeding, phlebitis or extravasation at intravenous site.

CRITICAL THINKING EXERCISE X

Part I. 1. Your state practice act, ANA standards, specialty organization standards (if you're in a specialty unit, like maternity), Joint Commission standards, unique standards of the facility where you're working. **2.** Promote communication, direct care and documentation, provide a record that can be used for evaluation and research, provide insurance companies with a record of care requirements. **3.** Expected outcomes (eg, dresses self without assistance by discharge); actual and potential problems (eg, Self-Care Deficit: Dressing); specific interventions (eg, have patient practice buttoning clothing three times a day; evaluation/progress notes (eg, able to button and unbutton clothing with minimal help). **4.** Patient's perception of priorities, understanding of the whole picture of problems, patient's prognosis and overall health status, expected length of stay or contact, presence of clinical guidelines or critical paths related to specific situation. **5.** Severe dyspnea. Severe breathing problems are top priority unless the patient is hemorrhaging. **6.** Knowing the overall discharge outcomes helps you decide which problems need to be given a high priority in order to be ready for discharge in a timely fashion. **Part II. 1.** Outcomes are used to direct interventions, motivate patients and caregivers, and evaluate progress. **2.** Outcome, indicator, goal, objective. **3.** Outcome and indicator. **4. a.** Report the problem to whoever is responsible for achieving the outcome. **b.** Develop and initiate a plan of care to treat the problem. **5.** All nurses are responsible for detecting and reporting patients who may require case management (ie, patients who may require extra resources to achieve the expected outcomes in a timely manner). **Part III. 1.** Measurable verbs help everyone to stay focused on observable data that will let you know how well the patient is progressing toward outcome achievement. For examples of measurable verbs, see page 152. **2. Subject:** Who is the person expected to achieve the goal? **Verb:** What actions must the person take to achieve the goal? **Condition:** Under what circumstances is the person to perform the actions? **Performance Criteria:** How well is the person to perform the actions? **Target Time:** By when is the person expected to be able to perform the actions? **3.** The following are incorrect. **a.** The verb isn't measurable. **c.** Nonspecific. How will we measure what is meant by "will improve"? **f.** No time frame listed; verb isn't measurable and observable. **i.** Verb isn't measurable. **4. a.** Will demonstrate healthy-looking gums, without redness or irritation by Jan 15. **b.** Will not demonstrate signs and symptoms of Impaired Skin Integrity in the rectal area and area will be kept clean. **c.** Will be able to communicate basic needs through use of flash cards and through an interpreter when required. **Part IV. a)** C, P **b)** A **c)** C **d)** C, P.

CRITICAL THINKING EXERCISE XI

Part I. 1. Classifying interventions into direct and indirect interventions allows you to examine nursing activities and time spent in direct contact with patients, and activities and time spent performing activities on behalf of the patient but away from the patient (eg, analyzing lab studies). **2.** See = What must be assessed or observed related to the intervention; do = what must be done; teach = what must be taught or reinforced; record = what must be recorded related to the intervention. **3.** What can be done about the cause(s) of this problem? What can be done to help this specific person achieve this specific outcome? **4.** See 1–5 at the top of page 165. **Part II. 1.** Monitor skin integrity, especially over bony prominences, with each position change. Post at bedside a schedule for turning every 2 hours, enlisting the client's maximum participation. Keep an air mattress on the bed. Ensure adequate vitamin C and protein intake. Keep sheets clean, dry, and unwrinkled. **2.** Preoperatively: Determine patient and family knowledge of coughing and deep breathing with incisional splinting. Teach as indicated and have patient return demonstration. Postoperatively: Monitor for incisional pain and medicate pm before pain is too intense. Teach the importance of asking for pain medication before pain is severe, changing positions, ambulating early, and coughing and deep breathing. Record pain level after medication is given. Record breath sounds q4h. Help client to cough and deep breath q2h the day of surgery and first postoperative day. **3.** Monitor daily bowel movements. Teach the relationship between exercise, diet, fluid intake, and bowel elimination. Develop a plan to increase roughage and fluid intake, and to increase exercise gradually (eg, using stairs instead of elevator). **Part III. 1.** PC: Extravasation, phlebitis, thrombus formation, fluid overload, infection. Plan: Follow hospital policies or standards for care of IV therapy. Monitor vital signs q4h. Monitor IV site for signs and symptoms of infection, extravasation, phlebitis, thrombus q4h. Instruct patient to report discomfort or swelling at IV site. **2.** PC: Hypoglycemia/hyperglycemia. Plan: Follow hospital policies or standards for care of diabetics. Record daily caloric intake. Record blood sugars q4h. Instruct patient to report symptoms of dizziness or "feeling funny" in any way. **3.** PC: Infection, blockage of the catheter, bleeding. Plan: Follow hospital policies and standards for Foley catheter care. Monitor temperature q4–8h. Monitor urine color, odor, and amount. Record intake and output q8h. Monitor meatus for drainage or bleeding. Instruct patient to report catheter or bladder discomfort. **Part IV.** Expected outcomes, actual and potential problems, specific interventions, evaluation/progress notes.

CRITICAL THINKING EXERCISE XII

1. a. No. **b.** Because it's the first time she's getting out of bed and you don't really know how she will respond. (See When Is It Safe to Delegate? on page 189). **2. a.** The nurse is accountable because nurses are accountable for outcomes of delegated care. **b.** The nurse could have assigned another aide to monitor the child or she could have clearly cautioned the mother not to leave her child unattended for any reason (rather, the mother should call if she needed to go to the bathroom or whatever). **3. a.** You perform a complete assessment and determine whether the patient is progressing as expected according to plan of care. For example, if the plan includes a critical path that states "chest tubes will be out by the second postoperative day," and the patient still has chest tubes, you've identified a variance in care. **b.** You should perform additional assessment to determine whether the delay is justified or whether actions need to be taken to improve the patient's likelihood of achieving the outcome. **c.** Additional assessments and interventions that may be required for the patient to progress may be omitted, resulting in harm to the patient or delays in recovery. **d.** If the patient is harmed, you may be accused of negligence. If there are delays in recovery, you may be accused of giving substandard care.

CRITICAL THINKING EXERCISE XIII

1. See "Six Purposes of Charting" on page 195. **2.** You'll be more accurate when the information is fresh in your mind. Charting what you've done often jogs your mind to recognize when you've forgotten to do something else you should have done. **3.** AIR-A: A—States she feels like she's choking, but is afraid to cough because of incisional pain. I—Instructed how to splint incision with a pillow. R—Coughed up gray mucus plug. Lungs clear. A—Stressed the importance of reporting pain to promote better breathing and coughing. **4. a.** It's judgmental and has no supporting evidence. **b.** It has no supporting evidence—states opinion, not facts. **5.** You should have drawn a line through the note, then written the word error, followed by your initials. Alternatively, you should have done whatever the policy at your school or clinical facility states.

CRITICAL THINKING EXERCISE XIV

Part I. 1) P. **2)** A. **3)** N. Insulin demand is affected by increased exercise. **4)** P. **5)** P. Fever and heat are also signs of infection. **Part II.** Continue the plan if the patient hasn't achieved outcomes, but you haven't identified any factors that impeded or enhanced care. Modify the plan when outcomes haven't been achieved, and you've identified factors that enhanced or impeded care. Terminate the plan if the patient has achieved outcomes and demonstrates ability to care for himself.

C R I T I C A L   T H I N K I N G   E X E R C I S E   X V

1. Information gained from these studies improves the quality and efficiency of patient care, and helps identify ways of improving nurses' job satisfaction. **2.** Considering all three types of evaluation—outcome (results), process (method), and structure (setting)—provides a comprehensive examination of care management. **3.** I'll follow policies and procedures carefully without skipping steps. I'll also pay attention to things that I'm doing that might make me prone to error and develop ways to prevent them (eg, ask people to wait when they want to talk to me and I'm pouring medications). I'll report things that make us all prone to error (eg, continually working with insufficient staff). I'll encourage my patients to take an active role in managing their health care. **4.** See Box 6.4 (page 219). **5.** Stay alert for error-prone situations. Take responsibility and report them to your manager. Find ways to build "safety nets" into procedures so that you can catch mistakes early or make sure the big mistakes don't happen. Work collaboratively to prevent mistakes; in complicated math calculations, get a colleague or pharmacist to double check your math.

appendix A

Four Roles of Advanced Practice Nurses (APNs)

Definition: Whereas *Registered Nurse* (RN) is the term used for nurses who have passed state board examinations after completing 2 to 4 years of undergraduate work, *Advanced Practice Nurse* (APN) is an "umbrella term" used for licensed registered nurses prepared at an *advanced degree level*. APNs function in any of the roles listed below. Certification requirements and authority to practice independently vary from specialty to specialty and state to state.

❏ **Clinical Nurse Specialists (CNSs)**[1]—Licensed registered nurses who have a master's or doctorate degree as a CNS and are expert clinicians in a specific nursing area, in terms of: a population (eg, pediatrics, geriatrics, women's health); a setting (eg, critical care, emergency room); a disease or medical subspecialty (eg, diabetes, oncology); a type of care (eg, psychiatric, rehabilitation); a type of problem (eg, pain, wounds, stress). In addition to providing direct patient care, CNSs influence patient outcomes by providing expert consultation for staff nurses, giving support in terms of education for nurses, and making improvements in health care delivery systems. Research about CNS practice shows improved outcomes such as: reduced hospital costs and length of stay; reduced frequency of emergency-room visits; improved pain management practices; increased patient satisfaction; and reduced medical complications in hospitalized patients.

❏ **Nurse Practitioners (NPs)**[2]—Licensed registered nurses with master's or doctorate degrees as nurse practitioners and advanced clinical experience, which enables them to diagnose and manage most common and many chronic illnesses, either independently or as part of a health care team. **NPs provide some care previously offered only by physicians and in most states have the ability to prescribe medications.** Working in collaboration with a physician, a nurse practitioner provides high-quality, cost-effective, and individualized care for the lifespan of a patient's special needs. **They focus mainly on health maintenance, disease prevention, counseling, and patient education in a wide variety of settings.** With a strong emphasis on primary care, nurse practitioners work within several specialties, including neonatology, nurse–midwifery, pediatrics, school health, family and adult health, women's health, mental health, home care, geriatrics, and acute care.

❏ **Certified Registered Nurse Anesthetists (CRNAs)**[3]—Licensed registered nurses with a master's degree in anesthesia. Provide anesthetics to patients in collaboration with surgeons, anesthesiologists, dentists, podiatrists, and other qualified health care professionals. When anesthesia is administered by a nurse anesthetist, it is recognized as the practice of nursing; when administered by an anesthesiologist, it is recognized as the practice of medicine. CRNAs administer approximately 65% of all anesthetics given to patients each year in the United States.

---

[2] Data from: American College of Nurse Practitioners. *What is a nurse practitioner?* Retrieved from: http://www.acnpweb.org/i4a/pages/index.cfm?pageid=3479

[3] Data from: American Association of Nurse Anesthetists. *Questions and answers: A career in nurse anesthesia.* Retrieved from: http://www.aana.com/becomingcrna.aspx?ucNavMenu_TSMenuTargetID=18&ucNavMenu_TSMenuTargetType= 4&ucNavMenu_TSMenuID=6&id=109

---

[1] Data from: Association of Clinical Nurse Specialists. *What is a clinical nurse specialist?* Retrieved from: http://www.nacns.org

❑ **Certified Nurse–Midwives (CNMs)**[4]—Licensed registered nurses with advanced academic degrees (certificate or master's degree in midwifery). Provide health care to women and newborns, focusing on the needs of individuals and families for physical care, emotional and social support, and for active involvement according to cultural values and personal preferences. **Laws and regulations governing the practice of nurse–midwifery and midwifery are rapidly changing.** Check with the regulatory agency in each state (usually the board of nursing, but also may be the boards of medicine, public health, medicine, midwifery, health arts, alternative health care, human resources, or health and environmental control).

[4]Data from: American College of Nurse–Midwives. *A career in midwifery.* Retrieved from: http://www.midwife.org/index.cfm

DEAD ON!! A Game to Promote Critical Thinking

Instructions: The point of this game is to be sure that you give key parts of thinking the time and attention they require, therefore promoting thinking that's more likely to be "dead on". Get 6 balls and put the letters **D, E, A, D, O, N,** on each one with indelible ink. Start with **the "D" ball,** and toss it to someone in the group. Ask the group to focus on answering the questions listed under **"D"** below. Once you have exhausted thoughts on **the "D" ball,** do the same for each of the remaining balls. Be sure to <u>stay focused</u> on the current ball. For example, if someone expresses <u>feelings</u> rather than <u>facts</u> with the first ball, point out that the rules are that emotions are addressed when **the "E" ball** is up for discussion.

D = Data
❏ What <u>data (facts)</u> do you have?
❏ What <u>other data</u> do you need?
❏ What <u>assumptions</u> have you made and what data might validate or negate them?

E = Emotions
❏ What emotions (gut reactions) are there (your own, others)?
❏ What's your intuition telling you, and what data might validate or negate it?
❏ How are values affecting thinking (yours, others)?

A = Advantages
❏ What's the vision, benefit(s), and most important desired outcome(s)?
❏ What are the specific advantages to <u>others</u> (benefits/outcomes)?

❏ What are the specific advantages to <u>you</u> (benefits/outcomes)?

D = Disadvantages
❏ What could go wrong (what are the risks)?
❏ What are the specific inconveniences/risks for <u>others</u>?
❏ What are the specific inconveniences/risks for <u>you</u>?
❏ What problems or issues <u>must</u> be addressed to get results?
❏ How much work will it take and do you have the necessary resources?

O = Out of the box
❏ Go out of the box—think of creative approaches!
❏ What can we do to decrease the disadvantages?
❏ What can we do to increase the likelihood of seeing the benefits?
❏ How can technology help?
❏ What research is there that might apply?
❏ What human resources are will to help?

N = Now what?
❏ What problems, risks, or issues <u>must</u> be addressed?
❏ Who are the key stakeholders (who will be most affected)?
❏ What professional, community, and informal resources can help?
❏ What's the plan (what interventions do you need to get results and avoid risks?
❏ What does all this imply?
❏ What did we miss when addressing the other balls? (Go through each of the balls again)

2003 R. Alfaro-LeFevre. Available at: www.AlfaroTeachSmart.com

Commonly Used NANDA Diagnoses Organized According to Gordon's Functional Health Patterns

Health Perception—Health Management
Growth & Development, Delayed
Health Maintenance, Ineffective
Management of Therapeutic Regimen, Ineffective
Risk for Injury
Infection, Risk for
Injury, Perioperative Positioning, Risk for
Risk for Aspiration
Swallowing, Impaired

Nutritional—Metabolic
Body Temperature, Risk for Imbalanced
Fluid Volume Deficit
Nutrition, Imbalanced: Less than Body Requirements
   Feeding Pattern, Ineffective Infant
   Swallowing, Impaired
Oral Mucous Membrane, Impaired
Skin Integrity, Impaired

Elimination
Constipation
Diarrhea
Urinary Incontinence, Stress
Urinary Incontinence, Total
Urinary Incontinence, Urge

Activity—Exercise
Activity Intolerance
Cardiac Output, Decreased
Disuse Syndrome
Home Maintenance Management, Impaired
Mobility, Impaired Physical
Ineffective Airway Clearance
Ineffective Breathing Patterns

Self-care Deficit, Bathing/Hygiene
Self-care Deficit, Dressing/Grooming
Self-care Deficit, Feeding
Self-care Deficit, Toileting

Sleep—Rest
Sleep Pattern Disturbance

Cognitive—Perceptual
Acute Pain
Chronic Pain
Chronic Confusion
Dysreflexia, Autonomic
Knowledge Deficit (specify)
Thought Processes, Impaired
Memory, Impaired
Unilateral Neglect

Self-Perception
Anxiety
Body Image, Disturbed
Fatigue
Fear
Powerlessness
Self-esteem Disturbance

Role—Relationship
Communication, Impaired
Grieving
Parenting, Impaired
Social Isolation

Sexuality—Reproductive
Sexuality Patterns, Ineffective

Coping—Stress Tolerance
Caregiver Role Strain
Coping, Ineffective
Post-Trauma Syndrome
Rape Trauma Syndrome
Self-mutilation, Risk for

Suicide, Risk for
Violence, Risk for

Value—Belief
Spiritual Distress

Good Learning Environments, Healthy Workplace Standards, and Establishing a Culture of Safety

What Makes a Good Learning Environment?

Students identify that the following make a good learning environment: (1) Staff and teachers are approachable and promote self-esteem and confidence, relating to learners with kindness, and showing genuine interest in them as people. (2) A good team spirit where everyone works together towards common goals in an atmosphere of trust and respect, making students feel they belong to a team. (3) High standards are maintained through the use of efficient and flexible approaches that are tailored to individuals, not tasks. (4) Teaching and learning are key features and an integral part of daily activities of the organization. (5) Staff and teachers who are keen to learn, and among whom ongoing development is actively promoted. Information is shared and learning opportunities are created and used well.[1]

What are Healthy Workplace Standards?

Standards for establishing and sustaining a healthy workplace environment form a foundation for creating a climate that fosters critical thinking by providing an atmosphere that's respectful, healing, and humane, These standards stress the need for: (1) Effective communication; (2) True collaboration; (3) Effective decision making; (4) Appropriate staffing; (5) Meaningful recognition; and (6) Authentic leadership. Having a safe and respectful environment requires maintaining *each* standard, because studies show that you don't get effective outcomes when any *one* standard is considered optional.[2]

Establishing a Culture of Safety

In a culture of safety, everyone feels responsible for safety and pursues it on a regular basis. Everyone— for example, nurses, physicians, and patient care technicians—looks out for one another and feels comfortable pointing out unsafe behaviors (eg, when hand-sanitation has been missed or when safety glasses should be worn). Safety takes precedence over egos or pressures to complete tasks with little help or time. The organization values and rewards such actions.

Recommended:

❑ Center for Disease Control and Prevention links for healthy workplace, violence and injury, prevention, and other topics. http://www.cdc.gov/

❑ Workplace Violence Prevention Position Statement. Retrieved May 8, 2006, from https://www.aacn.org/AACN/pubpolcy.nsf/Files/Workplace%20Violence%20Position%20Statement/$file/Workplace%20Violence%204.12.04.pdf

❑ AACN Testimony to the IOM Committee on Work Environment for Nurses and Patient Safety. Retrieved May 8, 2006, from http://www.aacn.org/aacn/pubpolcy.nsf/92712bceed60b1878825688e00776c1f/1138e880af4cafe788256cc60001ff73?OpenDocument

---

Source: R. Alfaro-LeFevre Workshop Handouts © 2006–2007

---

[1] Hand, H. (2006). Promoting effective teaching and learning in the clinical setting. *Nursing Standard, 20*(39), 55–63. Retrieved June 18, 2006, from http://www.nursing-standard.co.uk/archives/ns/vol20-39/pdfs/v20n39p5563.pdf

[2] American Association of Critical Care Nurses. (n.d.) Healthy work environment backgrounder. Retrieved May 8, 2006, from https://www.aacn.org/AACN/pubpolcy.nsf/Files/HWEPosStat/$file/HWE%20BG%20Color%206.21.04.pdf

Nursing Interventions Classification (NIC)
and Nursing Outcomes Classification (NOC) Examples

Examples of Nursing Interventions Classifications (NIC) Labels[1]

Abuse Protection Support	Bleeding Precautions	Hair Care
Acid-Base Management	Calming Technique	Hallucination Management
Acid-Base Monitoring	Cardiac Precautions	Immunization/Vaccination Management
Active Listening	Caregiver Support	Impulse Control Training
Activity Therapy	Case Management	Incident Reporting
Acupressure	Cast Care: Maintenance	Intravenous (IV) Therapy
Admission Care	Circulatory Precautions	Kangaroo Care
Airway Management	Code Management	Leech Therapy
Airway Suctioning	Cognitive Restructuring	Milieu Therapy
Allergy Management	Decision-Making Support	Mood Management
Amnioinfusion	Delegation	Multidisciplinary Care
Amputation Care	Dementia Management	Mutual Goal Setting
Analgesic Administration	Discharge Planning	Nail Care
Bed Rest Care	Documentation	Nausea Management
Behavior Management	Dying Care	Oral Health Maintenance
Bibliotherapy	Electrolyte Management	Oxygen Therapy
Biofeedback	Emergency Cart Checking	Pain Management
Birthing	Emotional Support	Patient Contracting
Bladder Irrigation	Endotracheal Extubation	

Examples of Nursing Outcomes Classification (NOC) Labels[2]

Acceptance: Health Status	Decision Making	Joint Movement: Passive
Adherence Behavior	Depression Control	Knowledge: Disease Process
Aggression Control	Dignified Dying	Leisure Participation
Ambulation: Walking	Distorted Thought Control	Loneliness
Ambulation: Wheelchair	Endurance	Medication Response
Anxiety Control	Family Coping	Memory
Asthma Control	Fear Control	Neglect Recovery
Blood Glucose Control	Fetal Status: Intrapartum	Newborn Adaptation
Body Image	Fluid Balance	Pain Control
Breastfeeding: Weaning	Grief Resolution	Quality of Life
Cardiac Pump Effectiveness	Growth	Risk Control
Caregiver Stressors	Health Beliefs	Safety Behavior: Personal
Caregiver Well-Being	Health Promoting Behavior	Self-Direction of Care
Circulation Status	Health Seeking Behavior	Self-Esteem
Coagulation Status	Hearing Compensation	Skeletal Function
Cognitive Ability	Behavior	Spiritual Well-Being
Comfort Level	Hope	Suffering Level
Community Competence	Hydration	Symptom Control
Concentration	Immunization Behavior	Thermoregulation

[1]For comprehensive list, see most up-to-date edition of: McClosky, J., & Bulechek, G. *Nursing interventions.* St. Louis, MO: Elsevier-Mosby.

[2]For comprehensive list, see most up-to-date edition of: Moorhead, S., Johnson, M., & Maas, M. *Nursing outcomes classification.* St. Louis, MO: Elsevier-Mosby.

Glossary

Accountable. Being responsible and answerable for something.

Advanced practice nurse (APN). *See* Four Roles of Advance Practice Nurses on page 247.

Advanced practice registered nurse (APRN). *See* Advanced practice nurse.

Affective domain outcomes. Measurable goals that deal with changes in attitudes, feelings, or values.

Analyze. To examine and categorize pieces of information to determine where they might fit into the whole picture.

Anticipatory. Expected or foreseen.

Assessment. The first step of the nursing process during which you gather and organize data (information) in preparation for the second step, Diagnosis.

Assessment tool. A printed or electronic form used to ensure that key information is gathered and recorded during Assessment.

Authority. The power or right to act, prescribe, or make a final decision.

Baseline data. Information that describes the patient's health before treatment begins (start-of-care data).

CareMap. *See* Critical pathway.

Care partner. *See* Unlicensed assistive personnel (UAP).

Care variance. *See* Variance in care.

Caring behavior. A way of acting that shows understanding and respect for others' ideals, values, feelings, needs, and desires.

Case management. An approach to patient care that aims to improve patient outcomes and satisfaction while reducing overall cost and length or incidence of hospital stays.

Client-centered outcome. A statement describing a measurable behavior of a client, family, or group that reflects the desired result of interventions (that the problem, or problems, are prevented, resolved, or controlled).

Client goal. *See* Client-centered outcome.

Clinical pathway. *See* Critical pathway.

Cognitive domain outcomes. Measurable goals that deal with acquiring knowledge or intellectual skills.

Competence. The quality of having the necessary knowledge and skill to perform an action in a safe and appropriate way, under various circumstances.

Critical. Characterized by careful and exact evaluation and judgment.

Critical pathway. A standard plan that predicts the course of recovery and day-by-day care required to achieve outcomes for a specific health problem within a specific time frame.

Cues. Pieces of information that prompt you to draw a conclusion about health status.

Data base assessment. Comprehensive data collected on initial contact with the patient to gain information about all aspects of the patient's health.

Data base form. *See* Assessment tool.

Defining characteristics. A cluster of cues (signs, symptoms, and risk [related] factors) often associated with a specific nursing diagnosis.

Definitive diagnosis. Most specific, most correct, diagnosis.

Definitive interventions. The most specific treatment required to prevent, resolve, or control a health problem.

Delegation. The transfer of responsibility for the performance of an activity while retaining accountability.

Depleted. Emptied wholly or in part; exhausted of.

Diagnose. To make a judgment and identify a problem or strength based on evidence from an assessment.

Diagnosis. (1) The second step of the nursing process. (2) The process of analyzing data and putting related cues together to make judgments about health status. (3) The opinion or judgment that's drawn after the diagnostic process is completed.

Diagnostic error. When a health problem has been overlooked or incorrectly identified.

Diagnostic reasoning. A method of thinking that involves specific, deliberate use of critical thinking to reach conclusions about health status.

Direct care interventions. Actions performed through interaction with patients (eg, helping someone out of bed, teaching someone about diabetes).

Direct data. Information gained directly from the patient.

Empathy. Understanding another's feelings or perceptions, but not sharing the same feelings or point of view (compare with Sympathy).

Etiology. Something known to cause a disease.

Evidence-based practice. Clinical practices that integrate the *best research* with *clinical expertise* and *patient values* to achieve the best outcomes. Requires knowing the strength of the evidence that supports your interventions.

Expedite. To speed up.

Focus assessment. Data collection that concentrates on gathering more information about a specific problem or condition.

Guidelines. Documents that delineate how care is to be provided in specific situations. *See* also Protocols, Policies, Procedures, Standards, and Standards of care.

Habits of inquiry. Thinking habits that enhance your ability to search for the truth (eg, following rules of logic).
Humanistic. *See* Caring behavior.

Indicators. Concrete, observable behaviors that can be observed to determine outcome achievement (eg, joint movement, absence of skin redness).
Indirect care interventions. Actions performed away from the patient but on behalf of a patient or group of patients. These actions are aimed at management of the health care environment and interdisciplinary collaboration.
Indirect data. Information gained from sources other than the patient (eg, someone's wife).
Inference. A conclusion drawn from a patient cue (or cues).
Intervention. An action performed to prevent or manage problems or to maximize comfort and human functioning.
Intuition. Knowing something without having supporting evidence.

Judgment. An opinion that's made after analyzing and synthesizing information.

Life processes. Events or changes that occur during one's lifetime (eg, growing up, aging, maturing, becoming a parent, moving, separations, losses).
Long-term goal. An objective that's expected to be achieved over a relatively long time period, usually weeks or months.

Medical diagnosis. A problem requiring definitive diagnosis by a qualified physician or advanced practice nurse.
Medical domain. Activities and actions a physician is legally qualified to perform or prescribe.
Medical orders. Interventions ordered by a physician or advanced practice nurse to treat a medical problem.
Medical process. The method physicians use to expedite diagnosis and treatment of diseases or trauma. The medical process focuses mainly on problems with structure and function of organs or systems.

Multidisciplinary plan. A plan that's developed collaboratively by key members of the health care team (eg, nursing, physical therapy, medicine).

Need. A requirement that, if fulfilled, reduces stress and promotes a sense of adequacy and well-being.
Nurse extender. *See* Unlicensed assistive personnel (UAP).
Nurse-prescribed intervention. An action a nurse may legally order or initiate independently.
Nursing assistant. *See* Unlicensed assistive personnel (UAP).
Nursing diagnosis. A clinical judgment about an individual, family, or community response to actual or potential health problems and life processes. Nursing diagnoses provide the basis for selection of nursing interventions to achieve outcomes for which the nurse is accountable. Nursing diagnoses often are called human responses because we, as nurses, focus on how people are responding to changes in health or life circumstances (eg, how they're responding to illness or to becoming a parent).
Nursing domain. Activities and actions a nurse is legally qualified to perform or prescribe.

Objective data. Information that's measurable and observable (eg, blood pressure, pulse, diagnostic studies).
Outcome. The result of prescribed interventions; usually refers to the desired result of interventions (ie, that the problem is prevented, resolved, or controlled) and includes a specific time frame for when the goal is expected to be achieved.

Palliative care. Care that alleviates pain and suffering but doesn't cure.
Patient care technician. *See* Unlicensed assistive personnel (UAP).
Policies. *See* Guidelines.
Primary care provider. The health care professional designated to be in charge of managing the patient's major medical problems (may be a physician, advance practice nurse, or physician's assistant).
Proactive. A way of thinking and behaving that accepts responsibility for one's actions and takes initiative to plan ahead to anticipate and prevent problems before they happen (comes from "act before").
Procedures. *See* Guidelines.
Prognosis. The predicted course or outcome of disease or trauma.

Protocols. *See* Guidelines.

Psychomotor outcomes. Measurable goals that deal with acquiring skills that require deliberate, specific muscle coordination to perform an activity (eg, walking with crutches).

Qualified. Having the knowledge, skill, and authority to perform an action.

Quality care. Cost-effective health care that increases the probability of achieving desired results and decreases the probability of undesired results.

Related factor. Something known to be associated with a specific diagnosis. *See* also Risk factor.

Risk factor. Something known to cause or contribute to a specific problem (eg, decreased vision contributes to Risk for Injury).

Risk (potential) diagnosis. A health problem that may develop if preventive actions aren't taken.

Sign. Objective data that indicate an abnormality.

Stakeholders. Those who are most affected by the plan of care, for example, patients, families, care-givers, and third-party payers.

Standard Care Plan. A preformulated plan that can be used as a guide to expedite development and documentation of a plan of care. *See* also Guidelines.

Standard of Care. A document outlining the minimal level of routine care provided for all patients in certain situations (focuses on what will be observed in the patient to let you know the care has been given). *See* also Guidelines.

Standard of Practice. A document outlining what the nurse will do in giving care in specific situations. *See* also guidelines given earlier. *See* also Guidelines.

Standard of Professional Performance. Statements that describe a competent level of behavior in the professional role.

Standards. Authoritative statements by which the nursing profession describes the responsibilities for which its practitioners are accountable. *See* also Guidelines.

Subjective data. Information the patient or client tells the nurse during Assessment (usually charted as "Patient states. . . .").

Sympathy. Sharing the same feelings as another (compare with Empathy).

Symptom. Subjective data that indicate an abnormality.

Syndrome diagnosis. A cluster of nursing diagnoses often associated with a specific situation or event.

Unlicensed assistive personnel (UAP). Someone without a license to practice nursing who is hired to assist nurses in care delivery. These individuals may have a variety of job titles (eg, nursing assistant, nurse extender, care partner, patient care technician) and have varied job descriptions and capabilities.

Variance in care. A case in which a patient hasn't achieved activities or outcomes by the time frame noted on a critical path. A variance in care triggers additional assessment to determine whether the delay is justified or whether actions need to be taken to improve the patient's likelihood of achieving the outcome.

Index

Page numbers followed by *b* indicate boxed material; page numbers followed by *f* indicate material in figures; page numbers followed by *t* indicate material in tables.

A

COMMON COMPLICATIONS RELATED TO TREATMENTS AND INVASIVE PROCEDURES

Anesthesia/Surgical Procedures:

Respiratory depression
Airways management problems
Aspiration
Atelectasis-pneumonia
Bleeding (internal or external)
Hypovolemia/shock
Infection/septic shock
Fluid/electrolyte imbalance
Thrombus/embolus
Paralytic ileus
Urinary retention
Incision complications (infection, poor healing, dehiscence/evisceration)
See also Angina/Myocardial Infarction, opposite.

Cardiac Catheterization/Invasive Monitoring:

Bleeding (internal or at insertion site)
Hemo-pneumothorax
Thrombus/embolus formation
Stroke
Infection/sepsis
See also Angina/Myocardial Infarction, opposite.

Chest Tubes/Thoracentesis:

Bleeding (internal or at insertion site)
Hemo-pneumothorax
Atelectasis
Chest tube malfunction/blockage
Infection/sepsis

Foley Catheter:

Infection/sepsis
Catheter malfunction/blockage
Bladder spasms

IV Therapy:

Bleeding (internal or at insertion site)
Air embolus
Phlebitis/thrombophlebitis
Infiltration/extravasation/tissue necrosis
Fluid overload
Infection/sepsis

Medications:

Adverse reactions (allergic response, exaggerated response, side effects)
Drug interactions
Overdose/toxicity

Nasogastric Suction:

Electrolyte imbalance
Tube malfunction/blockage
Aspiration
Bleeding

Paracentesis:

Bleeding (internal or at insertion site)
Paralytic ileus
Infection/sepsis

Skeletal Traction/Casts:

See also Fractures, opposite.